Gynecologic Radiation Therapy

Akila N. Viswanathan • Christian Kirisits
Beth E. Erickson • Richard Pötter
(Editors)

Gynecologic Radiation Therapy

Novel Approaches to Image-Guidance and Management

Springer

Akila N. Viswanathan, MD, MPH
Department of Radiation Oncology
Dana-Farber/Brigham and
Women's Cancer Center
Harvard Medical School
75 Francis Street L2
Boston, MA 02115
USA
aviswanathan@partners.org

Beth E. Erickson, MD
Department of Radiation Oncology
Medical College of Wisconsin Clinics
Froedtert Hospital
9200 W Wisconsin Ave.
Milwaukee, WI 53226
USA
berickson@mcw.edu

Christian Kirisits, ScD
Department of Radiotherapy
Vienna General Hospital
Medical University of Vienna
Währinger Gürtel 18-20
1090 Vienna
Austria
christian.kirisits@akhwien.at

Richard Pötter, MD
Department of Radiotherapy
Vienna General Hospital
Medical University of Vienna
Währinger Gürtel 18-20
1090 Vienna
Austria
Richard.poetter@akhwien.at

ISBN: 978-3-662-50156-6 ISBN: 978-3-540-68958-4 (eBook)

DOI: 10.1007/978-3-540-68958-4

Springer Heidelberg Dordrecht London New York

Softcover re-print of the Hardcover 1st edition 2011

Cover design: eStudioCalamar, Figueres/Berlin

Printed on acid-free paper

Springer is part of Springer Science+Business Media (www.springer.com)

Preface

The use of complex 3D imaging has significantly changed medicine in its approach to patients, particularly to those going under radiation. Over the past 30 years, the field of radiation oncology has evolved from reliance on pure 2D imaging to detailed visual analysis of tumor and complex structure surrounding it. This visualization has permitted more precise treatments in all areas of the body. For gynecologic therapy, the impact of imaging has changed treatment approaches over the past 10 years with the development of intensity modulated radiation therapy and image-guided brachytherapy. This text is a state-of-the-art presentation of the current thought and issues in the field of gynecologic imaging as applied to radiation oncology. Section 1 reviews general principles with regard to radiologic imaging. Section 2 applies imaging and discusses specific applications for external beam treatment planning. Sections 3 and 4 describe in detail image-guided brachytherapy. A highlight of this book is the diversity of institutional practical approaches presented from centers around the world.

This multi-institutional international collaboration has been a very fruitful endeavor and we hope it will improve the outcomes of gynecologic patients around the world. We wish to thank all of the authors, physicians, physicists, nurses, dosimetrists, support staff, and those providing care who made this work feasible, and of course, our patients for whom this work pertains.

Akila N. Viswanathan
Christian Kirisits
Beth E. Erickson
Richard Pötter

Contents

Part I

Radiological Imaging of Gynecologic Malignanies

1 Imaging of Gynecologic Malignancies

Jeffrey Olpin and Clare M. Tempany

1.1 Introduction

Gynecologic malignancies are an important cause of mortality and morbidity among women in the USA. Various imaging modalities have been developed over the past several decades that provide valuable clinical information regarding the presence and extent of uterine malignancies. Ultrasound (US) and computed tomography (CT) have been successfully employed as initial imaging modalities for the characterization of uterine malignancies. Positron emission tomography (PET) in combination with CT has emerged in recent years as a powerful tool in the assessment of more advanced, widely metastatic gynecologic malignancies. Magnetic resonance (MR) imaging is a robust imaging modality for the imaging of gynecologic malignancies, and is generally regarded as superior to CT in the staging of female pelvic malignancies. When available, MR should replace CT in the staging evaluation of patients with a known or suspected gynecologic malignancy. Significant advances in MR and CT have likewise led to increasing sophisticated radiation therapy treatment planning. These modalities provide state-of-the-art image guidance for both external beam and brachytherapy treatment, allowing for increasingly accurate and effective radiation dose delivery.

J. Olpin (✉)
University of Utah Hospitals & Clinics, 50 N Medical Dr # 1A71, Salt Lake City, UT, USA
e-mail: Jeffrey.olpin@hsc.utah.edu

C.M. Tempany
Department of Radiology, Brigham and Women's Hospital, 75 Francis St, Room L1-050, Boston, MA 02115
e-mail: Ctempanyafdhal@partners.org

A.N. Viswanathan et al. (eds.), *Gynecologic Radiation Therapy*,
DOI: 10.1007/978-3-540-68958-4_1, © Springer-Verlag Berlin Heidelberg 2011

1.2 Imaging Modalities

1.2.1 Ultrasound

Ultrasound has been commonly utilized as an initial imaging modality in the evaluation of patients with abnormal vaginal bleeding. Ultrasound offers several advantages as an initial imaging modality, including its widespread availability, relatively low cost, and lack of ionizing radiation. Over the years, ultrasound has evolved from simple A-mode to high-resolution, gray scale, real-time imaging. A-mode, or earliest type of ultrasound technique, only provided information as to the position and strength of a reflecting structure. M-mode, another simple ultrasound technique, provides rudimentary information regarding the changes of echo amplitude and position with time, and is most useful when assessing rapidly moving structures such as cardiac valves. B-mode is the mainstay of modern ultrasound imaging, which provides a real-time two-dimensional (2D) image of a scanned object. 2D images are obtained at a rate of 15–60 frames per second. Newer three-dimensional (3D) ultrasound techniques, with specialized transducers, can provide tumor volume measurements that are generally considered more accurate than conventional 2D thickness measurements, particularly in the detection of endometrial cancer.

Doppler ultrasound is another invaluable sonographic technique that provides dynamic vascular flow information. Two basic techniques of Doppler ultrasound are color flow and power mode Doppler. Color flow Doppler provides a color map to display information regarding the flow direction and velocity of moving blood within a vascular structure. Power mode Doppler also uses a color map to demonstrate the distribution of the amplitude of the Doppler signal. Power Doppler has the advantage of improved sensitivity for flow detection, but does not provide information regarding the flow direction or velocity.

Regarding ultrasound probe configuration, transabdominal and transvaginal probes are both utilized in the assessment of the female pelvis. Transabdominal sonography provides global visualization of the entire pelvis. Transvaginal sonography is a relatively newer technique that allows for the use of higher frequency transducers with resultant superior resolution of the uterus and its substructure. This technique is not as limited by patient size or uterine orientation. However, the technique is invasive, and generally requires a higher level of technical expertise. For the assessment of cervical and vaginal cancer, endorectal sonography is advantageous due to the orientation of the ultrasound image that is orthogonal to the ultrasound probe axis (Fig. 1.1).

1.2.1.1 Endometrial Carcinoma

Ultrasound is generally considered a first-line imaging modality in a suspected endometrial malignancy. Diffuse thickening of the endometrium is commonly seen in the setting of endometrial carcinoma. Endometrial thickening, defined as over 3–4 mm in women who are postmenopausal and not receiving exogenous estrogen, may be well defined and

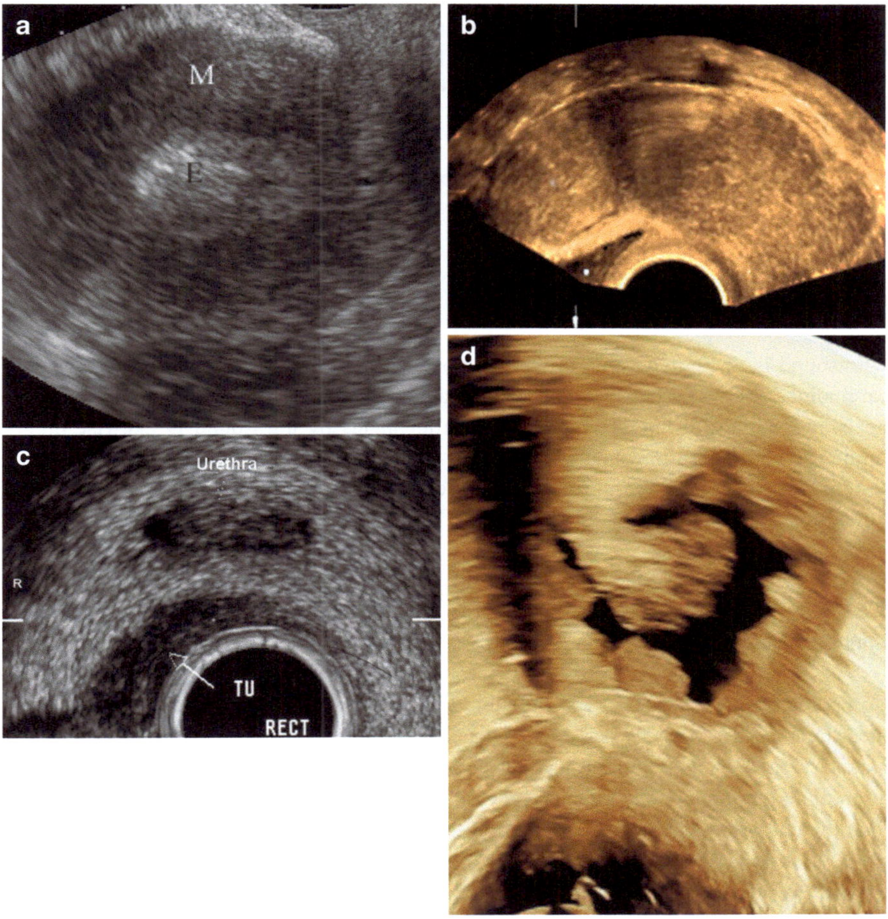

Fig. 1.1 (**a**) A transvaginal pelvic sonogram demonstrates diffusely thickening endometrium (E), as manifest by a centrally irregular, heterogeneous region of increased echogenicity, surrounded by the myometrium (M). The junctional zone is poorly visualized, and the degree of myometrial invasion is difficult to ascertain. Tumor involved the full thickness of the myometrium following total abdominal hysterectomy. (**b**) Vaginal endosonography (3D) of a bulky cervical cancer with infiltration of the uterine corpus (courtesy of A. Kratochwil, Medical University of Vienna). (**c**) Endosonography of a small vaginal cancer (7 mm thick) involving part of the vaginal circumference (20 mm) (courtesy of A. Kratochwil, Medical University of Vienna). (**d**) Coronal view from an endovaginal 3D ultrasound depicting extensive polypoid endometrial cancer within uterine cavity with minimal myometrial infiltration (courtesy of A. Kratochwil, Medical University of Vienna)

homogeneously echogenic on US, and may be indistinguishable from endometrial hyperplasia or polyps. Inhomogeneous endometrial echo-texture with poorly defined margins is generally more indicative of endometrial carcinoma (Fig. 1.1). Cystic changes of the endometrium may also be seen in the setting of endometrial hyperplasia and endometrial carcinoma.

3D sonography has been playing an increasingly important role in the assessment of endometrial pathology. In a recent study by Merce et al., 3D sonography in combination with power Doppler angiography was employed in an attempt to differentiate between endometrial carcinoma and endometrial hyperplasia in women with uterine bleeding. Various quantifiable parameters such as the vascularization index (VI), 3D power Doppler indices, and the intratumoral resistive index (RI) were found to be more useful than endometrial thickness for differentiating between hyperplasia and endometrial carcinoma [1]. These methods, while promising, have not been validated in large trials.

1.2.1.2 Cervical and Vulvo/Vaginal Carcinoma

Ultrasound is of limited value in the diagnosis and staging of cervical or vulvo/vaginal carcinomas, and is far better defined with magnetic resonance imaging (MRI). The diagnosis and staging of vulvar and vaginal malignancies by ultrasound is likewise highly limited. In Vienna, ultrasound is frequently used to determine the thickness of vaginal lesions, the diameter of cervical lesions, extent of parametrial invasion, as well as other tumor characteristics.

1.2.2 Computed Tomography

Computed tomography (CT) is a valuable imaging modality for assessing the extent of metastatic disease and for assessing the primary lesion in women with gynecologic malignancies (Fig. 1.2). Oral and intravenous contrast are routinely administered for the evaluation of abdominopelvic malignancies. Oral contrast is very important and must be taken in sufficient volume at least 1–2 h prior to the exam. A slice thickness of 2.5 mm is optimum for the characterization and staging of pelvic malignancies. 1,000 cc of oral contrast is typically administered, as well as 100–120 cc of intravenous contrast injected at a rate of 3–4 cc/s. Images are generally obtained during the portal venous phase with a typical scan delay of 50–70 s. Rectal contrast is often administered at the radiologist's discretion, and is particularly useful if direct invasion of tumor into the bowel is suspected.

1.2.2.1 Endometrial Carcinoma

Contrast-enhanced CT may demonstrate nonspecific areas of decreased attenuation in the endometrial cavity that may invade the myometrium. Endometrial carcinoma may present as a discrete mass or diffuse endometrial thickening on contrast-enhanced studies. Irregularity of the endometrial–myometrial interface suggests myometrial invasion. (Fig. 1.2a) However, CT is far less accurate than MR in its ability to reliably assess the degree of myometrial invasion or localized parametrial extension in disease confined to the pelvis [2]. CT is best reserved for evaluating regional lymph nodes and determining distant metastatic sites such as the lungs or liver.

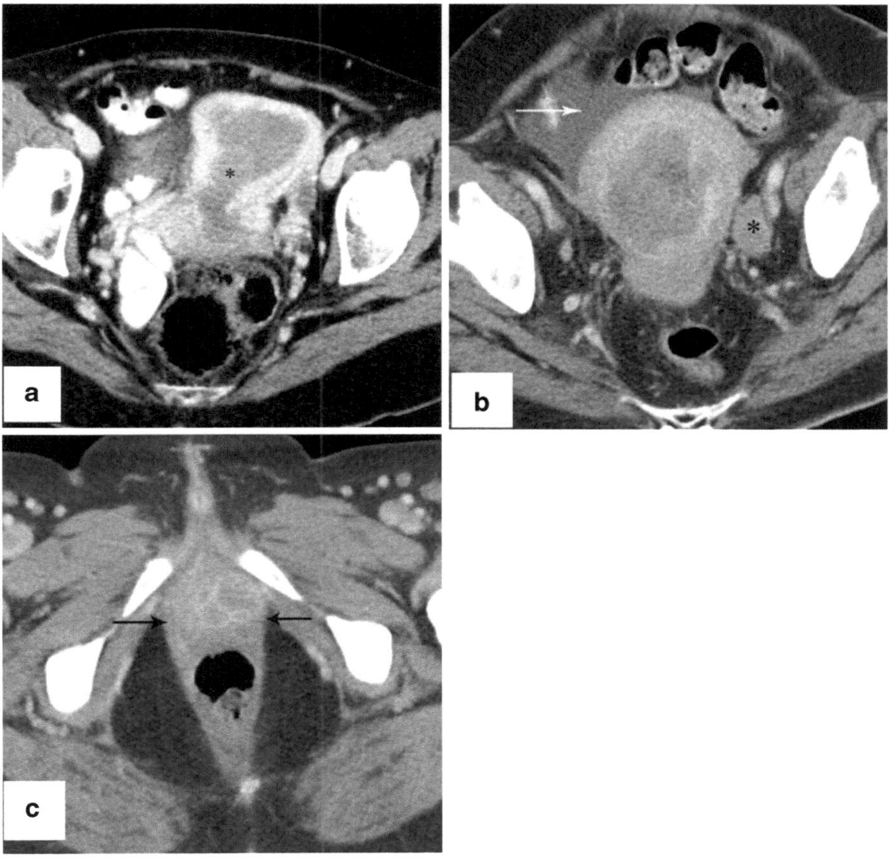

Fig. 1.2 (**a**) Endometrial carcinoma stage IB. Contrast-enhanced computed tomography (CT) demonstrates a soft-tissue attenuation endometrial mass (*) within the lower uterine segment. A fluid collection is noted proximal to the mass with resultant dilatation of the proximal uterus, indicative of uterine obstruction. Accurate assessment of the degree of myometrial invasion is inherently limited on CT. Pathologic review revealed less than 50% tumor involvement of the myometrium following hysterectomy. (**b**) Cervical carcinoma stage IIIC. Contrast-enhanced axial CT demonstrates a large, heterogeneous mass expanding the cervix. A small amount of ascites is noted anterior to the cervix (*arrow*). Parametrial lymphadenopathy is likewise noted (*). (**c**) Vulvar carcinoma. Contrast-enhanced CT scan demonstrates a multilobular, heterogeneous mass arising from the vaginal introitus, consistent with vulvar carcinoma

1.2.2.2 Cervical and Vulvar/Vaginal Carcinoma

The detection of suspected cervical, vaginal, or vulvar neoplasms is inherently limited by CT, as is the degree of localized cervical stromal or parametrial invasion (Fig. 1.2b and c). In a recent multicenter study jointly conducted by the American College of Radiology

Imaging Network (ACRIN) and Gynecologic Oncology Group (GOG), the level of reader agreement was low in the CT assessment of early invasive cervical cancer. MR imaging was significantly better than CT for tumor visualization and detection of parametrial involvement [3]. However, as in all gynecologic malignancies, regional nodes can be assessed as well as the liver and lungs as sites of potential metastatic disease. Nodes larger than 1 cm in short axis are generally considered abnormal [4].

1.2.3 PET and PET-CT

The use of 2-[fluorine 18]fluoro-2-deoxy-D-glucose (FDG) positron emission tomography (PET) combined with computed tomography (CT) for the evaluation of gynecologic malignancies is being increasing utilized. Combined PET-CT has largely replaced conventional PET since in-line PET-CT systems have become so widely available. PET-CT provides highly accurate localization of focal radiotracer uptake, which significantly improves the diagnostic accuracy compared with PET or CT alone.

1.2.3.1 Endometrial Carcinoma

There is avid FDG activity within the endometrium in the setting of endometrial carcinoma which, while nonspecific, frequently corresponds to endometrial thickening on conventional CT images. There is normal cyclic variation of endometrial FDG activity, which generally increases during menses, particularly in younger women. Detection of a mass or focal abnormality on MR/CT when combined with increased FDG uptake can increase the overall specificity of the individual modalities. The sensitivity of FDG-PET alone or FDG-PET plus MRI-CT is significantly higher than that of MRI-CT alone in overall lesion detection [5]. PET-CT is a useful modality for staging of endometrial carcinoma as well as evaluating response to therapy [6].

1.2.3.2 Cervical Carcinoma

PET-CT has been shown to be very effective for the staging of cervical cancer (Fig. 1.3). One report has shown sensitivity and specificity of 100% [7]. The technique has likewise been successfully employed to evaluate for early recurrence. PET has been shown to be more sensitive than MR or CT in the detection of para-aortic lymph node metastases in the setting of advanced cervical carcinoma [8]. A sensitivity and specificity of 100% and 99.7% respectively have been reported for the detection of metastatic lymph nodes greater than 5 mm [9].

The most common histologic subtype of cervical cancer is squamous cell carcinoma, which represents roughly 80% of primary cervical malignancies. Most cervical squamous

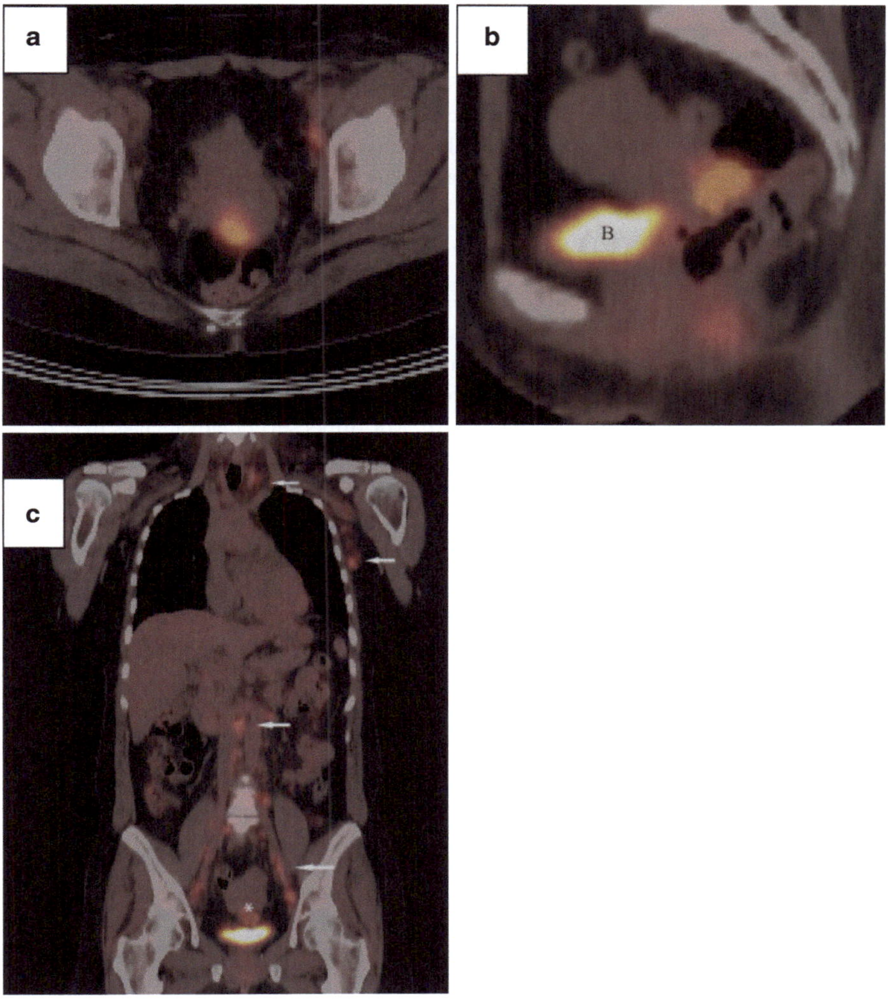

Fig. 1.3 (**a**) Cervical carcinoma. An axial section of a positron emission tomography-computed tomography (PET-CT) demonstrates intense metabolic activity within the cervix. The tumor extends to within several millimeters of the rectum. (**b**) Sagittal view demonstrating increased uptake in the urinary bladder, not to be confused with the cervical cancer. (**c**) PET-CT image demonstrates multiple bilateral iliac, paraaortic, left axillary, and left supraclavicular foci of intense metabolic activity, as well as the cervix (*), consistent with widespread nodal metastatic disease in a patient with stage IVB cervical cancer

cell carcinomas are FDG avid. FDG uptake is commonly seen in the adjacent vagina, uterus, bladder, or parametrial region in the setting of localized tumor extension. Normal physiologic FDG excretion into the endometrium and urinary bladder may result in false positive involvement. Complete bladder voiding prior to imaging is essential in order to avoid overcalling bladder involvement.

1.2.3.3 Vulvo/Vaginal Carcinoma

Primary and metastatic vaginal and vulvar carcinoma demonstrates avid uptake of FDG. As was previously described, physiologic FDG activity within a urine-filled bladder may obscure and/or overestimate the degree of vaginal or vulvar involvement.

1.2.4 Magnetic Resonance Imaging

MR has evolved as the gold standard for the noninvasive staging of gynecologic malignancies. MR is generally regarded as superior to ultrasound and CT in the evaluation of myometrial invasion and cervical involvement [10]. MR offers several advantages over other imaging modalities, including its inherent multiplanar capability, lack of ionizing radiation, and excellent soft-tissue contrast resolution. MR can provide highly accurate assessment of pelvic nodal involvement and the extent of local tumor invasion of other pelvic structures such as the parametria, vagina, or bladder and rectum. Other information, such as uterine orientation, tumor volume, concomitant ovarian pathology, or the presence of ascites can be readily ascertained by pelvic MR.

1.2.4.1 Scanner Hardware

Main Magnet

The strength of a magnet in an MR scanner is expressed by a unit of measurement referred to as a Tesla (T). Most modern MR scanners in clinical use range from 1.5–3T, which is roughly 30,000–60,000 times stronger than the earth's magnetic field. The higher field strength gives better overall signal-to-noise ratio (SNR), resulting in more accurate imaging.

Newer MR techniques, such as diffusion-weighted imaging (DWI), may potentially benefit from higher field strength pelvic imaging. Diffusion-weighted imaging (DWI) is a technique that exploits the differences in diffusion or movement of water molecules through various tissues, since water molecules diffuse at different rates through cancerous and normal tissue. Preliminary results in the use of diffusion-weighted imaging for predicting the histologic grade of endometrial carcinoma are promising [11].

There are several disadvantages associated with higher field strength pelvic imaging. While 3T imaging of the pelvis may provide better resolution of certain pelvic structures, 3T images tend to be noisier and are more susceptible to peristaltic artifacts because of the required longer imaging time. Additionally, susceptibility artifact from metallic clips in postoperative patients tends to be more pronounced at 3T imaging. Although the benefit of 3T abdominal imaging has been validated in hepatic and pancreatobiliary imaging, the benefit of higher field strength pelvic imaging has not yet been well established [12].

Scanner Configuration

Most conventional MR scanners are closed bore, in which the patient is placed into the tunnel of a relatively small diameter magnet. However, many claustrophobic or larger body habitus patients are unable to tolerate the relatively small diameter bore (60 cm) of a conventional 1.5 T scanner. In response to this subset of patients, several MR vendors have developed scanners in recent years with larger diameter bores and shorter bore lengths while maintaining a field strength of 1.5 T. Open-bore scanners are also available in which the patient lies between large horizontally or vertically oriented parallel magnets. However, one major disadvantage of the open-bore configuration is the inherently weaker magnetic field strength. State-of-the-art open MR scanners can only achieve a maximum field strength of around 1.0 T. Newer 3T magnets now have wider bore up to 70 cm and have a higher table weight limit of over 500 lb (225 kg) compared to the conventional 300 lb (135 kg).

Radiofrequency Coils

Radiofrequency (RF) coils function to both send and receive radiofrequency pulses in order to generate MR images. The body coil is a permanent circumferential coil that is incorporated into the scanner gantry that not only sends, but also receives RF signals when larger parts of the body are imaged. The body coil produces images with a large field of view, which is advantageous when imaging a large body part such as the abdomen. Surface coils are specially designed coils that conform to the specific body part that is being imaged. They are receiver-only coils that are placed immediately adjacent to an anatomic region of interest in order to maximize the signal-to-noise ratio. Phased array coils have become the standard coil of choice for pelvic imaging. These coils combine the strengths of surface coils with high signal-to-noise ratio and that of body coils with a large field of view. Newer endovaginal receiver-only coils permit high-resolution imaging of the cervix in order to more accurately assess early stage I cervical neoplasms [13]. Investigators have more recently performed diffusion-weighted MR imaging of the cervix utilizing an endovaginal coil in an attempt to more accurately detect early-stage disease [14].

MR Contrast Agents

Contrast agents can be divided into two broad categories: positive and negative contrast agents. Gadolinium is the most commonly employed intravenous positive MR contrast agent, which results in an increased signal intensity or "brighter" appearance of perfused tissue. Gadolinium is a lanthanide element that is paramagnetic in its trivalent state. When intravenously administered, it causes increased signal intensity on MR images by altering the local magnetic field of protons within the body. Pure gadolinium is toxic, but can be safely administered intravenously when chelated to other inert molecules such as diethylene triamine pentaacetic acid (DTPA).

Over the past few decades, gadolinium chelates have been safely administered to millions of patients with extremely uncommon side effects. However, nephrogenic systemic fibrosis (NSF) is a rare, but potentially debilitating disease that was first described in the literature in 2000 in association with IV gadolinium administration [15]. The disease occurs almost exclusively in patients with renal insufficiency who are exposed to IV gadolinium, and is characterized by multiorgan fibrosis of muscle, tendons, testes, cardiac atrium, lung, and dura mater. Renal function tests are now required for all patients with suspected moderate to severe renal insufficiency prior to gadolinium administration. Current recommendations suggest that gadolinium should be avoided in those patients with an estimated GFR (glomerular filtration rate) less than 40 mL/min. Low-dose gadolinium can be administered with caution to patients with a GFR between 40–60 mL/min if the benefits of a contrast-enhanced MR study outweigh the risks [16].

Negative contrast agents appear predominantly dark on MR, and are much less commonly utilized when compared to gadolinium-based compounds. Small particulate aggregates or superparamagnetic iron oxide (SPIO) particles are the most commonly used negative contrast agents. Recent advances in lymph-node avid MR contrast agents, such as ultrasmall super-paramagnetic iron oxide (USPIO) particles have revealed promising results in the detection of lymph node metastases in endometrial and cervical malignancies. While MR can be used to detect lymphadenopathy with a high degree of accuracy based on size criteria, nodes that are smaller than the size threshold may harbor metastatic deposits. USPIO particles have been successfully employed to differentiate between benign and metastatic lymph nodes. It has been well validated in the literature that USPIO particles are taken up in benign, reactive lymph nodes, whereas a little to no uptake of USPIO particles is seen in metastatic lymph nodes [17]. However, in the USA these compounds have not been approved by the FDA to date.

Imaging Protocol

Patients can be asked to fast for 4–6 h prior to the exam in order to limit motion artifact from bowel peristalsis. Alternatively, an antiperistaltic agent such as glucagon can be intramuscularly or intravenously administered in order to minimize peristalsis if necessary. Patients are encouraged to empty their bladder prior to imaging in order to minimize displacement of organs, which can result in ghosting and motion artifact from an excessively distended bladder. Patients are routinely imaged in the supine position using a pelvic phased array multichannel coil as previously described.

MR images obtained on virtually any MR examination can be classified into two broad categories: T1- and T2-weighted images. However, a fundamental tenet of MR imaging is that fluid is dark on T1-weighted images, whereas fluid is bright on T2-weighted images. The standard MR protocol for uterine and/or cervical malignancies includes axial T1-weighted spin-echo images with a large field of view of the entire pelvis in order to assess for pelvic lymphadenopathy and bone marrow changes.

T2-weighted images provide the optimal imaging of the uterine zonal and substructure anatomy. Furthermore, neoplastic processes are often better depicted on T2-weighted images, since cancerous tissues often demonstrate increased signal intensity on T2-weighted images due to the presence of edema. Small field of view multiplanar axial, sagittal, and coronal T2-weighted fast spin-echo images through the uterus are routine.

T1-weighted images after rapid injection of approximately 20 cc of Gadolinium contrast images axial or perpendicular to the long axis of the uterine corpus are frequently

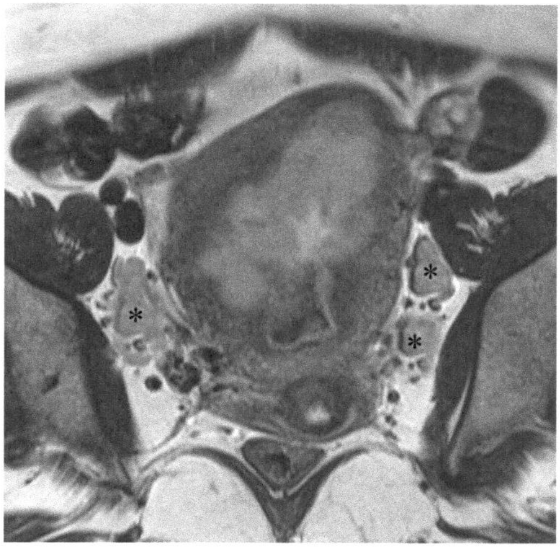

Fig. 1.4 Endometrial carcinoma stage IIIC. Axial T2-weighted MR demonstrates a large, intermediate signal mass expanding the uterine endometrium. Prominent parametrial lymphadenopathy is noted (*)

helpful in the assessment of myometrial invasion. Some investigators advocate the use of dynamic IV contrast enhancement for accurate evaluation of endometrial carcinoma in order to optimize visualization of the uterine zonal anatomy and the extent of tumor involvement [18]. This technique entails the serial acquisition of images through the uterine corpus at various time intervals following IV contrast administration.

1.2.4.2 Endometrial Carcinoma

In recent years, MRI has emerged as the gold standard in the staging of endometrial carcinoma (Fig. 1.4). MRI is significantly better than ultrasound or CT in the evaluation of both endocervical tumor extension and myometrial invasion [10]. The staging accuracy of endometrial carcinoma by MR has been reported to be between 85% and 93% [19, 20]. It has likewise been shown that dynamic IV contrast enhancement is a significantly more accurate means of assessing myometrial invasion when compared to conventional T2-weighted images [21]. As previously mentioned, diffusion-weighted imaging is a relatively new tool in the assessment of endometrial malignancies, which may potentially aid in the differentiation of benign and malignant conditions of the uterus [11]. The use of DWI in the evaluation of endometrial carcinoma has yet to be fully validated.

1.2.4.3 Cervical Carcinoma

As previously stated, MR remains the imaging gold standard for the most accurate imaging of cervical carcinoma (Fig. 1.5). The staging accuracy of cervical carcinoma by MR has been reported to range between 75% and 96% [19]. In a recent multicenter study by the ACRIN/GOG (American College of Radiology Imaging Network and the Gynecologic

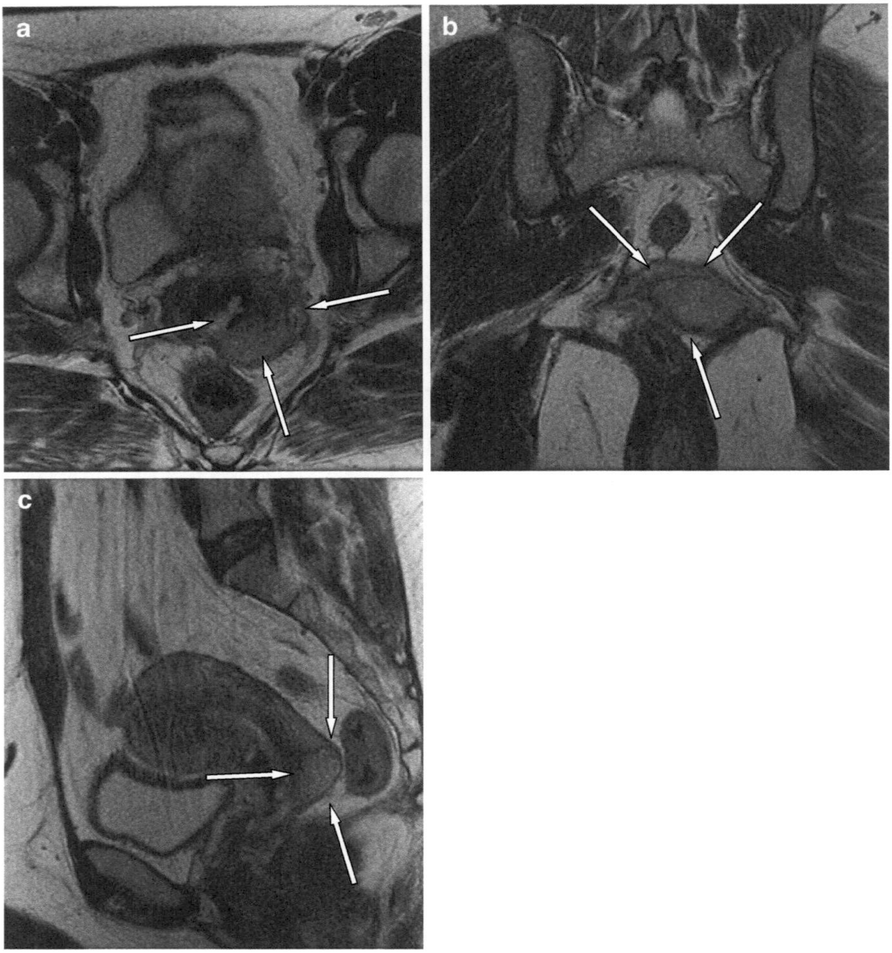

Fig. 1.5 Cervical carcinoma FIGO clinical stage IB1. Axial, coronal, and sagittal T2-weighted MR demonstrates a sharply marginated complex mass expanding the posterior lip of the cervix (*arrows*)

Imaging Group), experienced radiologists retrospectively compared the diagnostic performance and interobserver variability for both CT and MR in the pretreatment evaluation of early invasive cervical cancer. MR imaging was found to be significantly better than CT for tumor visualization and detection of parametrial invasion. In a study conducted by Hricak et al, 57 consecutive patients underwent pelvic MR prior to surgical staging. Overall, the accuracy of MR imaging in staging was 81% [22].

The MR protocol for the imaging of cervical carcinoma is similar to that for endometrial cancer. Cervical malignancies are best visualized on T2-weighted images. High-resolution, small field of view axial oblique T2-weighted images perpendicular to the long axis of the cervix are routine when assessing for parametrial invasion. Axial T1-weighted

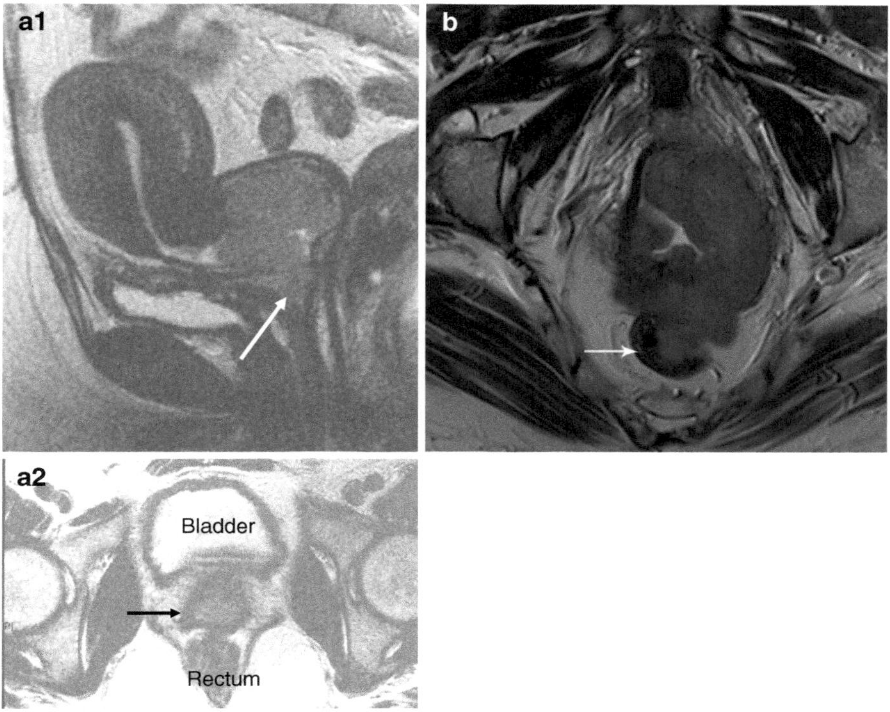

Fig. 1.6 (**a**) Cervical carcinoma stage IIA. (**a1**) Sagittal T2-weighted MR demonstrates a bulky, intermediate signal mass replacing the normal cervical stroma and with proximal vaginal extension (*arrow*). (**a2**) Axial T2-weighted MR of the same patient as in A. on a section that demonstrates tumoral involvement of the proximal vagina, bladder and rectum. (**b**) Cervical carcinoma stage IVA. Axial T2-weighted MR demonstrates a multilobular intermediate signal mass arising from the cervix. There is posterior extension of the mass with direct invasion of the anterior wall of the rectum (*arrow*)

images of the abdomen are routinely preformed in order to identify lymphadenopathy. MR images may also depict vaginal extension (Fig. 1.6).

MRI has proven to be an extremely useful tool not only for staging of cervical carcinoma, but also for monitoring treatment response and predicting clinical outcome. In a prospective study performed by Mayr et al., MR was performed on 34 patients with cervical cancer of various federation of gynecology and obstetrics (FIGO) stages before and after radiation therapy. Tumor volumetry (3D measurements) was obtained using T2-weighted images in order to quantify the tumor regression rate. Sequential tumor volumetry using MR imaging was found to be a very effective measure of the responsiveness of cervical cancer to irradiation [23]. MR imaging is more accurate and reproducible than exam under anesthesia (EUA) is also a safer and cheaper way to achieve a better staging result. Durfee et al. showed that MR directly alters management and most often will upstage cervical carcinomas [24].

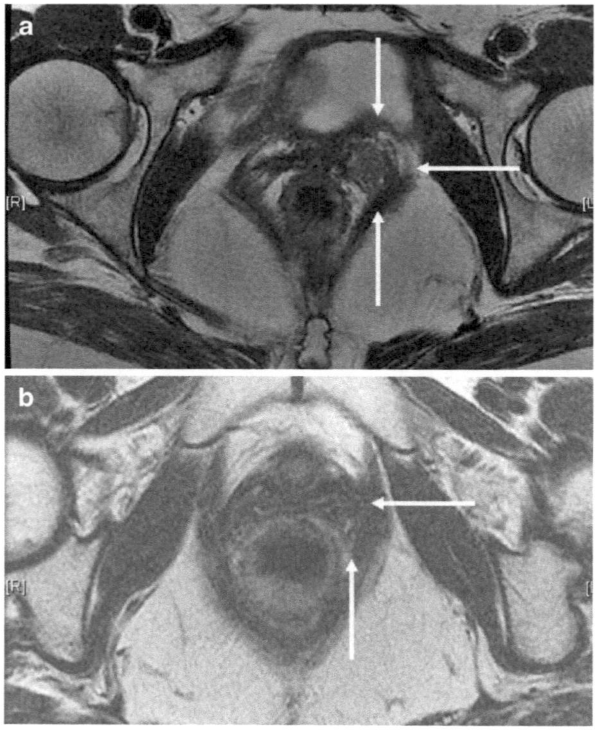

Fig. 1.7 Vaginal carcinoma. (**a**) Axial T2-weighted image demonstrates a mass arising from the left vaginal fornix that was clinically visible. (**b**) There has been a complete response after external beam radiation with concurrent chemotherapy followed by vaginal cylinder brachytherapy. An interstitial implant would have been required with residual thickening after external beam (*)

1.2.4.4 Vaginal and Vulvar Carcinoma

MR remains the primary imaging modality for the characterization and staging of vaginal and vulvar malignancies. MR can accurately depict the location and size of the tumor, degree of parametrial extension or pelvic sidewall involvement, degree of regional lymphadenopathy, and local spread of disease to the adjacent bladder or rectum (Fig. 1.7). Additionally, the signal characteristics of primary vaginal malignancies on MR have been shown to correlate with the histologic subtype of the tumor [25].

Primary vaginal tumors arise solely from the vaginal walls, and by definition cannot involve the external os superiorly or the vulva inferiorly. This distinction is important, since treatment options between vaginal and other adjacent cervical or vulvar neoplasms vary. MR has become an extremely valuable means of providing precise anatomic localization in order to differentiate between primary vaginal and nonvaginal malignancies [24]. MR has likewise become an essential component in surgical and radiation therapy planning. Patients who have an MRI and/or clinical exam after external beam radiation that shows a residual lesion measuring >5 mm require interstitial rather than vaginal cylinder brachytherapy.

1.3 Complications of Radiation Therapy

Since the advent of radiation therapy more than a century ago, significant technical advances have resulted in progressively effective radiation treatment with minimal complications. In spite of highly sophisticated delivery systems for the treatment of gynecologic neoplasms, complications can occur. More commonly, diffuse tissue edema with thickening of the bladder, rectum, sigmoid and small bowel loops are seen following radiation. Life-threatening complications from intracavitary radiation are uncommon. Iatrogenic fistulas are rare. Late complications can be evaluated with conventional retrograde cystourethrograms or barium studies, as can strictures of the rectosigmoid colon. Small bowel strictures are best evaluated with an upper GI with small bowel follow-through. CT has also proven to be very useful in the evaluation of various fistulas involving the lower pelvis.

Insufficiency fractures of the sacrum are another well-described complication of radiation therapy. These fractures typically involve the sacral aspect of the SI joint, followed by the pubic bones, and are best visualized on MR.

1.4 Summary

The techniques to noninvasively characterize gynecologic malignancies have evolved significantly over the past several decades. Diagnostic imaging will continue to be an essential component in the detection, staging, and pretreatment assessment of pelvic neoplasms. While ultrasound and CT continue to assist in the diagnosis of these disease entities, MR will undoubtedly remain the gold standard in the regional assessment of pelvic malignancies. However, PET-CT will undoubtedly continue to evolve as an indispensable tool in the workup of gynecologic malignancies, particularly in those individuals with widespread metastatic disease.

References

1. Merce LT, Alcazar JL, Lopez C, et al. Clinical usefulness of 3-dimensional sonography and power doppler angiography for diagnosis of endometrial carcinoma. J Ultrasound Med. 2007; 26:1279–87.
2. Hardesty LA, Sumkin JH, Hakim C, et al. The ability of helical CT to preoperatively stage endometrial carcinoma. AJR Am J Roentgenol. 2001;176:603–6.
3. Hricak H, Gatsonis C, Coakley FV, et al. Early invasive cervical cancer: CT and MR imaging in preoperative evaluation – ACRIN/GOG comparative study of diagnostic performance and interobserver variability. Radiology. 2007;245:491–8.
4. Hricak H, Yu K. Radiology in invasive cervical cancer. Am J Roentgenol. 1996;167:1101–8.

5. Chao A, Chang TC, Ng KK, et al. 18F-FDG PET in the management of endometrial cancer. Eur J Nucl Med Mol Imaging. 2006;33:36–44.
6. Kitajima K, Murakami K, Yamasaki E, et al. Accuracy of 18F-FDG PET/CT in detecting pelvic and paraaortic lymph node metastasis in patients with endometrial cancer. AJR Am J Roentgenol. 2008;190:1652–8.
7. Wong TZ, Jones EL, Coleman RE. Positron emission tomography with 2-deoxy-2-[(18)F] fluoro-D-glucose for evaluating local and distant disease in patients with cervical cancer. Mol Imaging Biol. 2004;6:55–62.
8. Jemal A, Siegel R, Ward E, et al. Cancer statistics, 2007. CA Cancer J Clin. 2007;57:43–66.
9. Sironi S, Buda A, Picchio M, et al. Lymph node metastasis in patients with clinical early-stage cervical cancer: detection with integrated FDG PET/CT. Radiology. 2005;238:272–9.
10. Kinkel K, Kaji Y, Yu KK, et al. Radiologic staging in patients with endometrial cancer: a meta-analysis. Radiology. 1999;212:711–8.
11. Tamai K, Koyama T, Saga T, et al. Diffusion-weighted MR imaging of uterine endometrial cancer. J Magn Reson Imaging. 2007;26:682–7.
12. Choi JY, Kim MJ, Chung YE, et al. Abdominal applications of 3.0-T MR imaging: comparative review versus a 1.5-T system. Radiographics. 2008;28:30.
13. deSouza N, Scoones D, Krausz T, et al. High-resolution MR imaging of stage I cervical neoplasia with a dedicated transvaginal coil: MR features and correlation of imaging and pathologic findings. Am J Roentgenol. 1996;166:553–9.
14. Charles-Edwards EM, Messiou C, Morgan VA, et al. Diffusion-weighted imaging in cervical cancer with an endovaginal technique: potential value for improving tumor detection in stage Ia and Ib1 disease. Radiology. 2008;249:541–50.
15. Cowper SE, Robin HS, Steinberg SM, et al. Scleromyxoedema-like cutaneous diseases in renal-dialysis patients. Lancet. 2000;356:1000–1.
16. Swaminathan S, Shah SV. New insights into nephrogenic systemic fibrosis. J Am Soc Nephrol. 2007;18:2636–43.
17. Rockall AG, Sohaib SA, Harisinghani MG, et al. Diagnostic performance of nanoparticle-enhanced magnetic resonance imaging in the diagnosis of lymph node metastases in patients with endometrial and cervical cancer. J Clin Oncol. 2005;23:2813–21.
18. Frei KA, Kinkel K, Bonel HM, et al. Prediction of deep myometrial invasion in patients with endometrial cancer: clinical utility of contrast-enhanced MR imaging – a meta-analysis and Bayesian analysis. Radiology. 2000;216:444–9.
19. Sala E, Wakely S, Senior E, et al. MRI of malignant neoplasms of the uterine corpus and cervix. AJR Am J Roentgenol. 2007;188:1577–87.
20. Manfredi R, Mirk P, Maresca G, et al. Local-regional staging of endometrial carcinoma: role of MR imaging in surgical planning. Radiology. 2004;231:372–8.
21. Seki H, Kimura M, Sakai K. Myometrial invasion of endometrial carcinoma: assessment with dynamic MR and contrast-enhanced T1-weighted images. Clin Radiol. 1997;52:18–23.
22. Hricak H, Lacey CG, Sandles LG, et al. Invasive cervical carcinoma: comparison of MR imaging and surgical findings. Radiology. 1988;166:623–31.
23. Mayr NA, Yuh WT, Magnotta VA, et al. Tumor perfusion studies using fast magnetic resonance imaging technique in advanced cervical cancer: a new noninvasive predictive assay. Int J Radiat Oncol Biol Phys. 1996;36:623–33.
24. Durfee SM, Zou KH, Muto MG, Sheets EE, Tempany CMC. The role of magnetic resonance imaging in treatment planning of cervical carcinoma. J Womens Imag. 2000;2:63–8.
25. Parikh JH, Barton DP, Ind TE, et al. MR imaging features of vaginal malignancies. Radiographics. 2008;28:49–63.

The Use of Sectional Imaging with CT and MRI for Image-Guided Therapy

2

Johannes C. Athanasios Dimopoulos and Elena Fidarova

2.1 Introduction

Sectional imaging is integrated in each link of the modern radiotherapy chain, from diagnostic procedures to target volume definition to treatment planning, dose delivery, and verification. While CT is widely used for modern EBRT, including intensity modulated radiotherapy (IMRT) and image-guided radiotherapy (IGRT), MRI represents the gold standard for IGBT for gynecological malignancies (see Chap. 5, Sect. 5.4).

High-precision radiotherapy techniques offer the option of enhancement of the therapeutic ratio, because the dose to the target is escalated and the normal organs are spared. However, in order to increase conformity, accurate target and organ delineation performed according to standardized protocols is required. Additionally, inter-/intrafraction variation due to tumor shrinkage and changes in dimensions and topography of the normal organs has to be taken into account, thus representing the main challenge for successful application of IGRT.

To reduce contouring uncertainties and to identify inter-/intrafraction variation with high accuracy, a radiation oncologist has to apply image acquisition protocols adapted to the needs of image-guided therapy, to analyze sectional images with particular attention to tumor regression, regions of potential tumor spread, and lymph nodes regions. This chapter aims to cover important issues of CT and MRI application for image-guided therapy.

J.C.A. Dimopoulos (✉)
Director of Department of Radiation Therapy, Metropolitan Hospital,
9 Ethn. Makariou and El. Venizelou, 18547 Athens, Greece
e-mail: adimopoulos@metropolitan-hospital.gr

E. Fidarova
Department of Radiotherapy, Vienna General Hospital, Medical University of Vienna,
Währinger Gürtel 18-20, 1090 Vienna, Austria
e-mail: Elena.fidarova@akhwien.at

A.N. Viswanathan et al. (eds.), *Gynecologic Radiation Therapy*,
DOI: 10.1007/978-3-540-68958-4_2, © Springer-Verlag Berlin Heidelberg 2011

2.2 General Technical Issues Regarding the Use of Sectional Imaging for Image-Guided Therapy

CT is the standard imaging modality for 3D conformal EBRT and IMRT of the pelvis. It provides information about the electron density of tissues that is required for the dose calculation algorithms of all the commercially available treatment planning systems. CT also lacks peripheral image distortion that is characteristic of MRI. Modern CT scanners obtain 64 slices for each turn of the gantry and offer the possibility of image acquisition of the entire abdomen and pelvis in less than 1 min. For in-room imaging, both multi-slice CT and cone-beam CT (CBCT) can be used. The new generation of accelerators is equipped with CBCT mounted on the gantry. This technical solution allows detecting individual variations under treatment conditions and their on-line correction [1, 2]. The use of such volumetric image-guidance has increased the demand for adaptive replanning [1].

MRI enables improved soft tissue depiction and gives detailed information about pelvic topography and tumor regression during radiotherapy [3–5]. It has to be noted though, that MRI is not routinely implemented for EBRT treatment planning mainly due to two major limitations: intrinsic spatial image distortion and missing electron density information [6, 7]. This implies that if MRI scans are used for treatment planning, tissue attenuation coefficients have to be assigned manually or a homogeneous attenuation has to be assumed within all image regions [6, 7]. An alternate option is co-registration and fusion of MR and CT images, which allow achieving desirable imaging information and creating optimal conditions for precise dose calculation [8, 9]. The problem of MR image distortions can be resolved by applying different image correction methods [10–13].

Low-field 0.2–0.5 T (Tesla) open MRI scanners offer improved patient accessibility and are suitable for claustrophobic patients [4]. However, the image quality of low-field scanners is not equivalent to the image quality of those with standard magnetic field strength of 1.5 T and higher. Therefore, scanners with 3 T are increasingly utilized in the radiology community. With higher field strength, the signal-to-noise ratio is increasing and the voxel volume can be reduced [14]. Image distortion is also increasing with increasing field strength [7]. Higher magnetic fields, like 7 and 8 T have been installed only in a few research centers as they present some technical challenges, e.g., the safety limits can be exceeded due to higher gradient amplitudes and radiofrequency power deposition [14]. Furthermore, they do not automatically produce better diagnostic images because of dielectric resonance effects [15].

2.3 Key Issues of Image Acquisition

Pelvic CT used for EBRT should be performed after administration of intravenous contrast agents. Additional improvement can be achieved by the use of oral iodine or barium-based contrast material. In the case of IGBT, intravenous contrast also assists in the identification of the superior border of the cervix due to visualization of the uterine vessels [16].

Retrograde application of bladder and rectal contrast before CT scanning improves delineation of these structures [16].

MR image acquisition protocols also need to be adapted to the needs of IGRT and IGBT. T2-weighted MRI sequences are considered the gold standard for IGRT and IGBT for gynecological malignancies [3, 4]. Vaginal contrast, e.g., with ultrasound gel, used for diagnostic scans improve visualization of the vaginal walls and lower parts of the cervix [4]. Bowel motion can be reduced by intravenous (e.g., *N*-Butylscopolan) or intramuscular (e.g., Glucagon chlorhydrate) drug administration. Use of MRI-compatible applicators and probes, vaginal packing impregnated with contrast agents (e.g., gadolinium, dilution 1:10) and a Foley catheter filled with contrast media (e.g., gadolinium, dilution 1:1) leads to clear visualization of relevant structures [4]. Only limited data about the impact of MR image orientation on contouring for IGBT is available [17]. However, current recommendations suggest using images orientated parallel and orthogonal to the applicator (sources) axes to obtain a "brachytherapy orientated view" (BOV) [18].

2.4 Issues of CT/MR Image Characteristics

CT scans provide information about topographic changes caused by tumor shrinkage, organ motion, and insertion of the brachytherapy applicator [19–21]. The normal organ contours (sigmoid colon, rectum, urinary bladder, vagina) as well as borders between organs and uterine parts (corpus, cervix) are often not clearly visible on native CT scans [22]. Improved visualization of these contours can be achieved by the use of contrast media, but even in this case organ walls are not clearly visualized [21]. Finally, the spatial relationship between the brachytherapy applicator, uterus (cervix, corpus), and surrounding organs becomes visible on CT images [4, 18, 21, 22].

However, there are some inherent limitations of CT for 3D delineation of relevant structures for IGRT and IGBT. The uterus is displayed as a homogenous organ located in the center of the true pelvis. Distinction between different patho-anatomical parts (corpus, cervix, tumor mass(es)), relies on indirect information about the topography of the endometrial cavity and uterine artery [16, 21, 23]. Parametrial ligaments and uterine arteries can be identified on CT with a wide variation of shapes and thicknesses [16, 21, 23]. Accurate detection of tumor and parametrial infiltration on CT is challenging compared to MRI [21, 24, 25]. CT provides limited information about radiation changes and distinction between cervix and residual disease (within the parametria and the uterus) [16, 21].

MRI appears to discriminate soft tissue and tumor in the pelvis and has the capability of imaging in multiple planes, as compared to CT [26]. A comparison between MR and CT as imaging modalities used for IGBT, revealed no significant differences in volume sizes and DVH parameters for the organs at risk (OAR), but for target volumes, CT-based contouring significantly overestimated the contour width when compared to MRI (Fig. 2.1) [16].

Information essential to improve IGRT and IGBT, like tumor extent, topography, and regression, as well as topography of patho-anatomical structures, is provided by MRI

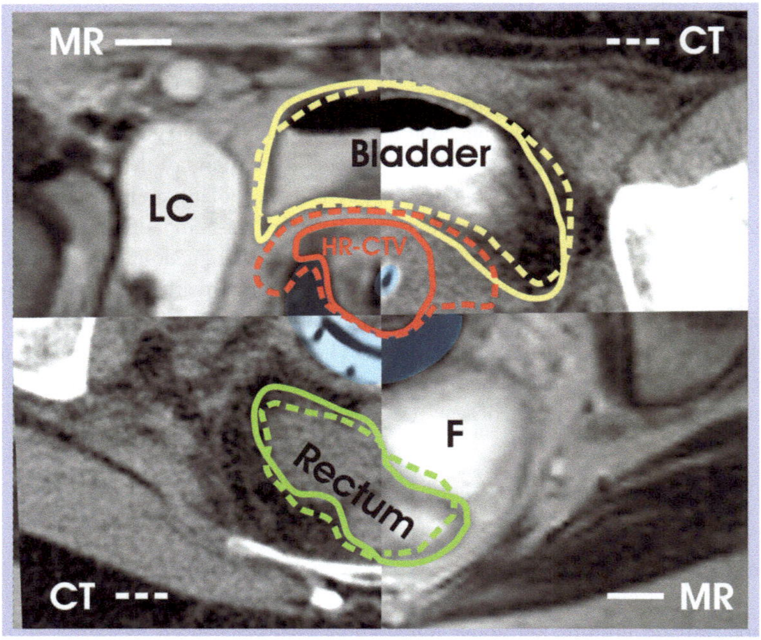

Fig. 2.1 Image fusion between axial computed tomography (CT) and magnetic resonance (MR) scans at time of brachytherapy. Bladder, rectum, and High Risk (HR) Clinical Target Volume (CTV) are contoured (CT – *dotted line*, MR – *solid line*). Organs at risk (OAR) contours deviate only slightly, whereas HR CTV is larger on CT, especially in lateral directions. Blue transparent color indicates tandem-ring applicator, which is depicted as a homogeneous black structure in magnetic resonance imaging (MRI). On the contrary, details of the applicator (source channel, holes for needles) are clearly visible on a CT scan (LC, lymphocyst after laparoscopic lymph node staging; F, free fluid in the pouch of Douglas)

[3, 4, 27–29]. A systematic analysis of MRI findings before EBRT and at the time of brachytherapy with the applicator in place, provided information helpful to reduce uncertainties regarding the definition of gross target volume (GTV), clinical target volume (CTV), and patho-anatomical structures (Fig. 2.2) [4]. Finally, it has been shown that the parametrial space, as the region of potential tumor spread, can be defined on axial MR images based on visible radiological criteria [4].

The most important image characteristics, as well as the pearls and pitfalls of CT and MRI for image-guided therapy are summarized in Table 2.1.

2.5 The Issue of Lymph-Node Delineation for High-Precision and Image-Guided EBRT

The detection of pathologic enlarged lymph nodes with sectional imaging is of major importance for IGRT. The precision of CT and MRI for the detection of lymph node

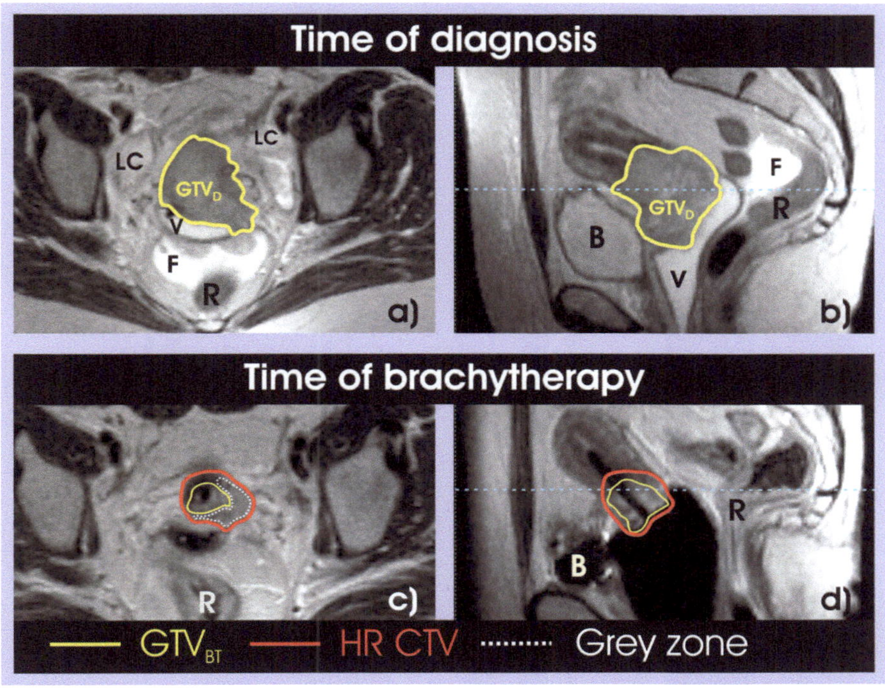

Fig. 2.2 MRI scans of a patient with FIGO IIB cervical cancer at time of diagnosis ((**a**) – axial plane, (**b**) – sagittal plane) and at time of brachytherapy ((**c**) – axial plane, (**d**) – sagittal plane). Tumor at time of diagnosis (GTV_D), which replaces the uterine cervix (**a**, **b**) and invades the left parametrium (**a**), is depicted as a homogeneous intermediate signal intensity mass. At the time of brachytherapy, HR CTV consists of high signal intensity residual tumor (GTV_{BT}), intermediate signal intensity "grey zones" and low signal intensity cervical tissue (**c**, **d**). *Dotted blue line* on sagittal images represents the level at which the correspondent axial scan was obtained (LC, lymphocyst after laparoscopic lymph node staging; F, free fluid in the pouch of Douglas; V, vagina contrasted with ultrasound gel; B, bladder; R, rectum)

metastasis is comparable [30–32]. Since both imaging modalities rely on size criteria (short axis >1 cm) for the detection of pathologic lymph nodes, the sensitivity of these methods is rather low, ranging between 40% and 70% [33–35]. Lymph node specific MRI contrast agents, e.g., ultrasmall particles of iron oxide (USPIO), show the potential of improving sensitivity for the prediction of lymph node metastasis. In the study of Rockall et al. the sensitivity increased from 29% using standard size criteria, to 93% using USPIO criteria based on a node-by-node approach, and from 27% to 100% based on a patient-by-patient approach [34]. FDG PET/CT is more accurate in identifying nodal metastases as the nodes do not need to be enlarged to be PET/CT positive. The reported sensitivity and specificity of PET/CT is within a range of 50–75% and 90–99% respectively [36–38].

Table 2.1 General characteristics with pearls and pitfalls of computed tomography (CT) and magnetic resonance (MR) for the different stages of image-guided therapy

	General characteristics					
	Soft tissue depiction	Image acquisition	Contrast media	Multiplanar imaging	Radiation exposure	Scanning time
MRI	Superior quality on T2-weighted sequences	Specific protocols required	Not obligatory needed	without reconstruction	No	Long
CT	I nferior quality	Specific protocols required	Recommended	only with reconstruction	Yes	Short
	Diagnostic scan					
	Tumor detection	**Parametrial invasion**	**Invasion of organs**	**Invasion of vagina**	**LN status**	**Recurrence detection**
MRI	Estimation of dimensions within 0.5 cm compared to pathology specimen. Detection of endocervical growth and uterine corpus invasion is possible	High accuracy for: –Distinction between stromal and parametrial invasion –Estimation of degree of parametrial invasion	High accuracy in prediction of infiltration of surrounding organs	High accuracy in predicting vaginal invasion, if vaginal contrast is used (e.g., ultrasound gel)	CT and MRI have similar inaccuracy in detecting LN metastases	Dynamic contrast-enhanced MRI enables differentiating tumor recurrence from radiation fibrosis
CT	Inaccurate estimation of tumor dimensions even with contrast enhancement and inability to detect uterine corpus invasion	Low accuracy in distinction between parametrial tumor spread and normal parametrial tissue	Early invasion of bladder and rectum is not reliably detectable	Low accuracy in predicting vaginal infiltration, especially at early stages	CT and MRI have similar accuracy in detecting LN metastases	CT is of low predictive value for differentiation between radiation fibrosis and recurrence

	IGRT scans (in addition to information gained from diagnostic scans)	
	Tumor regression	Organ changes
MRI	Accurate quantitative estimation of tumor regression during the entire course of radiotherapy is possible. Distinction between macroscopic visible (residual) tumor mass(es), pathologic residual tissue including edema, inflammation, fibrosis and tumor cells ("grey zones"), and surrounding tissue possible	Reliable detection of changes in organ position and volume possible
CT	Quantitative estimation of tumor regression not reliable. Distinction between macroscopic visible (residual) tumor mass(es), pathologic residual tissue ("grey zones"), and surrounding tissue not possible	Reliable detection of changes in organ position and size possible

	Brachytherapy scans				
	Target definition	Parametrial invasion	Invasion of organs	Invasion of vagina	Applicator depiction
MRI	Different parts of HR CTV [GTV = macroscopic tumor mass(es), ("grey zones") and cervix] are detectable	Detection of macroscopic tumor and residual pathologic tissue within the parametria possible	Detection of residual organ involvement possible	Detection of residual vaginal involvement possible	Inferior quality on T2-weighted sequences
CT	Different parts of HR CTV are not detectable	Reliable detection of macro-scopic tumor and residual pathologic tissue within the parametria not possible	Detection of residual organ involvement not always possible	Detection of residual organ involvement not always possible	Superior quality – Different parts of the applicator (e.g., source channel, wholes) are visible

Table 2.2 Location of assessed lymph nodes in relation to adjacent blood vessels

LN group		Average distance (range), mm[a]		
		Chao et al. [41]	Taylor et al. [43][b]	Diniwell et al. [42][c]
Common iliac	Right	12 (5–16)	–	–
	Left	16 (6–22)	–	–
	Ventral	0.3 (0–2)	–	–
	Not specified	–	7	7 (3–21)
External iliac	Medial	–	7	–
	Anterior	–	7	–
	Lateral	Right 16 (11–22)[d] Left 14 (7–17)[d]	15	–
	Not specified	–	–	7 (3–10)
Internal iliac		–	5	7 (3–14)
Obturator		–	3	8 (4–19)
Inguinal	Right	17 (7–28)	–	–
	Left	15 (8–23)	–	–
Para-aortic	Distal	–	–	9 (4–23)
	Ventral	2 (0–6)	–	–
	Right	9 (6–15)	–	–
	Left	22 (10–45)	–	–

[a]All distances were rounded
[b]At least 90% of LN covered by the given margin
[c]90% of LN was localized within given distance
[d]Relative to pelvic side wall

Some recent studies focused on the definition of guidelines for the delineation of the pelvic nodal target volume [39, 40]. Table 2.2 summarizes the margins proposed by different authors [41–43]. Chao and Lin suggested guidelines for IMRT of gynecological tumors based on lymphangiogram-assisted CT lymph-node delineation [41]. The authors recommend margins of 15–20 mm, with some modifications. Diniwell and colleagues used MRI scans with the contrast agent ferumoxtran-10 to investigate the nodal pelvic CTV [42]. In their study a 3D margin of 9–12 mm around the blood vessels and a margin of 22 mm medial to the pelvic sidewall were required to cover 90% of nodal tissue in 90% of patients [42]. Taylor et al. used MRI with iron oxide particles as a contrast agent and generated five CTVs with modified margins of 3–15 mm around the iliac vessels [43]. Appropriate lymph node coverage was achieved when a modified margin of 7 mm was used. Vilarino-Varela et al. confirmed these results [44].

The margins proposed by the recent RTOG consensus guidelines for delineation of the CTV for postoperative pelvic IMRT are mainly in agreement with the findings of Taylor et al. [39]. To draw a conclusion about the clinical impact of the suggested margins, we await the results of the ongoing multicenter RTOG-0418 on postoperative pelvic IMRT for the treatment of gynecologic malignancies. In the mean time, the issue of margins for pelvic IMRT should be viewed cautiously.

2.6 The Issue of Tumor Volume Regression and Organ Motion for IGRT and IGBT

The magnitude of tumor volume regression influences organ topography and, consequently the dosimetric parameters in pelvic IMRT [3, 5, 45–47]. Van de Bunt et al. [5] used MRI to investigate whether a replan of IMRT after delivering 30 Gy results in dose reduction to the bowel. DVH analysis demonstrated that bowel dose decreased significantly in those cervical cancer patients who had tumor regression >30 cm^3 on MRI. Dimopoulos et al. found that during EBRT ~50% of patients had a tumor volume reduction of >30 cm^3 on MRI, in ~40% a reduction of >40 cm^3 occurred and ~30% had a reduction of >50 cm^3. It was also shown that a significant tumor volume decrease (of some 25–30%) has to be expected during the last third of EBRT [3]. Lee et al. have studied changes in position and volume of the cervix during the course of both EBRT and high dose rate (HDR) brachytherapy using CT [20]. They estimated that 50% of tumor regression occurs after ~30 Gy and that it takes about 21 days to achieve it [20]. Available data advocate the adaptation of IMRT plan after the third week of treatment. The benefit of more frequent replanning for patients with rapid tumor response should be addressed in future treatment planning studies.

The impact of topographical organ changes between fractions on internal PTV margins for IMRT of cervical cancer was investigated by van de Bunt et al. by using weekly MR imaging [47]. The largest margins had to be applied in anterior and posterior directions (24 and 17 mm respectively), while margins of 12, 16, 11, and 8 mm were sufficient in right lateral, left lateral, superior, and inferior directions, respectively [47]. Taylor and Powell proposed an asymmetrical internal margin with CTV–PTV expansion of the uterus, cervix, and upper vagina of 15 mm anteriorly posteriorly, 15 mm superiorly inferiorly, and 7 mm laterally and expansion of the nodal regions and parametria by 7 mm in all directions [46]. Currently it seems that there is not enough evidence to suggest any widely applicable recommendations regarding the appropriate individualized internal PTV margin. Its adaptation shall be addressed with caution taking in consideration one's own experience.

During fractionated IGBT, the time-related topography between tumor/target and OAR is also taken into consideration (Fig. 2.3) [48, 49]. In a recent MRI-based study, measurements of volumes encompassing GTV at the time of brachytherapy (GTV_{BT}) and "grey zones" showed that tumor regression during HDR brachytherapy appeared to have some impact on organ topography as well [3]. The mean volume was reduced from 16 to 10 cm^3 between first and the second fractions with later minor reduction from 9 to 8 cm^3 between third and fourth fractions [3].

2.7 Conclusion

Both CT and MRI are widely used for image-guided radiotherapy of gynecological malignancies. CT is a standard imaging modality for treatment planning of EBRT, while MR represents the modality of choice for IGBT. MRI provides detailed information about

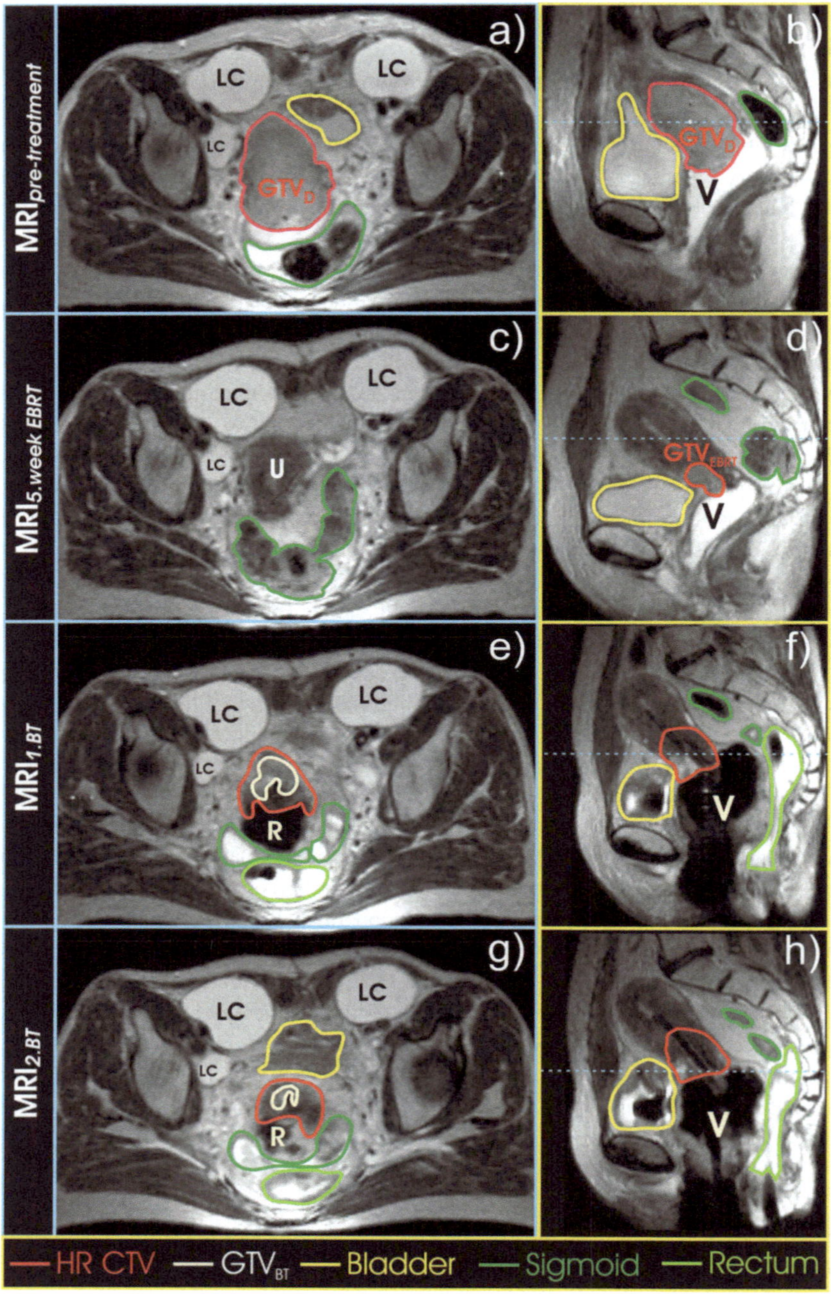

MRI pre-treatment
MRI 5.week EBRT
MRI 1.BT
MRI 2.BT
a)
b)
c)
d)
e)
f)
g)
h)
LC
U
R
V
GTV D
GTV EBRT
HR CTV
GTV BT
Bladder
Sigmoid
Rectum

Fig. 2.3 MRI scans of a patient with FIGO IIB cervical cancer at different time points of definitive radiochemotherapy. At diagnosis, a bulky tumor of cervix with proximal infiltration of both parametria is visible (GTV_D) (**a, b**). Significant tumor regression occurred during external beam radiotherapy (EBRT) and at the fifth week of treatment only small residual tumor of the anterior cervical lip is present (**d**). The axial scan at the fifth week (**c**) is taken at the same level, according to bony landmarks, as the pretreatment scan (**a**). It reveals normal uterine corpus and no evidence of tumor (**c, d**). At time of first (**e, f**) and second (**g, h**) BT further reduction of tumor is seen. *Dotted blue line* on sagittal images represents the level at which the correspondent axial scan was obtained (LC, lymphocyst after laparoscopic lymph node staging; GTV_D, gross tumor volume at diagnosis; V, vagina contrasted with ultrasound gel (**b, d**) or with packing impregnated with gadolinium (**f, h**); U, uterine corpus; R, ring)

tumor extension and enables accurate monitoring of tumor regression and organ movement during the entire course of IGRT and IGBT. Less precise information about tumor extension, tumor regression, and internal changes of organ and tumor topography can be obtained with CT. CTV margins for successful coverage of relevant lymph node regions derived from CT and MRI are comparable. The use of repetitive sectional imaging with treatment plan adaptation leads to reduction of the dose to the bowel during IGRT. Characteristics of tumor/target at diagnosis and at different time points of EBRT, which are essential for successful IGBT, are provided with higher accuracy by MRI.

Finally, it has to be stressed that IGRT has a potential not only to apply higher doses and to reduce margins around the tumor, but also to assure that interfraction variation in organ motion and patient setup are taken into account. Reduction of radiotherapy-related morbidity, improvement of locoregional control, and quality of life might be potential benefits of using repetitive imaging for IGRT. Those endpoints should be evaluated in future prospective randomized trials.

References

1. Tanyi JA, Fuss MH. Volumetric image-guidance: does routine usage prompt adaptive re-planning? An institutional review. Acta Oncol. 2008;47:1444–53.
2. Verellen D, De RM, Tournel K, et al. An overview of volumetric imaging technologies and their quality assurance for IGRT. Acta Oncol. 2008;47:1271–8.
3. Dimopoulos J, Schirl G, Baldinger A, Helbich T, Pötter R. MRI Assessment of Cervical Cancer for Adaptive Radiotherapy. Strahlenther Onkol. 2009;185:282–7.
4. Dimopoulos JC, Schard G, Berger D, et al. Systematic evaluation of MRI findings in different stages of treatment of cervical cancer: potential of MRI on delineation of target, pathoanatomic structures, and organs at risk. Int J Radiat Oncol Biol Phys. 2006;64:1380–8.
5. van de Bunt L, van der Heide UA, Ketelaars M, de Kort GA, Jurgenliemk-Schulz IM. Conventional, conformal, and intensity-modulated radiation therapy treatment planning of external beam radiotherapy for cervical cancer: the impact of tumor regression. Int J Radiat Oncol Biol Phys. 2006;64:189–96.
6. Chen Z, Ma CM, Paskalev K, et al. Investigation of MR image distortion for radiotherapy treatment planning of prostate cancer. Phys Med Biol. 2006;51:1393–403.

7. Khoo VS, Joon DL. New developments in MRI for target volume delineation in radiotherapy. Br J Radiol. 2006;79 Spec No 1:S2–15.
8. Kessler ML. Image registration and data fusion in radiation therapy. Br J Radiol. 2006;79 Spec No 1:S99–108.
9. Veninga T, Huisman H, van der Maazen RW, Huizenga H. Clinical validation of the normalized mutual information method for registration of CT and MR images in radiotherapy of brain tumors. J Appl Clin Med Phys. 2004;5:66–79.
10. Doran SJ, Charles-Edwards L, Reinsberg SA, Leach MO. A complete distortion correction for MR images: I. Gradient warp correction. Phys Med Biol. 2005;50:1343–61.
11. Fransson A, Andreo P, Potter R. Aspects of MR image distortions in radiotherapy treatment planning. Strahlenther Onkol. 2001;177:59–73.
12. Reinsberg SA, Doran SJ, Charles-Edwards EM, Leach MO. A complete distortion correction for MR images: II. Rectification of static-field inhomogeneities by similarity-based profile mapping. Phys Med Biol. 2005;50:2651–61.
13. Tanner SF, Finnigan DJ, Khoo VS, Mayles P, Dearnaley DP, Leach MO. Radiotherapy planning of the pelvis using distortion corrected MR images: the removal of system distortions. Phys Med Biol. 2000;45:2117–32.
14. Payne GS, Leach MO. Applications of magnetic resonance spectroscopy in radiotherapy treatment planning. Br J Radiol. 2006;79 Spec No 1:S16–26.
15. Norris DG. High field human imaging. J Magn Reson Imaging. 2003;18:519–29.
16. Viswanathan AN, Dimopoulos J, Kirisits C, Berger D, Potter R. Computed tomography versus magnetic resonance imaging-based contouring in cervical cancer brachytherapy: results of a prospective trial and preliminary guidelines for standardized contours. Int J Radiat Oncol Biol Phys. 2007;68:491–8.
17. Petric P, Dimopoulos J, Kirisits C, Berger D, Hudej R, Potter R. Inter- and intraobserver variation in HR CTV contouring: intercomparison of transverse and paratransverse image orientation in 3D-MRI assisted cervix cancer brachytherapy. Radiother Oncol. 2008;89:164–71.
18. Potter R. Modern imaging in Brachytherapy. In: Gerbaulet A, Potter R, Mazeron JJ, Meertens H, Van LE, editors. The GEC ESTRO Handbook of Brachytherapy. Brussels: European Society for Therapeutic Radiology and Oncology; 2002. p. 123–51.
19. Beadle BM, Jhingran A, Salehpour M, Sam M, Iyer RB, Eifel PJ. Cervix regression and motion during the course of external beam chemoradiation for cervical cancer. Int J Radiat Oncol Biol Phys. 2009;73:235–41.
20. Lee CM, Shrieve DC, Gaffney DK. Rapid involution and mobility of carcinoma of the cervix. Int J Radiat Oncol Biol Phys. 2004;58:625–30.
21. Potter R, Haie-Meder C, Van LE, et al. Recommendations from gynecological (GYN) GEC ESTRO working group (II): concepts and terms in 3D image-based treatment planning in cervix cancer brachytherapy-3D dose volume parameters and aspects of 3D image-based anatomy, radiation physics, radiobiology. Radiother Oncol. 2006;78:67–77.
22. Saarnak AE, Boersma M, van Bunningen BN, Wolterink R, Steggerda MJ. Inter-observer variation in delineation of bladder and rectum contours for brachytherapy of cervical cancer. Radiother Oncol. 2000;56:37–42.
23. Foshager MC, Walsh JW. CT anatomy of the female pelvis: a second look. Radiographics. 1994;14:51–64.
24. Vick CW, Walsh JW, Wheelock JB, Brewer WH. CT of the normal and abnormal parametria in cervical cancer. AJR Am J Roentgenol. 1984;143:597–603.
25. Walsh JW, Goplerud DR. Prospective comparison between clinical and CT staging in primary cervical carcinoma. AJR Am J Roentgenol. 1981;137:997–1003.
26. Hricak H, Lacey CG, Sandles LG, Chang YC, Winkler ML, Stern JL. Invasive cervical carcinoma: comparison of MR imaging and surgical findings. Radiology. 1988;166:623–31.

27. Hatano K, Sekiya Y, Araki H, et al. Evaluation of the therapeutic effect of radiotherapy on cervical cancer using magnetic resonance imaging. Int J Radiat Oncol Biol Phys. 1999;45: 639–44.
28. Mayr NA, Magnotta VA, Ehrhardt JC, et al. Usefulness of tumor volumetry by magnetic resonance imaging in assessing response to radiation therapy in carcinoma of the uterine cervix. Int J Radiat Oncol Biol Phys. 1996;35:915–24.
29. Mayr NA, Taoka T, Yuh WT, et al. Method and timing of tumor volume measurement for outcome prediction in cervical cancer using magnetic resonance imaging. Int J Radiat Oncol Biol Phys. 2002;52:14–22.
30. Kim SH, Choi BI, Lee HP, et al. Uterine cervical carcinoma: comparison of CT and MR findings. Radiology. 1990;175:45–51.
31. Kim SH, Choi BI, Han JK, et al. Preoperative staging of uterine cervical carcinoma: comparison of CT and MRI in 99 patients. J Comput Assist Tomogr. 1993;17:633–40.
32. Yang WT, Lam WW, Yu MY, Cheung TH, Metreweli C. Comparison of dynamic helical CT and dynamic MR imaging in the evaluation of pelvic lymph nodes in cervical carcinoma. AJR Am J Roentgenol. 2000;175:759–66.
33. Manfredi R, Mirk P, Maresca G, et al. Local-regional staging of endometrial carcinoma: role of MR imaging in surgical planning. Radiology. 2004;231:372–8.
34. Rockall AG, Sohaib SA, Harisinghani MG, et al. Diagnostic performance of nanoparticle-enhanced magnetic resonance imaging in the diagnosis of lymph node metastases in patients with endometrial and cervical cancer. J Clin Oncol. 2005;23:2813–21.
35. Scheidler J, Heuck AF. Imaging of cancer of the cervix. Radiol Clin North Am. 2002;40: 577–90, vii.
36. Kitajima K, Murakami K, Yamasaki E, et al. Accuracy of 18F-FDG PET/CT in detecting pelvic and paraaortic lymph node metastasis in patients with endometrial cancer. AJR Am J Roentgenol. 2008;190:1652–8.
37. Loft A, Berthelsen AK, Roed H, et al. The diagnostic value of PET/CT scanning in patients with cervical cancer: a prospective study. Gynecol Oncol. 2007;106:29–34.
38. Park JY, Kim EN, Kim DY, et al. Comparison of the validity of magnetic resonance imaging and positron emission tomography/computed tomography in the preoperative evaluation of patients with uterine corpus cancer. Gynecol Oncol. 2008;108:486–92.
39. Small Jr W, Mell LK, Anderson P, et al. Consensus guidelines for delineation of clinical target volume for intensity-modulated pelvic radiotherapy in postoperative treatment of endometrial and cervical cancer. Int J Radiat Oncol Biol Phys. 2008;71:428–34.
40. Taylor A, Rockall AG, Powell ME. An atlas of the pelvic lymph node regions to aid radiotherapy target volume definition. Clin Oncol (R Coll Radiol). 2007;19:542–50.
41. Chao KS, Lin M. Lymphangiogram-assisted lymph node target delineation for patients with gynecologic malignancies. Int J Radiat Oncol Biol Phys. 2002;54:1147–52.
42. Dinniwell R, Chan P, Czarnota G, et al. Pelvic lymph node topography for radiotherapy treatment planning from ferumoxtran-10 contrast-enhanced magnetic resonance imaging. Int J Radiat Oncol Biol Phys. 2009 Jul 1;74:844–51.
43. Taylor A, Rockall AG, Reznek RH, Powell ME. Mapping pelvic lymph nodes: guidelines for delineation in intensity-modulated radiotherapy. Int J Radiat Oncol Biol Phys. 2005;63: 1604–12.
44. Vilarino-Varela MJ, Taylor A, Rockall AG, Reznek RH, Powell ME. A verification study of proposed pelvic lymph node localisation guidelines using nanoparticle-enhanced magnetic resonance imaging. Radiother Oncol. 2008;89:192–6.
45. Lim K, Chan P, Dinniwell R, et al. Cervical cancer regression measured using weekly magnetic resonance imaging during fractionated radiotherapy: radiobiologic modeling and correlation with tumor hypoxia. Int J Radiat Oncol Biol Phys. 2008;70:126–33.

46. Taylor A, Powell ME. An assessment of interfractional uterine and cervical motion: implications for radiotherapy target volume definition in gynecological cancer. Radiother Oncol. 2008;88:250–7.
47. van de Bunt L, Jurgenliemk-Schulz IM, de Kort GA, Roesink JM, Tersteeg RJ, van der Heide UA. Motion and deformation of the target volumes during IMRT for cervical cancer: what margins do we need? Radiother Oncol. 2008;88:233–40.
48. Haie-Meder C, Potter R, Van LE, et al. Recommendations from Gynecological (GYN) GEC-ESTRO Working Group (I): concepts and terms in 3D image based 3D treatment planning in cervix cancer brachytherapy with emphasis on MRI assessment of GTV and CTV. Radiother Oncol. 2005;74:235–45.
49. Kirisits C, Potter R, Lang S, Dimopoulos J, Wachter-Gerstner N, Georg D. Dose and volume parameters for MRI-based treatment planning in intracavitary brachytherapy for cervical cancer. Int J Radiat Oncol Biol Phys. 2005;62:901–11.

The Physics of CT and MR Imaging

3

Robert Hudej and Uulke A. Van der Heide

3.1 Introduction to CT

Computed tomography (CT) [1] effectively eliminates many of the limitations of conventional film radiography. In contrast to film radiography, CT images accurately depict in three-dimensional (3D) internal anatomical structures. Additionally, due to the low ratio between scattered and primary X-ray photons, CT images depict better low contrast resolution, enabling the differentiation between similar tissues. Even though CT has a lower spatial resolution than radiography and lower soft-tissue contrast than MRI, the described advantages make it a reliable and valid imaging modality for 3D brachytherapy.

In this chapter, basic principles of CT image generation and some practical imaging aspects with respect to 3D gynecological brachytherapy are described.

3.1.1 CT Basics

In the third generation of CT scanners, the X-ray beam from the X-ray tube is collimated into a fan-beam, encompassing the entire patient's width. An array of solid-state detectors rests on the opposite side of the patient and rigidly connects with the X-ray tube so that they both rotate around the patient. In all modern body CT scanners, the patient steadily moves through the gantry while the tube and detectors continuously rotate with sub-second rotation times. In this way the X-ray tube and detectors follow a spiral path with respect to the patient, commonly called a spiral CT.

R. Hudej (✉)
Department of Radiophysics, Institute of Oncology Ljubljana, Zaloska 2, 1000 Ljubljana, Slovenia
e-mail: rohudej@onko-i.si

U.A. Van der Heide
Department of Radiotherapy, UMC Utrecht, Heidelberglaan 100, Utrecht, The Netherlands
e-mail: u.a.vanderheide@umcutrecht.nl

A.N. Viswanathan et al. (eds.), *Gynecologic Radiation Therapy*,
DOI: 10.1007/978-3-540-68958-4_3, © Springer-Verlag Berlin Heidelberg 2011

Each element of the detector array measures the attenuated intensity of the primary beam, which is the measure of the average linear attenuation coefficient along the ray path between the source and the detector. The combined signal from the whole array forms a projection of attenuation coefficients of the imaged volume at that particular sampling angle. During one rotation, the signal on the detector array is typically sampled 1,000–2,000 times, and the same number of projections per rotation at different angles is obtained. The imaged volume is then divided into 3D rectangular boxes, called voxels, and for each voxel a relative absorption coefficient, called CT number in Hounsfield units, is calculated from the obtained projections with a filtered back projection reconstruction method [2].

3.1.2 Artifacts

Beam hardening causes shading, a common CT artifact. This appears as a hypointense region behind thicker bone regions or implants. Streaking artifacts appear in CT images due to inconsistent detector measurements, caused by patient motion or by the presence of metal, when the measured intensity is below the detection limit. Due to the properties of the filtered back projection reconstruction algorithm, these inconsistencies appear in the image as streaks.

3.1.3 Practical Aspects

During the development of CT imaging protocols for gynecological brachytherapy, special care has to be taken in order to obtain CT images with a slice thickness as small as 1 mm, which enables accurate applicator reconstruction. At the same time, images have to demonstrate an acceptable signal-to-noise ratio so that the tissue depiction quality enables accurate contouring. Moreover, depiction quality can be significantly reduced due to the streaking artifacts caused by the metal applicators. It is therefore advisable to use CT compatible plastic applicators or applicators with maximally reduced metal quantity (e.g., needles without metal obturators during imaging).

3.2 Introduction to MRI

When magnetic resonance imaging (MRI) [3–5] is applied in radiotherapy, some specific issues must be addressed. For example, sequences may be applied that are not common in a diagnostic setting; patient positioning and immobilization procedures that are used in the actual treatment may also be required during imaging; and the geometrical accuracy of images is of greater importance than for diagnostic use. In this chapter, we address some of these issues and discuss the considerations that play a role in developing imaging protocols suitable for application in gynecologic radiotherapy.

3.2.1 MRI Basics

A key feature of MRI is that a large variety of tissue contrasts can be achieved by simply varying scan parameters. While a comprehensive description of contrast mechanisms falls outside the scope of this chapter, we will discuss the T1 and T2 processes as the most fundamental examples of how soft tissue contrast on MRI is achieved.

In equilibrium, nuclear spins of the scanned material are oriented along the direction of the applied static magnetic field (B_0). When the spin system is excited by an external radio-frequency (RF) pulse, called the 90° pulse, the spins flip to a plane transverse to the B_0 axis. After the pulse, spins start to relax back to the direction of B_0 with the relaxation time T1. This process is called longitudinal relaxation or spin–lattice relaxation. During this process, nuclear spins precess around the B_0 axis with an angular frequency, called the Larmor frequency ω_0. Because the precise angular frequency depends on the local environment of the nuclei, after the 90° pulse is applied, the phase of the spins gradually spreads. If at some point in time T, after the 90° pulse, a 180° pulse is applied, the spins flip and their phases start to converge. Then at time 2T, called echo time (TE), the realignment of the spins is at least partially restored and an "echo" signal in the receiver coil is induced. Because of the molecular interactions, the coherence of the spins in the transverse plane is gradually lost. This mechanism is called transverse relaxation or spin–spin relaxation with the corresponding relaxation time T2. The 180° pulses can be applied several times in a sequence, each time producing the echo signal. When the signal is reduced enough as a consequence of the spin–lattice and spin–spin relaxation, the initial spin system in the transverse plane is restored with another 90° pulse. The time between two successive 90° pulses is called the repetition time (TR).

The sensitivity of the MR signal to T1 or T2 can be modified by changing TR and TE. A combination of a long repetition time (TR >> T1) and an echo time TE that is on the order of T2 results in an image that is sensitive to variations in T2 (T2-weighted image). A TR that is on the order of T1 or a bit shorter in combination with a TE << T2 results in a T1-weighted image. As T1 and T2 are properties of a particular tissue, the resulting images exhibit excellent soft tissue contrast.

3.2.2 MRI Sequences for Gynecologic Imaging

In addition to the two above-mentioned RF pulses, different MRI techniques include different additional pulses combined in a specific sequence that is simply called a MRI sequence. There are many different MRI sequences implemented in each MRI scanner, but in principle, the imaging sequences that are used for diagnosis of gynecologic tumors are also used in radiotherapy (Table 3.1).

T2-weighted sequences (spin echo, fast spin echo, gradient spin echo) are an important part of any imaging protocol, because tumors can be well distinguished from the surrounding soft tissues. Because of their long repetition time (TR is several seconds on a 1.5 T scanner, see Table 3.1), the overall scan time can be quite long. In order to keep the scanning time within a reasonable time frame, a limited number thick slices are scanned, resulting in

Table 3.1 Common MRI scan parameters for specified sequences

Sequence	TE [ms]	TR [ms]	Flip angle	Slices	Thickness [mm]	Gap [mm]	FOV [cm]	Matrix	Fat suppression
T2 spin echo	100	3,000	90	30	4	0.5	32 × 32	512 × 512	
SPACE	131	1,500	150	176	1	0	40 × 40	386 × 384	
T_1-thrive	2.7	5.5	10	100	3	−1.5[a]	40 × 40	512 × 512	SPIR
bSSFP	2.9	5.8	50	100	3	−1.5[a]	34 × 34	512 × 512	

[a]A negative gap implies overlapping slices

a limited field of view, or a limited resolution in the out-of-plane direction respectively. For this reason, typically separate scans in axial, sagittal, and coronal planes are acquired. While this solution is satisfactory for diagnostic purposes, it represents a disadvantage in radiotherapy since treatment planning software does not always support the use of data sets that are not axially sliced.

T1-weighted sequences (spin echo, fast spin echo, gradient spin echo) give a high signal in fat tissue while contrast in other tissues is relatively low. These sequences can be successfully applied for representation of gadolinium contrast or for representation of copper sulfate markers, used for the applicator active channel identification. All the limitations, characteristic of T2-weighted sequences, apply also to T1-weighted sequences.

Possible solutions for the described limitations are 3D sequences to speed up acquisition of T1 or T2-weighted scans, and allow a better spatial resolution in all directions. Various MRI manufactures bring them to the market under different names, such as VISTA, SPACE, XETA for T2 contrast and Thrive, FAME or VIBE for T1 contrast. The pulse sequences of a 3D scan are similar to slice-based 2D scans, but rather than exciting a single slice at a time, the entire volume is excited. While this approach results in a high isotropic resolution accompanied by a large field of view, subtle changes in contrast may occur. A balanced sequence, such as a balanced steady-state free precession (bSSFP) sequence or true fast imaging with steady-state precession (TrueFISP) sequence is another way to speed up the acquisition of a volume, allowing a higher spatial resolution. However, this technique comes at the cost of reduced contrast, because both T1 and T2 are represented in the image. Nevertheless, such a sequence can be very useful for applicator reconstruction for brachytherapy planning [6].

3.2.3 MRI Artifacts

In contrast to CT images, MR images are prone to artifacts that result in distortion of the geometry. The inhomogeneity of the static magnetic field, B_0, can cause substantial distortions of an image, particularly toward the edges of the field of view. These effects are small for 1.5 and 3.0 T scanners, but can be significant for open scanners, in particular at low magnetic field [7, 8].

More important in clinical practice are susceptibility artifacts. They are caused by differences in magnetic susceptibility between soft tissue and air or metal or plastic objects. These differences result in a distortion of the magnetic field (Fig. 3.1a) causing shifts in the location of the tissues on the image. The shifts are particularly large close to the body surface [7] and near brachytherapy applicators, if their magnetic susceptibility differs from tissue. These artifacts can be minimized by using steep field gradients for position encoding. An important additional, although trivial cause of deformation of the body contour, is the use of external receiver coils on the patient.

Motion artifacts due to patient and/or organ movement, can be a significant issue in MRI, especially when sequences with long acquisition times are used. The motion results in overall image blurring with ghost images of the moving tissue (Fig. 3.1b). In gynecologic

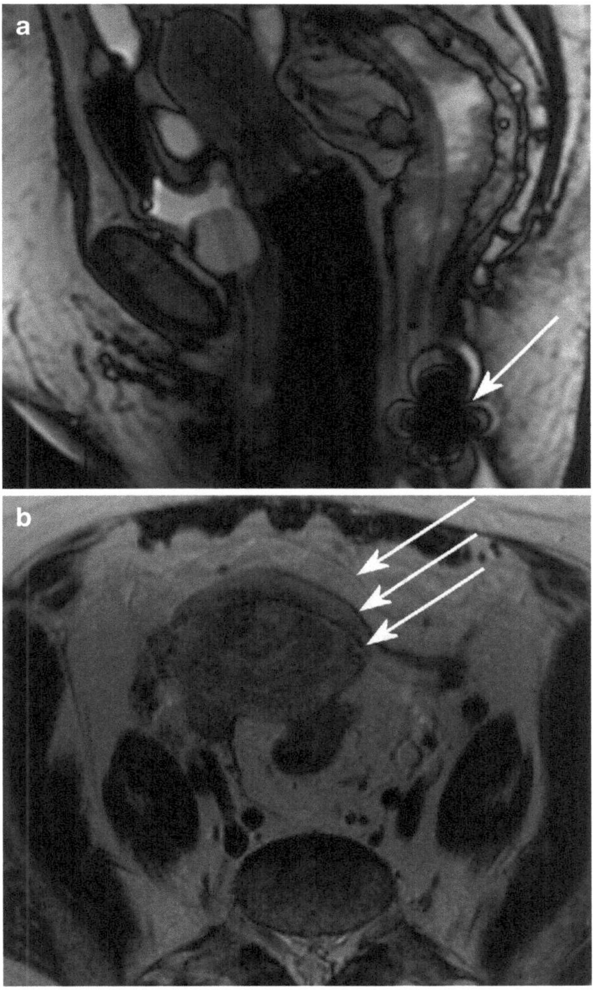

Fig. 3.1 (**a**) TrueFISP image with a pronounced susceptibility artifact caused by the presence of a metallic seed (*white arrow*). (**b**) T2 spin echo image with a characteristic motion artifact. Organ motion results in the appearance of ghost images of that organ (*white arrows*)

brachytherapy the whole patient movement during MRI can be significantly reduced if the patient is still under spinal or general anesthesia, administered before the applicator insertion. Additionally, it is recommended to administer antispasmodic medication before the MRI scan in order to suppress bowel movement.

3.2.4 Heating

The RF radiation used in MRI pulse sequences results in energy deposition in tissue, which may lead to a local temperature increase in the patient. The specific absorption rate (SAR) is related to the specific pulse sequence. For short repetition times in combination with 90° pulses, SAR limits are easily exceeded. The SAR can be reduced by reducing the flip angle from 90° to smaller angles, but this has an impact on the contrast of the image. Alternatively, the repetition time can be increased, but this increases the overall scan time. Thus, SAR limits have an impact on the sequences that can be used.

In MRI-guided brachytherapy, the RF radiation and switching of magnetic field gradients can cause heating of the tips of conducting guidewires and catheters [9]. In a conductive circuit, such as a guidewire, a current can be induced, which causes heating because of the ohmic resistance. If a resonant condition exists in a circuit, this heating can become problematic. If a length of a wire or needle is approximately half the wavelength of the RF radiation, it can function as a resonant antenna, resulting in heating particularly at the tip. This wavelength is determined by the frequency of the RF and the electric properties of the tissues surrounding the needle. While many studies identify the factors related to RF heating of catheters and needles, no clear guidelines exist to formulate safe practice.

3.3 Conclusion

In gynecologic brachytherapy, 1.5T MRI is becoming the imaging method of choice due to its good image resolution and superior soft tissue contrast, compared to more conventional CT imaging. Significant resources are still being invested in improvement of imaging sequences with the purpose of increasing the signal-to-noise ratio and the reduction of imaging times. The introduction of 3T MRI in clinical practice in selected centers indicates that higher magnetic fields may improve the image quality even further under the condition that new and efficient imaging sequences are employed, which are able to mitigate the increased susceptibility artifacts and the increased specific absorption rate in the tissue. Further work in this area is needed and will be of great interest.

References

1. Kalender WA. Computed tomography: fundamentals, system technology, image quality, applications. Munich: Publicis MCD Verlag; 2000.
2. Natterer F. The mathematics of computerized tomography (classics in applied mathematics, 32). Philadelphia: Society for Industrial and Applied Mathematics; 2001.
3. Haacke EM et al. Magnetic resonance imaging: physical principals and sequence design. New York: Wiley; 1999.
4. MR Technology information portal: http://www.mr-tip.com Accessed on 13th July 2010.
5. The Basics of MRI: http://www.cis.rit.edu/htbooks/mri/ Accessed on 13th July 2010.
6. Haack S, Nielsen SK, Lindegaard JC, Gelineck J, Tanderup K. Applicator reconstruction in MRI 3D image-based dose planning of brachytherapy for cervical cancer. Radiother Oncol. 2009;91:187–93.
7. Moerland MA et al. Analysis and correction of geometric distortions in 1.5 T magnetic resonance images for use in radiotherapy treatment planning. Phys Med Biol. 1995;40:1651–64.
8. Mah D et al. MRI simulation: effect of gradient distortions on three-dimensional prostate cancer plans. Int J Radiat Oncol Biol Phys. 2002;53:757–65.
9. Dempsey MF et al. Investigation of the factors responsible for burns during MRI. J Mag Res Imag. 2001;13:627–31.

The Use of Positron Emission Tomographic Imaging for Image-Guided Therapy

4

Elizabeth Kidd and Perry Grigsby

4.1 Introduction

As the ability to perform three-dimensional (3D) treatment planning for cervical cancer critically depends on accurately defining the areas of disease, FDG-PET (fluorodeoxy-glucose-positron emission tomography) represents an important tool for radiation treatment planning. FDG-PET provides valuable information for cervical cancer about the extent of the primary tumor and areas of lymph node metastasis, thereby aiding in target delineation. Additionally, FDG-PET/CT combines the benefits of anatomic and functional imaging. The functional aspects of FDG-PET offer significant prognostic information, which could guide treatment modifications, such as boosting more metabolically active tumor regions. FDG-PET is an imaging tool used routinely for radiation treatment planning, for both external radiation and brachytherapy.

4.2 FDG-PET and External Radiation Treatment Planning

In an era of targeted radiotherapy, accurately defining the areas of disease becomes critically important, as the tissues outside of the target volume will not receive therapeutic radiation doses. Research has shown that over the course of treatment, there can be significant movement of the uterus and cervix, which can affect treatment planning. In particular, it has been found that changes in rectal filling may affect cervical position, while bladder filling has more impact in uterine body position [1]. Other researchers have suggested

E. Kidd (✉)
Department of Radiation Oncology, Stanford University Cancer Center, 875 Blake Wilbur Drive, Stanford, CA 94305
e-mail: ekidd@stanford.edu

P. Grigsby
Mallinckrodt Institute of Radiology, Washington University, 4511 Forest Park, Suite 200, St. Louis, MO, 63108, USA
e-mail: pgrigsby@radonc.wustl.edu

A.N. Viswanathan et al. (eds.), *Gynecologic Radiation Therapy*,
DOI: 10.1007/978-3-540-68958-4_4, © Springer-Verlag Berlin Heidelberg 2011

significant variability in cervical tumor volume during treatment [2]. Lim et al. also noticed great variability in the way cervical tumors regress during radiation and that the process seemed to be influenced by cellular radiosensitivity and proliferation [3], which might suggest an added benefit of the functional information provided by FDG-PET.

Variability in contouring among radiation oncologists is known to be a factor that may adversely affect treatment delivery [4]. A significant decrease in inter- and intra-observer variation in tumor contouring has been shown by incorporating functional imaging, in particular with FDG-PET fusion [5–7]. For cervical cancer, defining the extent of the primary tumor is important for radiation treatment planning and overall prognosis. Miller and Grigsby have established that primary cervix tumor volume can be accurately determined using FDG-PET, and that this PET-defined cervical tumor volume predicts progression-free and overall survival [8]. This 40% isocontour size has been validated with MRI [9] and pathologically correlated for early stage cervical cancer [10]. Better target delineation is key to decreasing the volume of normal tissue irradiated, as this could also allow for higher doses and possibly better tumor control. It has been estimated that approximately 60% of cancer patients undergoing imaging with FDG-PET have potential changes in target volume and/or dose distribution parameters [11].

Besides providing valuable information about the extent of the primary cervix tumor, FDG-PET also has a high sensitivity and specificity for detecting lymph node metastasis [12–15] (Fig. 4.1). One study found that PET/CT has a sensitivity of 100% and a specificity of 99.7% for detecting cervical cancer lymph nodes larger than 5 mm [16]. In contrast, CT and MRI both rely on size criteria for lymph node diagnosis and therefore lack the ability to identify metastasis in normal size lymph nodes and are only moderately sensitive for detecting cervical cancer nodal metastasis [17].

Although lymph node status is not part of cervical cancer staging, lymph node findings are critical for prognosis and treatment planning. Studies have shown a strong correlation between lymph node status on FDG-PET and overall survival [18]. Additionally, radiation treatment field size might require modification, based on the additional information provided by FDG-PET, so that involved lymph nodes are included and treated with an adequate margin. At Washington University in St. Louis, cervical cancer patients with FDG-avid para-aortic lymph nodes have their radiation treatment field expanded to include the para-aortic lymph nodes and are treated with curative intent (Fig. 4.2). It has been shown that involved para-aortic nodes can be safely dose escalated to 60 Gy using IMRT [19–21]. Using FDG-PET

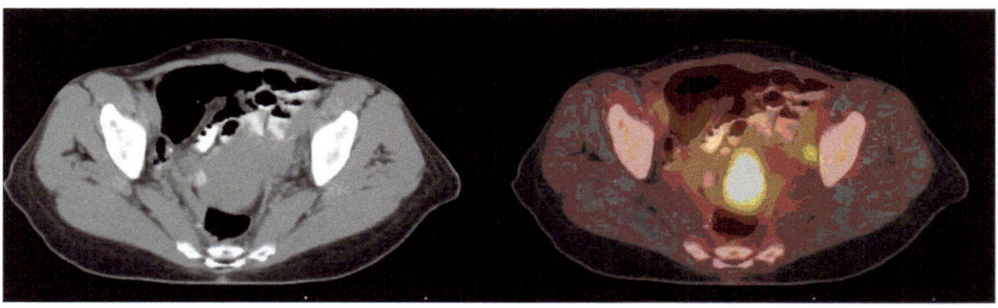

Fig. 4.1 CT and PET/CT axial images showing a comparison of identifying the cervix and local lymph node without and with the aid of FDG-PET imaging

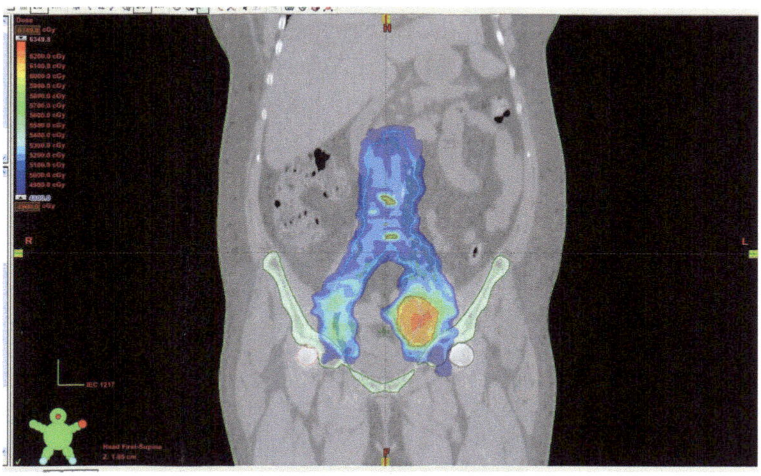

Fig. 4.2 Expanded treatment field to include FDG-avid para-aortic lymph nodes. The PET-positive pelvic and para-aortic lymph nodes are shown in orange, while the general pelvic and para-aortic lymph node region is shown in blue and green

data, dose escalation to involved lymph nodes based on size has also been investigated [22]. FDG-PET can greatly affect treatment field size and dose for cervical cancer patients.

At Washington University, all cervical cancer patients undergo a FDG-PET simulation, using a hybrid PET/CT scanner, as well as a CT simulation for localization and alignment marks. To minimize bladder activity, all gynecologic patients undergoing an FDG-PET, have a Foley catheter in the urinary bladder before receiving FDG, receive 20 mg intravenous furosemide before or after the FDG injection, and have intravenous fluids (1,000–1,500 mL of 0.9% or 0.45% saline) during the study. Serum blood glucose levels are maintained at about 100 mg/dL and the FDG-PET is deferred if blood glucose concentration exceeds 200 mg/dL. Delaying PET imaging for 1 hour after FDG injection improves the sensitivity for detection of nodal metastasis in cervical cancer.

The PET/CT and CT simulation images are registered using point and anatomic matching [23, 24]. The fused PET/CT images allow for easy contouring of the metabolically active primary cervix tumor and involved lymph nodes, for potential boosting or dose augmentation. Using the volumetric tool from Siemens e.soft ® software to create a region of interest encompassing the tumor, the maximaum standardized uptake value (SUV) of the FDG-avid cervix tumor can be determined. The volume created by the 40% threshold of the maximum SUV defines the metabolically active primary cervix tumor (MTV cervix), as described previously [8](Fig 4.3). This 40% threshold volume has been validated by imaging and pathology, as discussed above. (Fig. 4.3).

To reduce inter- and intra-observer variability in target delineation, some institutions use auto-delineation methods based on a certain percentage of the maximum standardized uptake value (SUV) or tumor-to-background ratio [25–28]. Of note, PET parameters can vary between facilities, scanners, or different time intervals between FDG injection and imaging, which can affect auto-contouring methods.

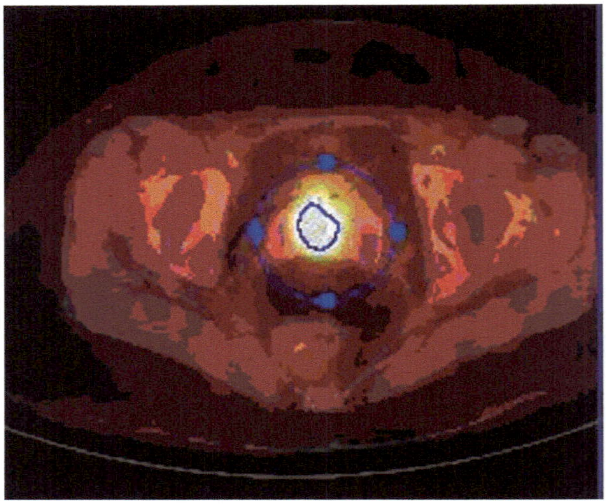

Fig. 4.3 Axial FDG-PET images showing the 40% threshold, within the region of interest, used for defining the MTV (metabolic target volume) cervix for radiation treatment planning

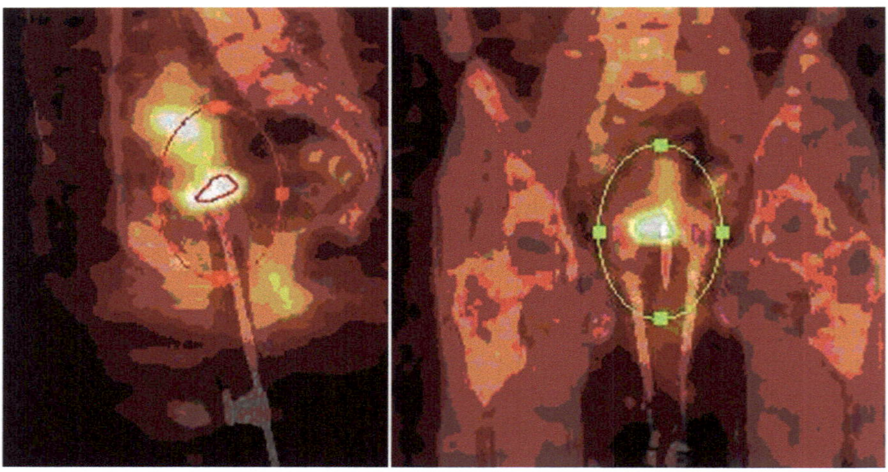

Fig. 4.4 Sagittal, and coronal FDG-PET/CT images of a cervical cancer patient with a tandem and ovoids in place. The larger red and green ovals define the region of interest, while the thicker-rimmed, more irregular-shaped structure is the 40% isocontour or MTV cervix

4.3 FDG-PET and Brachytherapy

Image-guided three-dimensional (3D) brachytherapy is a new approach for cervical cancer that is rapidly replacing 2D methods. FDG-PET has specific advantages by clearly defining the primary cervical tumor in relation to surrounding structures and the brachytherapy implant (Fig. 4.4). Initially, using FDG-PET before PET/CT was developed and before there were CT or MRI compatible applicators readily available, we performed PET-based brachytherapy by placing small sealed tubes of FDG into the applicators (2.5 mCi/mL for the ovoids and 0.75 mCi/mL for the tandem; each tube contained about 0.25 mL). Therefore, at that time with PET only there was no need to fabricate CT compatible applicators to prevent artifacts with imaging. Today, PET/CT is utilized instead of PET alone and CT and MRI applicators are readily commercially available, which makes the need for using tubes of FDG as “dummy” markers unnecessary. FDG-PET cervical brachytherapy demonstrates the 3D spatial relationship of the cervical tumor to the tandem and ovoid applicators, bladder, and rectum. Using 3D brachytherapy, such as with FDG-PET/CT, allows easy delineation and monitoring of the primary cervix tumor in relation to the brachytherapy implant and the surrounding normal tissues. In an initial small study involving 11 patients, Malyapa et al. found that in comparing the 3D information provided by FDG-PET to 2D methods, the maximal bladder and rectum doses were higher while the

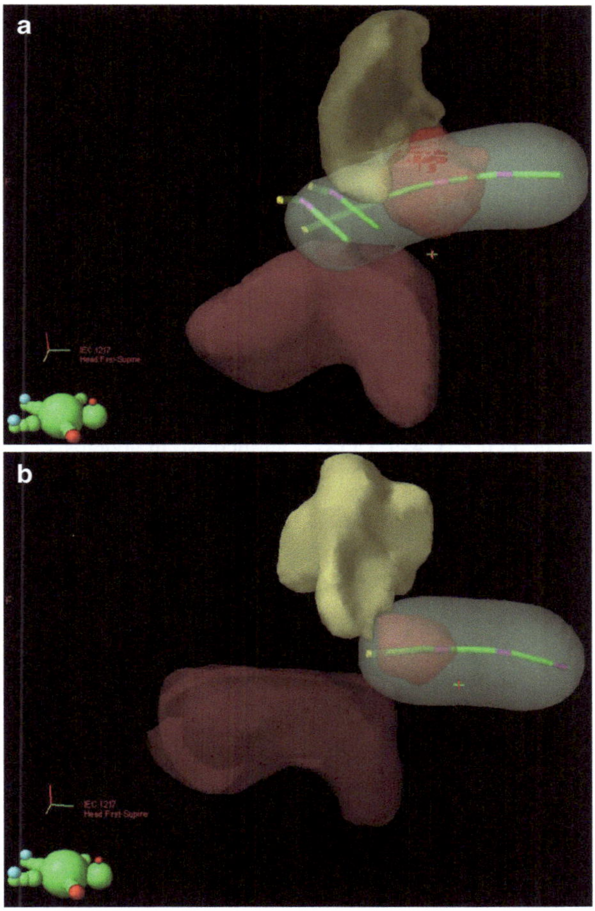

Fig. 4.5 Comparison of fraction 1 tandem and ovoids (**a**) and fraction 5 tandem only (**b**) FDG-PET guided brachytherapy, where red is the FDG-avid cervix tumor, bright green with purple the tandem and ovoid source positions, yellow alone is the bladder, brown the rectum, and light green the 6.5 Gy target isodose surface

minimal dose to the FDG-avid tumor dose was lower than the point A dose [29]. Lin et al. confirmed these results with additional patients and also looked at how the cervical target coverage changed during the course of radiation treatment [30]. Sequential FDG-PET 3D brachytherapy allows evaluation of changes in tumor dimension and adjacent organs and thereby facilitates possible optimization of dose coverage without increasing toxicity.

There has also been research evaluating adaptive brachytherapy treatment planning for cervical cancer using FDG-PET. With optimizing the planning for the FDG-avid tumor volume and maintaining the same dose levels to the bladder and rectum, higher percentages of tumor coverage and increased dose to point A could be achieved [31] (Fig. 4.5). FDG-PET guided brachytherapy for cervical cancer has the potential for improving primary tumor coverage while possibly allowing more sparing of normal tissues.

4.4 Functional Imaging and Radiation Treatment Planning

FDG-PET has the added value of the functional information provided by the imaging. Functional or metabolic imaging demonstrates certain features of the malignant phenotype that distinguish tumor from non-tumor cells, but also provides valuable prognostic information. For cervical cancer, the amount of FDG uptake by the primary tumor serves as a biomarker for risk of lymph node involvement, treatment response, and overall survival [32]. The prognostic value of FDG uptake has also been shown in other cancers [33]. Research has also shown that the variability of the FDG uptake across individual cervical tumors also has prognostic value [34]. The prognostic value of both high and heterogeneic FDG uptake suggests the possible value of dose-painting or boosting particular subvolumes of the cervical tumor.

Other promising aspects of PET relate to the use of different isotopes, such as for hypoxia or proliferation. In an initial study, using PET with ^{60}Cu-ATSM to identify hypoxic cervical tumors, it was found that the tracer uptake was correlated with overexpression of VEGF, EGFR, CA-9, COX-2, an increase in apoptosis and a significantly poorer 4-year overall survival [35]. PET imaging with these or other novel isotopes could have future impact on radiation treatment planning.

References

1. Taylor A, Powell ME. An assessment of interfractional uterine and cervical motion: Implications for radiotherapy target volume definition in gynecological cancer. Radiother Oncol. 2008;88:250–7.
2. Mayr NA, Yuh WT, Taoka T, et al. Serial therapy-induced changes in tumor shape in cervical cancer and their impact on assessing tumor volume and treatment response. AJR Am J Roentgenol. 2006;187:65–72.
3. Lim K, Chan P, Dinniwell R, et al. Cervical cancer regression measured using weekly magnetic resonance imaging during fractionated radiotherapy: radiobiologic modeling and correlation with tumor hypoxia. Int J Radiat Oncol Biol Phys. 2008;70:126–33.

4. Weiss E, Hess CF. The impact of gross tumor volume (GTV) and clinical target volume (CTV) definition on the total accuracy in radiotherapy theoretical aspects and practical experiences. Strahlenther Onkol. 2003;179:21–30.
5. Caldwell CB, Mah K, Ung YC, et al. Observer variation in contouring gross tumor volume in patients with poorly defined non-small-cell lung tumors on CT: the impact of 18FDG-hybrid PET fusion. Int J Radiat Oncol Biol Phys. 2001;51:923–31.
6. Fox JL, Rengan R, O'Meara W, et al. Does registration of PET and planning CT images decrease interobserver and intraobserver variation in delineating tumor volumes for non-small-cell lung cancer? Int J Radiat Oncol Biol Phys. 2005;62:70–5.
7. Steenbakkers RJ, Duppen JC, Fitton I, et al. Reduction of observer variation using matched CT-PET for lung cancer delineation: a three-dimensional analysis. Int J Radiat Oncol Biol Phys. 2006;64:435–48.
8. Miller TR, Grigsby PW. Measurement of tumor volume by PET to evaluate prognosis in patients with advanced cervical cancer treated by radiation therapy. Int J Radiat Oncol Biol Phys. 2002;53:353–9.
9. Grigsby PW. PET and PET/CT in Cervical and Uterine Cancer. In: Wahl RL, Beanlands RSB, editors. Principles and Practices of PET and PET/CT. 2nd ed. Philadelphia: Lippincott; 2008. p. 348–54.
10. Showalter TN, Miller TR, Huettner P et al. 18F-fluorodeoxyglucose-positron emission tomography and pathologic tumor size in early-stage invasive cervical cancer. Int J Gynecol Cancer. 2009 Nov; 19:1412-4.
11. Guha C, Alfieri A, Blaufox MD, et al. Tumor biology-guided radiotherapy treatment planning: gross tumor volume versus functional tumor volume. Semin Nucl Med. 2008;38:105–13.
12. Choi HJ, Roh JW, Seo SS, et al. Comparison of the accuracy of magnetic resonance imaging and positron emission tomography/computed tomography in the presurgical detection of lymph node metastases in patients with uterine cervical carcinoma: a prospective study. Cancer. 2006;106:914–22.
13. Grigsby PW, Dehdashti F, Siegel BA. FDG-PET evaluation of carcinoma of the cervix. Clinical Positron Imaging. 1999;2:105–9.
14. Narayan K, Hicks RJ, Jobling T, et al. A comparison of MRI and PET scanning in surgically staged loco-regional advanced cervical cancer: potential impact on treatment. Int J Gynecol Canc. 2001;11:263–71.
15. Rose PG, Adler LP, Rodriguez M, et al. Positron emission tomography for evaluating para-aortic nodal metastasis in locally advanced cervical cancer before surgical staging: a surgico-pathologic study. J Clin Oncol. 1999;17:41–5.
16. Sironi S, Buda A, Picchio M, et al. Lymph node metastasis in patients with clinical early-stage cervical cancer: detection with integrated FDG PET/CT. Radiology. 2006;238:272–9.
17. Bellomi M, Bonomo G, Landoni F, et al. Accuracy of computed tomography and magnetic resonance imaging in the detection of lymph node involvement in cervix carcinoma. Eur Radiol. 2005;15:2469–74.
18. Grigsby PW, Siegel BA, Dehdashti F. Lymph node staging by positron emission tomography in patients with carcinoma of the cervix. J Clin Oncol. 2001;19:3745–9.
19. Esthappan J, Mutic S, Malyapa RS, et al. Treatment planning guidelines regarding the use of CT/PET-guided IMRT for cervical carcinoma with positive paraaortic lymph nodes. Int J Radiat Oncol Biol Phys. 2004;58:1289–97.
20. Esthappan J, Chaudhari S, Santanam L, et al. Prospective clinical trial of positron emission tomography/computed tomography image-guided intensity-modulated radiation therapy for cervical carcinoma with positive para-aortic lymph nodes. Int J Radiat Oncol Biol Phys. 2008;72:1134–9.
21. Mutic S, Malyapa RS, Grigsby PW, et al. PET-guided IMRT for cervical carcinoma with positive para-aortic lymph nodes-a dose-escalation treatment planning study. Int J Radiat Oncol Biol Phys. 2003;55:28–35.

22. Grigsby PW, Singh AK, Siegel BA, et al. Lymph node control in cervical cancer. Int J Radiat Oncol Biol Phys. 2004;59:706–12.
23. Macdonald DM, Lin LL, Biehl K, et al. Combined intensity-modulated radiation therapy and brachytherapy in the treatment of cervical cancer. Int J Radiat Oncol Biol Phys. 2008;71:618–24.
24. Mutic S, Dempsey JF, Bosch WR, et al. Multimodality image registration quality assurance for conformal three-dimensional treatment planning. Int J Radiat Oncol Biol Phys. 2001;51: 255–60.
25. Black QC, Grills IS, Kestin LL, et al. Defining a radiotherapy target with positron emission tomography. Int J Radiat Oncol Biol Phys. 2004;60:1272–82.
26. Daisne JF, Duprez T, Weynand B, et al. Tumor volume in pharyngolaryngeal squamous cell carcinoma: comparison at CT, MR imaging, and FDG PET and validation with surgical specimen. Radiology. 2004;233:93–100.
27. Davis JB, Reiner B, Huser M, et al. Assessment of 18F PET signals for automatic target volume definition in radiotherapy treatment planning. Radiother Oncol. 2006;80:43–50.
28. Nestle U, Kremp S, Schaefer-Schuler A, et al. Comparison of different methods for delineation of 18F-FDG PET-positive tissue for target volume definition in radiotherapy of patients with non-Small cell lung cancer. J Nucl Med. 2005;46:1342–8.
29. Malyapa RS, Mutic S, Low DA, et al. Physiologic FDG-PET three-dimensional brachytherapy treatment planning for cervical cancer. Int J Radiat Oncol Biol Phys. 2002;54:1140–6.
30. Lin LL, Mutic S, Low DA, et al. Adaptive brachytherapy treatment planning for cervical cancer using FDG-PET. Int J Radiat Oncol Biol Phys. 2007;67:91–6.
31. Lin LL, Mutic S, Malyapa RS, et al. Sequential FDG-PET brachytherapy treatment planning in carcinoma of the cervix. Int J Radiat Oncol Biol Phys. 2005;63:1494–501.
32. Kidd EA, Siegel BA, Dehdashti F, et al. The standardized uptake value for F-18 fluorodeoxyglucose is a sensitive predictive biomarker for cervical cancer treatment response and survival. Cancer. 2007;110:1738–44.
33. Berghmans T, Dusart M, Paesmans M, et al. Primary tumor standardized uptake value (SUVmax) measured on fluorodeoxyglucose positron emission tomography (FDG-PET) is of prognostic value for survival in non-small cell lung cancer (NSCLC): a systematic review and meta-analysis (MA) by the European Lung Cancer Working Party for the IASLC Lung Cancer Staging Project. J Thorac Oncol. 2008;3:6–12.
34. Kidd EA, Grigsby PW. Intratumoral Metabolic Heterogeneity of Cervical Cancer. Clin Cancer Res. 2008;14:5236–41.
35. Grigsby PW, Malyapa RS, Higashikubo R, et al. Comparison of molecular markers of hypoxia and imaging with (60)Cu-ATSM in cancer of the uterine cervix. Mol Imaging Biol. 2007;9:278–83.

Part II

Clinical Utility of Imaging for External Beam Radiation

Image-Guidance in External Beam Planning for Locally Advanced Cervical Cancer

5

Karen Lim, Michael Milosevic, Kristy Brock, and Anthony Fyles

5.1 Introduction

Cervix cancer remains a serious health problem among women worldwide despite advances in management [1]. While non-bulky early stage disease can be treated with surgery, chemoirradiation remains the mainstay of management for more advanced stages, with locoregional failure rates approaching 20–30% at 5 years [2]. The morbidity and mortality associated with such events is substantial and salvage therapies remain limited. The acute and late toxicity associated with concurrent chemo-radiation can be significant and is largely a function of the volume of normal tissues irradiated and dose delivered [3].

The advent of conformal radiotherapy techniques and technology has allowed for more normal tissue sparing and sparked interest in the use of intensity-modulated radiotherapy (IMRT) for the treatment of cervix cancer. While planning studies have predicted substantial organ at risk (OAR) sparing, the clinical outcomes have been more modest. The rates of grade 2 gastrointestinal (GI) toxicity experienced by patients undergoing IMRT for either definitive cervix cancer or post-operative cervix/endometrial cancer have ranged from 10 to 85% [4–8]. Roeske et al. noted that many of their whole-pelvis IMRT patients developed acute toxicity at a rate comparable to those treated with conventional pelvic fields [5]. The reasons for this wide range are multifactorial, in part due to differences in target volumes and the smaller amount of bowel within the pelvis for definitive cervix cancer versus post-operative cases, as well as different planning margins used by the different groups. Gerszten et al. noted that the inability to clearly define areas at risk by computed tomography (CT) criteria resulted in generous planning target volumes (PTVs), which closely approximated traditional large pelvic fields [4]. Additionally, the current incomplete understanding of the complex tumor and normal organ motion and deformation dynamics influences PTV

K. Lim (✉), M. Milosevic, K. Brock, and A. Fyles
Department of Radiation Oncology, Princess Margaret Hospital,
610 University Ave, Toronto, ON, M5G 2M9, Canada
e-mail: Karen.Lim@sswahs.nsw.gov.au; Michael.Milosevic@rmp.uhn.on.ca;
Kristy.Brock@rmp.uhn.on.ca; Anthony.Fyles@rmp.uhn.on.ca

A.N. Viswanathan et al. (eds.), *Gynecologic Radiation Therapy*,
DOI: 10.1007/978-3-540-68958-4_5, © Springer-Verlag Berlin Heidelberg 2011

margins and conformal treatment strategies, which impacts the volume of normal tissues irradiated [9]. In order to optimize treatment volumes for cervix cancer patients, high-quality soft tissue discrimination within the pelvis is essential. The different imaging modalities used for this purpose have already been covered in previous chapters; however, magnetic resonance imaging (MRI) remains the optimal modality for this purpose.

5.2 Tumor Volume Regression

Tumor volume regression during radiotherapy can be substantial, with up to an 80% volume reduction by the time 45–50 Gy has been delivered [10–12]. The pattern and rate of tumor regression is highly variable from patient to patient and may be asymmetric [13].

As the tumor regresses, normal tissues can move into the high-dose region, increasing acute toxicity (Fig. 5.1). It can also alter the position of target tissues, resulting in geographical target miss (Fig. 5.2).

5.3 Tumor Motion

Numerous studies have documented tumor motion using various imaging modalities, focusing mainly on the cervix and uterus. Attempts to characterize this motion using orthogonal X-rays [14–16], CT [17–20], and MRI [21–23] have been limited by poor

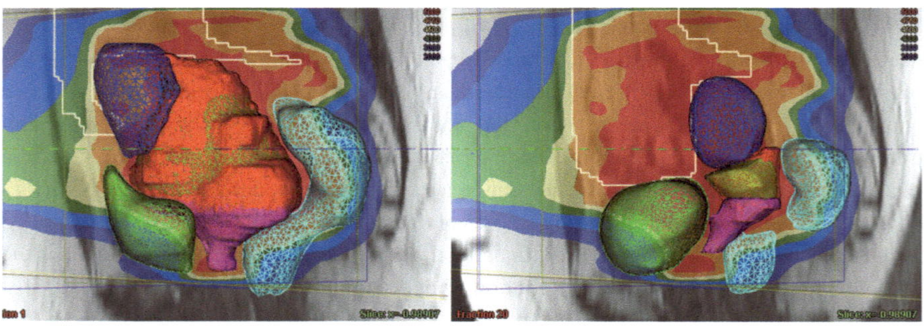

Fig. 5.1 Sagittal T2-weighted images taken from Pt A at the start of external beam radiotherapy (*left*) and at week 4 of treatment (*right*). GTV (*red mesh*), cervix (*khaki mesh*), uterus (*dark blue mesh*), upper vagina (*pink mesh*), bladder (*green mesh*), rectosigmoid (*cyan mesh*), and small bowel (*pale yellow contour*). Theoretical dose color wash from a conformal IMRT plan is overlaid over both images (5,000cGy = red; 4,750cGy = orange; 4,500cGy = yellow; 4,000cGy = green; 3,000cGy = light blue; 2,000cGy = dark blue). The initial gross tumor volume of almost 200cc regressed markedly by the fourth week of treatment. As a result, small bowel (*yellow contour*) now occupies a major portion of the high-dose region

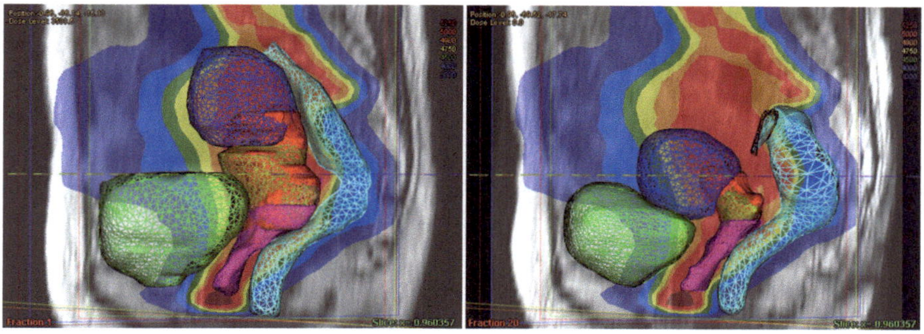

Fig. 5.2 Sagittal T2-weighted images taken from Pt B at the start of external beam radiotherapy (*left*) and at week 4 of treatment (*right*). GTV (*red mesh*), cervix (*khaki mesh*), uterus (*dark blue mesh*), upper vagina (*pink mesh*), bladder (*green mesh*), rectosigmoid (*cyan mesh*), and small bowel (*pale yellow contour*). Theoretical dose color wash from a conformal IMRT plan is overlaid over both images (5,000cGy = red; 4,750cGy = orange; 4,500cGy = yellow; 4,000cGy = green; 3,000cGy = light blue; 2,000cGy = dark blue). As treatment progressed, tumor regression resulted in the uterus changing from a relatively upright position to an anteverted one. This caused a portion of uterus to be under-dosed (Adapated from [27]. Courtesy of Elsevier Ltd.)

soft tissue definition and/or the infrequency of imaging. Different methodologies have been used to determine uterus and/or cervix motion including point of interest analysis (using tumor surrogates like fiducial markers [14–16] or anatomical landmarks [21, 23]), center of mass [19], and overlapping clinical target volume (CTV) analysis [18, 22]. The use of tumor surrogates (e.g., fiducial gold seeds inserted under direct vision) usually limits analysis to only the cervix and the fiducials themselves can fall out or shift as the tumor shrinks and deforms. CT scans provide more soft tissue information (uterus and cervix) but discrimination between other components of the CTV is poor. MRI provides the most soft tissue detail and has been used to comprehensively explore inter- and intra-fraction motion of the cervix and uterus during radiotherapy [21]. Chan et al. found intra-fraction organ motion to be relatively small (<10 mm) but inter-fraction motion ranged up to several centimeters, implying that large margins would be required to compensate for this motion unless daily imaging correction was used. Most of the organ motion studies to date have described translational changes in orthogonal planes (*x*/*y*/*z*). A few studies have assessed the motion of related CTV such as parametrial tissue or vagina in the definitive cervix setting. Taylor et al. did examine the range of vaginal motion using two consecutive MR scans during treatment for a mixed group of cervix and endometrial cancer patients [24]. They found the inter-fraction motion of the vagina to range up to 10 mm in the anterior–posterior direction (Table 5.1). As a consequence of the large range of inter-fraction tumor motion measured by these studies, margin recommendations across the literature have generally ranged from 10 to 24 mm [7, 14–17, 19, 21, 22, 24].

Table 5.1 Magnetic resonance imaging (MRI) studies looking at uterus and cervix motion in cervix cancer patients

Author (year)	Van de Bunt (2008)		Chan (2008)		
Number of patients [median age (range)]	n = 20 (not stated)		n = 20 [47 years (33–70)]		
Methods	Cervix cancer		Cervix cancer		
	MRI baseline & weekly		MRI & cine MRI – done baseline & weekly during standard EBRT		
	Target motion not directly measured. Margins required to encompass GTV & CTV from week to week used as a surrogate for target shifts		Point of interest study – uterine fundus, uterine canal & cervical os		
Inter-fraction motion	GTV	CTV	Uterine fundus	Uterine canal	Cervical os
Sup/inf (mm)	Sup = 4	Sup = 11	CC = 24.4	CC = 15.7	CC = 11.3
	Inf = 8	Inf = 8			
Ant/post (mm)	Ant = 12	Ant = 24	AP = 14.5	AP = 13.1	AP = 11.2
	Post = 14	Post = 17			
Left/right (mm)	Rt = 12	Rt = 12	–	–	–
	Lt = 11	Lt = 6			
Comments	Bladder & bowel prep. not specified		Bladder & bowel prep. specified		
	CTV-PTV margins recommendation:		Suggested inter-fraction margins – fundus (10–40 mm); canal (10–25 mm), os (10–15 mm)		
	Ant = 24 mm; Post = 17 mm; Rt = 12 mm; Lt = 16 mm; Sup = 11 mm; Inf = 8 mm		Intra-fraction motion measured from 11,564 cine MRI frames Suggested intra-fraction margins- fundus (10 mm), canal (50 mm), os (5 cm)		

GTV, gross tumor volume; CTV, clinical target volume; PTV, planning target volume; MRI, magnetic resonance imaging; EBRT, external beam radiotherapy; CC, cranio-caudal; AP, anterior-posterior

5.4 Organ Motion

Surrounding normal tissue motion has been poorly characterized in the literature in relation to the treatment of cervix cancer. While inherently it is understood that bladder and rectal filling might have some impact on neighboring tumor motion, correlations in most studies to date have been weak [21, 25]. This, in part, may arise from the lack of separation of patients into groups with different uterus positions. From work done at our institution, the impact of bladder filling on uterus position is more marked in patients with anteverted uteri compared to those with upright or retroverted uteri Taylor et al. demonstrated a strong correlation between bladder volume and uterine fundus displacement (superior-inferior) in a cohort of gynecological patients who underwent MR imaging on two consecutive days [24]. The difficulty with using organ volume change or point of interest (POI) shift to try and describe organ motion is that neither is necessarily representative of the motion occurring at the surface interface between the critical structure and the tumor target.

5.5 Deformation

In an attempt to characterize the motion of the surrounding normal tissues more accurately, our group has used in-house deformation software [26] and weekly MR images of patients undergoing external beam radiotherapy to model the inter-fractional geometrical changes of the bladder and rectum as well as the gross tumor volume, cervix, uterus, and upper vagina. Twenty patients were studied and confirmed the large range in motion experienced by many of these structures. The combined Euclidean vector motion of the bladder, rectosigmoid, and uterus ranged up to 3.2, 4.0, and 4.5 cm, respectively. Most of this motion occurred in the anterior–posterior and superior–inferior directions. Left–right motion was generally less than 0.5 cm for all structures modeled (Fig. 5.3).

All of these patients were instructed on the use of a bladder and bowel preparation prior to and during treatment. Despite this instruction, the variation in bladder and rectal filling was substantial. For the entire group, mean bladder volume was 105.7cc ± 124.9 (range 8.8–693.1cc) and mean rectosigmoid volume was 70.2cc ± 34.9 (range 24.8–175.9cc). While the benefits of controlling organ filling are well recognized in the prostate literature, for cervical cancer, this remains a controversial issue. Both Chan et al. [21] and Van de Bunt et al. [25] felt that controlling bladder and rectal filling was unlikely to yield significant reductions in inter-fraction margin sizes given the weak correlations seen in their studies. However, the benefits of stringent bladder and rectal filling have not been prospectively analyzed in cervix cancer patients where active interventions (such as getting the patient to partially empty an overly full bladder or evacuate a gas-filled rectum prior to treatment) were undertaken if it was seen that these organs were not in-line with planning dimensions.

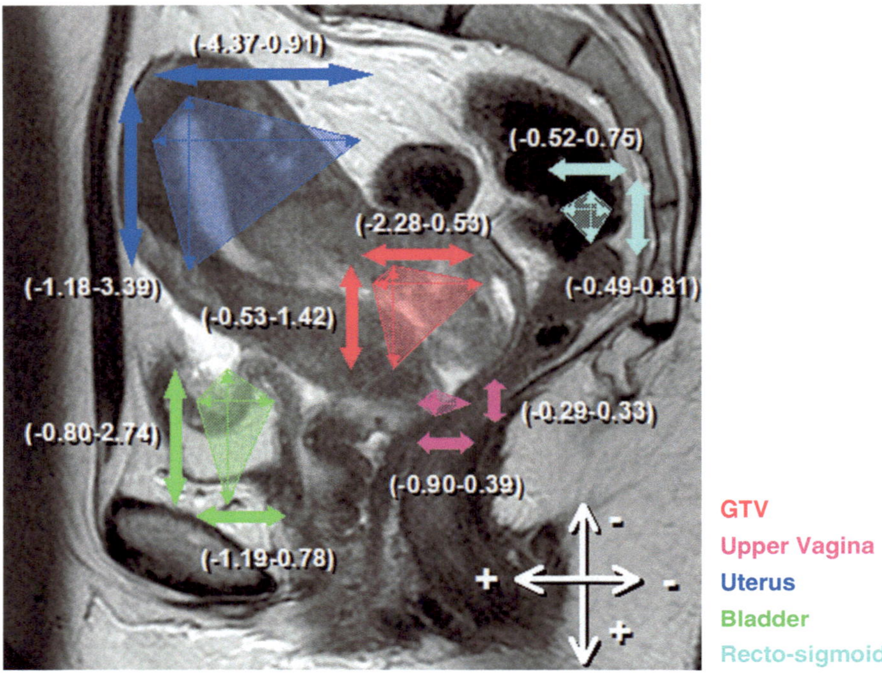

Fig. 5.3 Sagittal T2-weighted MR image of a cervix cancer patient with the range of AP (anterior–posterior) and SI (superior–inferior) inter-fraction motion for all 20 patients. Negative values refer to the posterior and superior direction, measurements in centimeter

5.6 Use of Image Guidance

Based on the above data, any conformal IMRT treatment for cervix cancer would require routine daily soft tissue image guidance during treatment to verify target positioning. Work from our institution has demonstrated marked changes in tumor target positioning during treatment, which would not have been appreciated clinically without the aid of prospective imaging (Figs. 5.4–5.6).

These cases highlight the dangers associated with the use of conformal treatment fields without daily soft tissue image guidance. The various modalities available for image guidance have been covered extensively in previous chapters. Unfortunately, all of them have their limitations from either a resource availability or imaging quality perspective. Without doubt, MRI provides the best soft tissue discrimination of targets within the pelvis, but availability is often limited in many treatment centers and would require moving the patient from the treatment position. In-room CT provides planning quality images and good soft tissue contrast without needing to move the patient from the treatment position, but availability is again limited. Cone-beam CT and helical

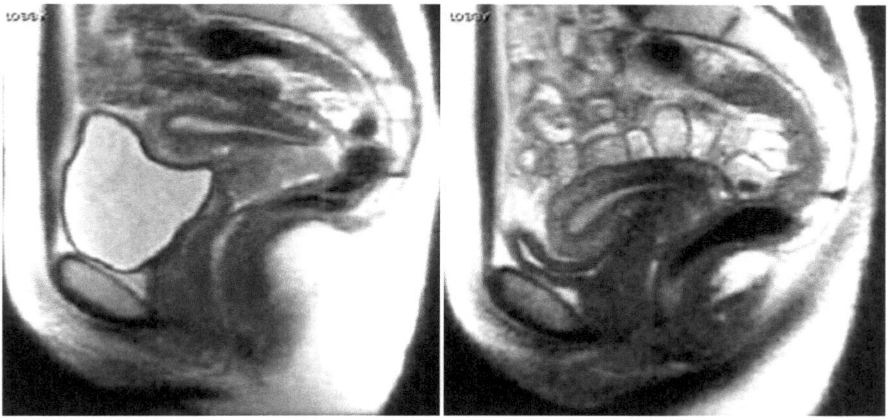

Fig. 5.4 Sagittal T2-weighted images of Pt C taken 1 week apart during external beam radiotherapy. It is apparent that the uterus position in this patient was strongly influenced by bladder filling (Adapated from [28]. Courtesy of Elsevier Ltd.)

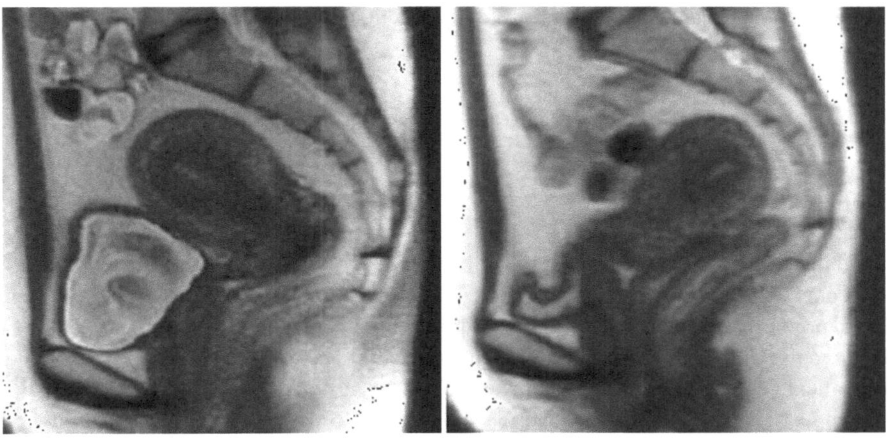

Fig. 5.5 Sagittal T2-weighted images of Pt D taken 1 week apart during external beam radiotherapy. Here the patient demonstrated marked change in the uterus position (anteverted to retroverted) with no relationship to bladder filling. This patient subsequently reverted to an anteverted uterus position on the following week's scan

tomotherapy both offer the advantages of relatively fast imaging with the patient in the treatment position. Unfortunately, image quality can be poor depending on various patient and machine factors. In very thin patients, the lack of intra-abdominal fat results in poor discrimination between the various tissue planes of their pelvic organs. Due to the wide separation in very large patients, online images may also demonstrate artifact which masks the location of the cervix and uterus. Modification of machine parameters such as the mA used and incorporation of image filtering will improve image quality in

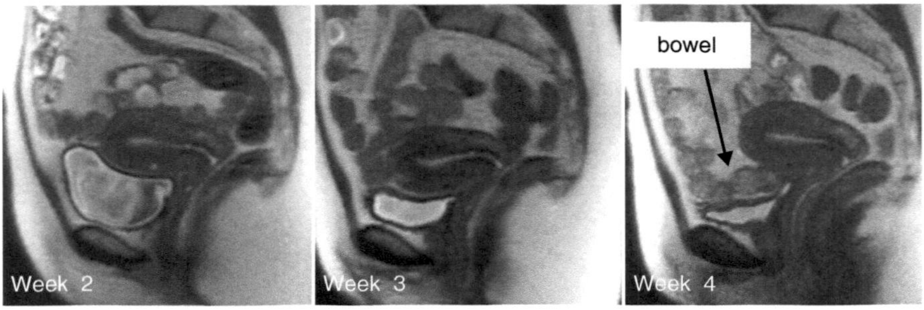

Fig. 5.6 Sagittal T2-weighted images of Pt E taken 1 week apart during external beam radiotherapy. It appears that uterus position is influenced by bladder filling in week 2 and 3. However in week 4 the interposition of a loop of small bowel between the empty bladder and the uterus caused the uterus to be shifted superiorly similar to the effect of a full bladder

some patients. However, other artifacts, such as those caused by bowel gas, result in degraded image quality, which is difficult to compensate for even with hardware or software modifications.

5.7 Significance

From the current literature, it is expected that IMRT would provide significant OAR sparing compared to standard WPRT or EFRT. However, these planning studies have been based primarily on imaging at one point in time without organ motion or tumor regression factored in. The studies have also varied in their definitions of CTV, the margins used, and the patient population (radical vs. adjuvant following hysterectomy). Clinical studies have shown OAR sparing to be less than planning studies predicted, suggesting that current IMRT margins may be too generous. Understanding the complex interplay between tumor and adjacent normal organ motion dynamics in the context of elastic, deformable structures rather than single points is essential if smaller IMRT margins are to be used.

It is the inoperable locally advanced cervix cancer patient who is most at risk of treatment toxicity due to large RT volumes and concurrent chemotherapy, and who stands to benefit most from IMRT. Local recurrence rates of 20–30% for these patients indicate that there is room for improvement. The ability of IMRT to reduce normal tissue toxicity GI, genitourinary (GU), bone marrow (BM) would allow for more aggressive locoregional therapy (concomitant boost, dose escalation) and/or systemic therapy. This in turn has the potential to enhance tumor control and long-term survival. Image guidance and individualized adaptive strategies, driven by future technological advances, will play an essential role in the management of this cancer.

References

1. Eifel PJ et al. Time course and outcome of central recurrence after radiation therapy for carcinoma of the cervix. Int J Gynecol Cancer. 2006;16(3):1106–11.
2. Eifel P et al. Pelvic irradiation with concurrent chemotherapy versus pelvic and para-aortic irradiation for high-risk cervical cancer: an update of radiation therapy oncology group trial (RTOG) 90-01. J Clin Oncol. 2004;22(5):872–80.
3. Kirwan J et al. A systematic review of acute and late toxicity of concomitant chemoradiation for cervical cancer. Radiother Oncol. 2003;68(3):217–26.
4. Gerszten K et al. Feasibility of concurrent cisplatin and extended field radiation therapy (EFRT) using intensity-modulated radiotherapy (IMRT) for carcinoma of the cervix. Gynecol Oncol. 2006;102(2):182–8.
5. Roeske JC et al. A dosimetric analysis of acute gastrointestinal toxicity in women receiving intensity-modulated whole-pelvic radiation therapy. Radiother Oncol. 2003;69(2):201–7.
6. Beriwal S et al. Early clinical outcome with concurrent chemotherapy and extended-field, intensity-modulated radiotherapy for cervical cancer. Int J Radiat Oncol Biol Phys. 2007;68(1): 166–71.
7. Kavanagh BD et al. Clinical application of intensity-modulated radiotherapy for locally advanced cervical cancer. Semin Radiat Oncol. 2002;12(3):260–71.
8. Salama JK et al. Preliminary outcome and toxicity report of extended-field, intensity-modulated radiation therapy for gynecologic malignancies. Int J Radiat Oncol Biol Phys. 2006;65(4): 1170–6.
9. Ahamad A et al. Intensity-modulated radiation therapy after hysterectomy: comparison with conventional treatment and sensitivity of the normal-tissue-sparing effect to margin size. Int J Radiat Oncol Biol Phys. 2005;62(4):1117–24.
10. Lim K et al. Cervical cancer regression measured using weekly magnetic resonance imaging during fractionated radiotherapy: radiobiologic modeling and correlation with tumor hypoxia. Int J Radiat Oncol Biol Phys. 2008;70(1):126–33.
11. Mayr NA et al. Method and timing of tumor volume measurement for outcome prediction in cervical cancer using magnetic resonance imaging. Int J Radiat Oncol Biol Phys. 2002; 52(1):14–22.
12. Nam H et al. The prognostic significance of tumor volume regression during radiotherapy and concurrent chemoradiotherapy for cervical cancer using MRI. Gynecol Oncol. 2007;107(2): 320–5.
13. Mayr NA et al. Serial therapy-induced changes in tumor shape in cervical cancer and their impact on assessing tumor volume and treatment response. AJR Am J Roentgenol. 2006;187(1):65–72.
14. Kaatee RS et al. Detection of organ movement in cervix cancer patients using a fluoroscopic electronic portal imaging device and radiopaque markers. Int J Radiat Oncol Biol Phys. 2002;54(2):576–83.
15. Lee CM, Shrieve DC, Gaffney DK. Rapid involution and mobility of carcinoma of the cervix. Int J Radiat Oncol Biol Phys. 2004;58(2):625–30.
16. Yamamoto R et al. High dose three-dimensional conformal boost (3DCB) using an orthogonal diagnostic X-ray set-up for patients with gynecological malignancy: a new application of real-time tumor-tracking system. Radiother Oncol. 2004;73(2):219–22.
17. Buchali A et al. Impact of the filling status of the bladder and rectum on their integral dose distribution and the movement of the uterus in the treatment planning of gynecological cancer. Radiother Oncol. 1999;52(1):29–34.
18. Lee JE et al. Interfractional variation of uterine position during radical RT: weekly CT evaluation. Gynecol Oncol. 2007;104(1):145–51.

19. Li XA et al. Interfractional variations in patient setup and anatomic change assessed by daily computed tomography. Int J Radiat Oncol Biol Phys. 2007;68(2):581–91.
20. Beadle B.M et al. Cervix regression and motion during the course of external beam chemoradiation for cervical cancer. Int J Radiat Oncol Biol Phys. 2009;73(1):235–41. Epub 2008 May 29.
21. Chan P et al. Inter- and intrafractional tumor and organ movement in patients with cervical cancer undergoing radiotherapy: a cinematic-MRI point-of-interest study. Int J Radiat Oncol Biol Phys. 2008;70(5):1507–15.
22. van de Bunt L et al. Motion and deformation of the target volumes during IMRT for cervical cancer: what margins do we need? Radiother Oncol. 2008;88:233–40.
23. Huh SJ, Park W, Han Y. Interfractional variation in position of the uterus during radical radiotherapy for cervical cancer. Radiother Oncol. 2004;71(1):73–9.
24. Taylor A, Powell MEB. An assessment of interfractional uterine and cervical motion: Implications for radiotherapy target volume definition in gynecological cancer. Radiother Oncol. 2008;88(2):250–7.
25. van de Bunt L et al. Conventional, conformal, and intensity-modulated radiation therapy treatment planning of external beam radiotherapy for cervical cancer: The impact of tumor regression. Int J Radiat Oncol Biol Phys. 2006;64(1):189–96.
26. Brock KK et al. Accuracy of finite element model-based multi-organ deformable image registration. Med Phys. 2005;32(6):1647–59.
27. Lim K et al. Pelvic Radiotherapy for cancer of the cervix: is what you plan actually what you deliver? Int J Radiat Oncol Biol Phys. 2009; 74(1):304–12.
28. Lim K et al. Consensus Guidelines for Delineation of Clinical Target Volume for Intensity-Modulated Pelvic Radiotherapy for the Definitive Treatment of Cervix Cancer. Int J Radiat Oncol Biol Phys. 2010 May 14.

6 Physics Perspectives on the Role of 3D Imaging

Dietmar Georg and Christian Kirisits

6.1 Introduction

Whole pelvic radiotherapy (WPRT) followed by a boost to the tumor has been a standard component of definitive radiotherapy for locally advanced cervix cancer for many years. Besides treating the primary site, WPRT is used to sterilize subclinical metastatic disease in the pelvic lymph nodes. The current standard for WPRT is a conformal external radiotherapy technique (3D-CRT), such as a four-field box, based on three-dimensional (3D) sectional imaging.

WPRT treatments based on a 3D-CRT technique result in irradiating large volumes of small and large bowel, rectum, and bladder. Therefore, gastrointestinal and genitourinary symptoms are among the most important acute and chronic toxicities in these patients [1, 2]. To improve complication-free disease control, various advanced EBRT approaches have been proposed that allow delivering adequate doses to both tumor and areas of lymphatic drainage, while at the same time sparing normal structures. These techniques are based on improved immobilization, the use of intensity modulations, and the use of image guidance for patient setup verification [e.g., 3–5].

6.2 Advanced Photon Beam Therapy for Whole Pelvic Irradiations

Intensity modulated radiation therapy (IMRT) is an approach that increases the conformity of the high-dose region in three dimensions to the shape of irregular and concave target volumes. Additionally, steep dose gradients created via computerized treatment plan optimization limit the dose to surrounding normal tissues. Several treatment plan

D. Georg (✉) and C. Kirisits
Department of Radiotherapy, Vienna General Hospital,
Medical University of Vienna, Währinger Gürtel 18–20, 1090 Vienna, Austria
e-mail: dietmar.georg@akhwien.at; christian.kirisits@akhwien.at

A.N. Viswanathan et al. (eds.), *Gynecologic Radiation Therapy*,
DOI: 10.1007/978-3-540-68958-4_6, © Springer-Verlag Berlin Heidelberg 2011

comparisons illustrate the potential benefit for organs at risk (OAR), such as small bowel, rectum, and bladder, through improved dose distributions [6–9]. Furthermore, an IMRT-based simultaneous integrated boost technique for WPRT including the boost for the tumor site has been evaluated in terms of dosimetry and radiobiology [10]. Clinical series treating pelvic gynecologic malignancies with IMRT show a reduction in treatment-related toxicity by decreasing the incidence of acute gastrointestinal side effects [11–14].

In most departments, external beam therapy (EBT) treatment planning is based on pretreatment imaging. The clinical target (CTV) and planning target volumes (PTV) are based on a static simulation imaged prior to treatment. However, the tumor volume changes its location, shape, and volume during the course of treatment. Weekly magnetic resonance (MR) imaging showed the need of anisotropic margins that can exceed 10 mm in order to cover the uterus movement [15]. Tumor shrinkage by 46% after 30 Gy and more than 60% after 45 Gy are reported in literature [9, 16, 17]. 3D conformal techniques, using dose plateaus with appropriate margins seem to be appropriate for target coverage. However, the change of topography involves also the organs at risk. Adaptation to the actual situation could substantially decrease the dose to healthy tissue [18]. When applying steep dose gradients in three dimensions with advanced techniques, the various interfraction effects such as motion and deformation of the tumor and changes in organ filling need to be considered carefully in order to avoid underdosage of the target and excessive doses to OAR.

The primary OARs for WPRT are the rectum, the bladder and the bowel structures. For younger patient receiving WPRT irradiation of the ovaries can lead to castration [19]. Total doses of 5 Gy have been reported as critical [20]. Ovarian transposition is a feasible method to protect the ovaries. Nevertheless, the radiation oncologist needs to pay special attention to the ovarian dose, especially if advanced techniques are applied that increase the out-of-field dose [21].

Although IMRT enables improved OAR sparing of the primary OARs through computerized treatment plan optimization, several issues related to these OARs need to be considered. Most importantly, the critical structures to be spared are the organ wall and not the organ filling. However, organ filling and consequently the location of the organ wall can change between fractions. Due to the vicinity of the rectum to the uterus large parts of the rectal wall are included in the PTV and it is only possible to spare those parts of the rectal wall that are not included in the PTV. IMRT enables sparing the anterior part in the concavity of the typical PTV for cervix cancer, but the sparing effect of the bladder and its filling must not be confused with the sparing effect of the bladder wall. Finally, it has been shown in several studies that a full and/or large bladder reduces small bowel exposure, because an increase in bladder volume pushes the small bowel upward, i.e., out of the primarily irradiated volume [8]. Another option for moving bowel structures out of the irradiated area is to use a bellyboard and prone positioning of the patient [3, 22].

Dose-volume-histograms (DVHs) depend on the delineation protocol. For organs like the bladder, the whole OAR is usually contoured while rectum and bowels are only partly defined. For delineation of bowel structures different strategies have been used. For example, Roeske et al. and Liu et al. defined the peritoneal cavity below L4–L5 (excluding rectum and bladder) as small bowel region, while Portelance et al. outlined all individual loops [12, 13, 23]. For these reasons, it is not straightforward to compare DVH and dose volume objectives for bowel structures that drive IMRT planning.

The above-mentioned issues are well known, but the technology (including hardware and software) to study inter- and intra-fraction organ movement and deformation for pelvic targets has only recently become available. Therefore, it has been difficult to draft recommendations for delineation of OAR and the assessment of DVHs for WPRT. Today, OAR delineation and the interpretation of the DVH remain based on whole organ contouring on the "snapshot" Computed Tomography (CT) at the time of treatment planning.

6.3 Image Guidance for External Beam Therapy

Interfraction setup variations are taken into account via margins around the CTV to construct the planning target volume (PTV). For 3D-CRT of cervix cancer, several portal imaging studies have addressed the issue of repositioning accuracy and its consequences on the definition of margins [e.g., 24, 25]. The use of electronic portal imaging systems, an early form of image guidance, has become standard clinical practice for conformal radiotherapy since the 1990s. Other groups have evaluated external marker-based systems for patient setup verification of WPRT for gynecologic malignancies [5].

Today it is generally acknowledged that advanced radiotherapy techniques, such as IMRT, require precise patient immobilization and image guidance for treatment planning and delivery. Treatment delivery units combined with imaging equipment have become commercially available. Although developments like linear accelerators with integrated cone-beam CT (CBCT) or tomotherapy have pushed image-guided radiation therapy (IGRT), the image quality of X-ray based imaging technology suffers from its low soft-tissue contrast. In a recent study about delineation of the prostate gland, the impact of the limited CBCT image quality on interobserver variations was evaluated [26]. As an example, Figure 6.1 illustrates cone-beam CT (CBCT) images of a cervix cancer

MR, which is known to be superior in terms of soft-tissue contrast, has been intensively used for repetitive imaging studies to quantify interfraction and intra-fraction organ motion for cervix cancer patients [15, 27, 28]. This is of particular importance because the CTV for gynecological patients consists of multiple structures that exhibit complex changes during the course of radiotherapy. Non-isostropic margins around the GTV and the CTV have been recommended. From a study of weekly MR scans of 20 patients, van de Bunt et al. concluded that for the construction of a meaningful CTV, margins of 12–14 mm are need in anterior and posterior (AP) direction, about 12 mm in lateral direction, and 4 and 8 mm in superior and interior (SI) direction [15]. For CTV to PTV expansion, 15 mm or more is needed in AP and SI directions, while 7–10 mm suffice in the lateral direction [15, 28]. Although rectal filling and bladder filling alter the position of the cervix and uterine body, whether measures to control the filling status may overcome this is not clear.

Inspired by the superior image quality of MR, a dedicated MR linac for image guided radiation therapy (IGRT) has been proposed [29]. Based on this concept, Kerhof et al. presented the concept of online MR-guided external beam radiation (EBT) of cervical cancer [18].

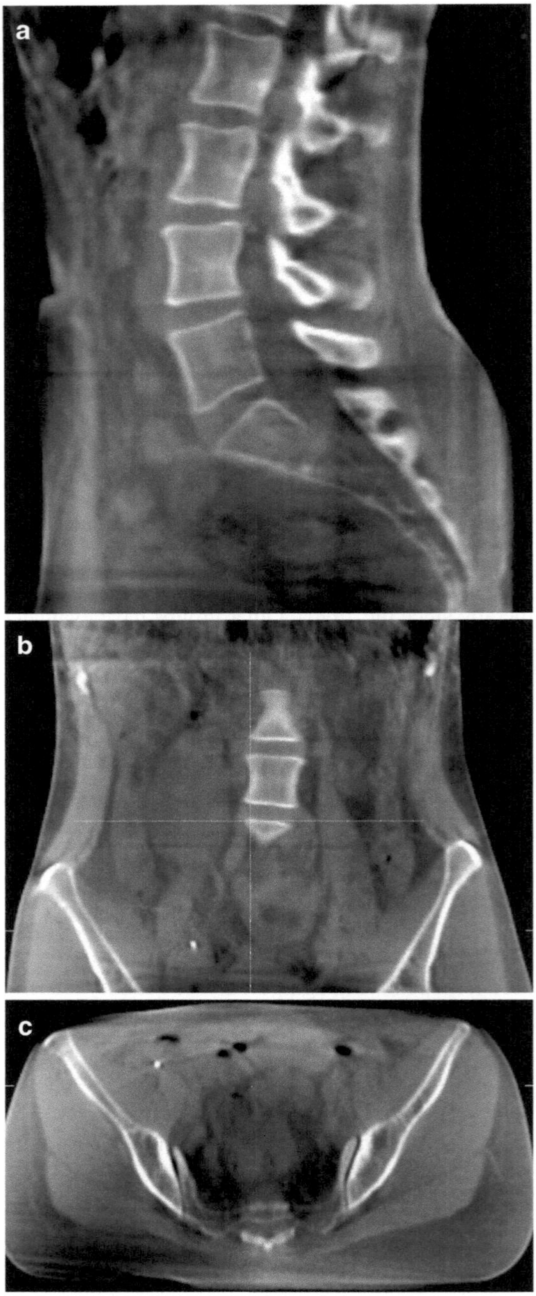

Fig. 6.1 Example of a cone-beam CT (CBCT) image of a cervix cancer patient for image guided external beam therapy (EBT). (**a**) Sagittal view, (**b**) coronal view, (**c**) axial view

This treatment planning study found that compared to commonly applied pretreatment image-based planning, weekly online planning significantly reduced irradiated volumes of bladder, rectum, bowel, and sigmoid. Figure 6.2 shows a CT-based treatment plan in relation to the actual topography visualized by repetitive MR imaging, and possible plan adaptation.

6.4 External Beam Therapy as an Alternative to Intracavitary Brachytherapy

Stimulated by recent technological developments, external beam therapy (EBT) has challenged brachytherapy (BT) and vice versa in several treatment planning and clinical studies regarding the management of gynecological cancers [30–33]. For example, tomotherapy boost was compared with a simple BT technique based on a Suit–Fletcher applicator [33]. Molla et al. reported on 15 patients who received an IMRT boost on a dedicated linac [32]. The conclusions drawn from these investigations were that inversely planned IMRT allows better sparing of OAR and generates more homogenous dose distributions. These studies were biased because advanced EBRT was predominantly compared with simple BT techniques. In addition, important concepts such as the need of margins in EBRT to account for setup and internal motion were not always considered in depth. In general, a dose homogeneity comparison between EBT and BT for gynecologic RT is not meaningful. For BT a large part of the highest dose volume (>200% of prescription dose) is located within the applicator, the vaginal packing, and directly in the gross tumor volume (GTV). Furthermore, the substantial clinical experience with image-guided BT cannot be neglected [34, 35]. Thus, it cannot be assumed a priori that the dose distribution throughout a boost volume needs to be homogenous. In contrary, the high doses delivered to the central part of the GTV and CTV might be even essential for the success of this treatment modality.

More recent studies tried to compare high-tech EBRT against high-tech brachytherapy for locally advanced cervix cancer [36, 37]. Similar to inversely planned EBRT, BT was also planned using manual or computerized optimization and sophisticated applicator technology was considered. For example, Georg et al. [37] challenged inversely planned EBT with photons (IMRT) and protons (IMPT) to deliver the highest possible dose to the PTV while respecting D_{1cc} and D_{2cc} limits from BT, assuming the same fractionation (4×7 Gy). For this purpose, nine patients were selected and treated either with intracavitary, combined interstitial/intracavitary or complex interstitial BT. Margins (3 and 5 mm) were added to the brachytherapy CTV to construct an EBRT PTV. If IMRT was limited to D_{2cc} and D_{1cc} from BT, the minimal dose that covered 90% (D90) of the HR-PTV and IR-PTV (according to GEC-ESTRO recommendations) was lower for EBT. On the other hand, volumes receiving 60 Gy (in EQD_2) were approximately twice as large for IMRT compared to BT (Table 6.1). In summary, it was found that for cervix cancer boost treatments, both IMRT and IMPT seem to be inferior to advanced BT. Figure 6.3 shows a comparison of dose distribution for the boost volume for image-guided BT, and IMRT with photons and protons. It must be mentioned although image guided brachytherapy (IGBT) has become the "golden" standard for delivering boost treatments to gynecological targets, there might be patients who are not eligible for BT.

Table 6.1 Characteristics of the 3 Gy per boost fraction volume, which is an estimate for the 60 Gy total dose volume

$V_{3\,Gy}$ [cm^3]	Mean ± standard deviation	Min	Max	No > 600 cm^3	No < 450 cm^3
BT	325 ± 105	206	501	0	7/8
$IMXT_{5\,mm}$	681 ± 258	519	1187	5/8	0
$IMPT_{5\,mm}$	502 ± 144	347	741	1/8	3/8

BT, brachytherapy; $IMXT_{5mm}$, intensity modulated photons with 5mm margins; $IMPT_{5mm}$, intensity modulated protons with 5mm margins

6.5 Issues Related to Combined WPRT and Brachytherapy Boost

The addition of external beam dose to the brachytherapy boost has been a major point of discussion. Using a conventional 3D conformal technique (e.g., four-field box) the dose distribution in the center of the treated volume is homogenous according to the International Commission on Radiation Units & Measurements (ICRU) recommendation (–5% to +7% [38]). This homogenous dose plateau is located at the region of the CTV at brachytherapy, the posterior part of the bladder, the anterior part of the rectum, and the parts of the sigmoid close to the uterus. Therefore, the DVH values related to the GTV and CTV and the most exposed parts of the OAR (D_{2cc}, $D_{0.1cc}$) are directly added to the prescribed dose of the external beam plan [39]. In the case of IMRT, the dose distribution can show a more inhomogeneous dose distribution, with dose peaks distributed within the OARs. However, these dose regions are not primarily placed in the dose regions of interest for the brachytherapy and total dose/volume parameters (i.e., anterior rectum wall, posterior bladder wall). When adding external beam dose distributions with brachytherapy plans these issues have to be considered. For certain techniques, it seems appropriate to add one single reference dose for IMRT to the brachytherapy dose values, while other approaches leading to substantial uncertainties have to be analyzed in detail.

Several studies have focused on comparing advanced EBT with standard or advanced BT. Unfortunately, fewer studies focus on "intelligent" combinations of advanced EBT and advanced BT. One basic question to be addressed is whether image-guided adaptive BT can utilize the dose reduction in OAR that can be achieved with high-tech EBT, in order to further improve the therapeutic ratio and consequently outcome. Image-guided and adaptive EBT and BT are both often not done in an integrated fashion, but independent from each other. Instead of comparing them, future studies should focus on combining advanced EBT and advanced BT by utilizing inherent advantages of both options, in order to fully exploit the potential of advanced radiotherapy. Such activities are compromised by the lack of availability of commercial treatment planning systems in which composite EBT and BT plans can be fully integrated. The substantial change of topography when inserting the brachytherapy applicators makes it impossible to use rigid registration techniques. Voxel to voxel tracking with deformable registration is currently one of the most interesting topics for further developments.

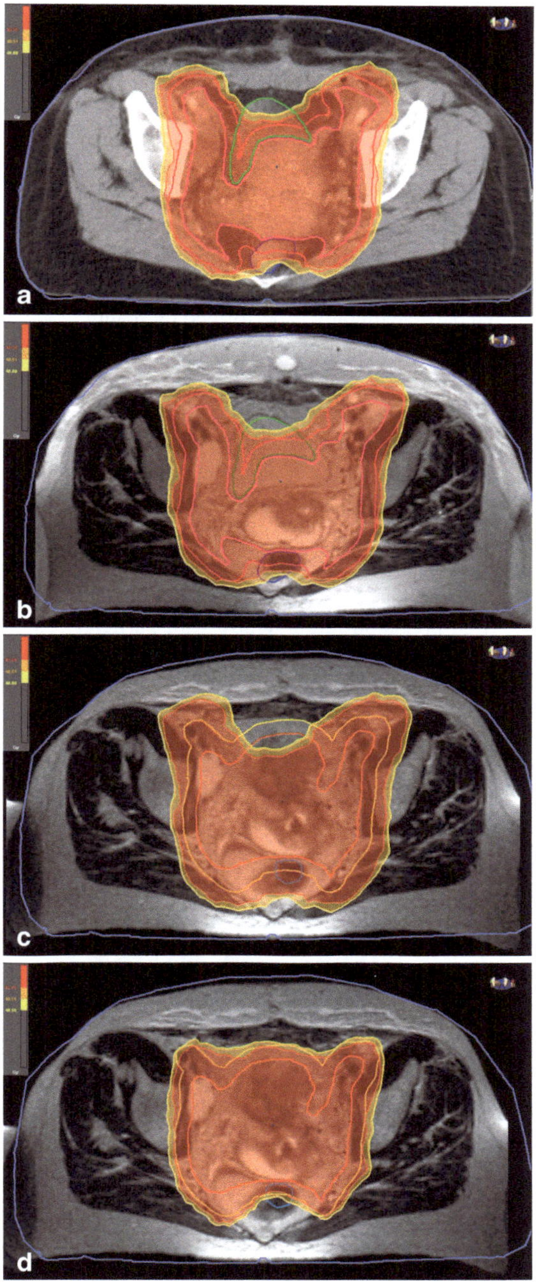

Fig. 6.2 This set of images illustrate the changes in topography between the planning CT (**a**), a magnetic resonance imaging (MRI) taken on the same day (**b**), and an MRI from third week of external beam treatment (**c**). Yellow and orange isodose lines correspond to 90% and 95% dose, respectively. The clinical target volume (CTV) and planning target volume (PTV) used for the initial plan are drawn in *magenta* and *red*, respectively. While changes between CT and MRI before treatment are smaller, substantial deviations can be observed for week 3. The anterior part of the CTV is even outside of the 90% isodose line. (**d**) This shows an adapted plan, taking into account the changes in topography

6.6 Particle[1] Therapy for Whole Pelvic Irradiations

Proton and ion beam therapies are known to offer dosimetric advantages because of their superior physical characteristics. Typical DVHs of OAR for proton therapy (PT), when compared to IMRT with photons are similar in the high-dose region while low- and medium-dose regions show improved OAR sparing with protons.

Similar to IMRT with photons, computerized treatment plan optimization through inverse planning is becoming available for particle therapy. The delivery of intensity modulated particle therapy is performed by scanning the beam across the field and by changing the penetration depth through active or passive energy variation. Equipment for planning and delivering a scanned particle beam is becoming commercially available. Figure 6.4 illustrates a typical dose distribution for whole pelvic radiotherapy for 3D-CRT, passively scattered protons, and inversely planned IMRT with photons and protons.

Only a small series of cervix cancer patients has been treated with carbon ions, and for a small number of patients, protons were used as a boost modality [40, 41]. The rather sparse clinical experience available today is still based on the so-called passive scattering techniques where the pencil beam of the accelerator is scattered to produce a spread-out-Bragg-peak that covers the PTV.

High-precision radiotherapy with particles requires special considerations. Any anatomical changes at the time of treatment delivery compared to the time of treatment planning may have a significant impact on the range of particles. Therefore, weight loss and

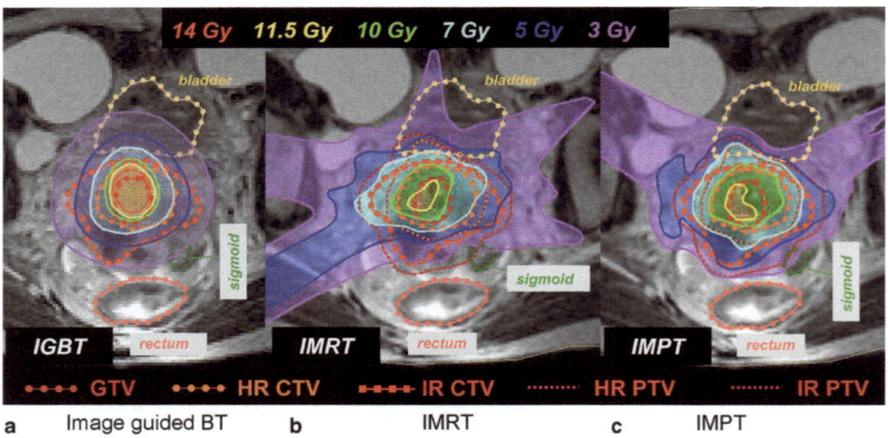

Fig. 6.3 Typical isodose distributions for boost treatment for cervix cancer. (**a**) image-guided brachytherapy (IGBT), (**b**) intensity modulated radiotherapy (IMRT), and (**c**) intensity modulated proton therapy (IMPT)

[1] Within this chapter, particle therapy is restricted to the therapeutic use of charged particles much heavier than electrons.

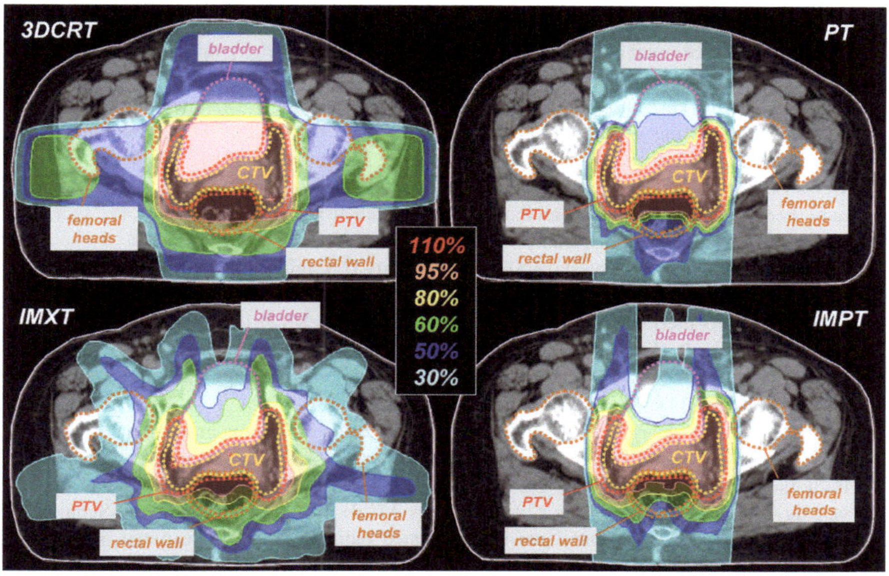

Fig. 6.4 Comparison of typical dose distributions for 3D conformal treatment (3D-CRT), intensity modulated photon treatment (IMXT), proton therapy (PT), and intensity modulated proton therapy (IMPT). In addition to target conformity, the total volume treated to low-dose values, and high- and low-dose regions within organs at risk (OAR) are of interest

changes in the filling status of an organ are critical. Image guidance for verifying setup and anatomy is imperative for particle therapy. Inter-fraction variations during the course of ion beam therapy for locally advanced cervix carcinoma have been addressed by Kato et al. [41]. Initially these authors based the whole pelvic and the boost treatment on two different planning CT data sets. Based on their early experience they proposed an adaptive approach with multiple planning CTs and a CTV for the local boost that was modified twice in order to account for tumor shrinkage and to further improve OAR sparing.

The challenge remains to construct a composite treatment plan from individual treatment plans that are based on different topography, with similar difficulties as discussed above when combining advanced EBT and advanced BT techniques.

References

1. Corn BW, Lanciano RM, Greven KM, et al. Impact of improve irradiation technique, age, and lymph node sampling on the severe complication rate of surgically staged endometrial cancer patients: A multivariate analysis. J Clin Oncol. 1994;12:510–5.
2. Perez CA, Breaux S, Bedwinek JM, et al. Radiation therapy alone in the treatment of carcinoma of the uterine cervix Radiation therapy alone in the treatment of carcinoma of the uterine cervix. II. Analysis of complications. Cancer. 1984;54:235–46.

3. Adli M, Mayr NA, Kaiser HS, Skwarchuk MW, Meeks SL, Mardirossian G, et al. Does prone positioning reduce small bowel dose in pelvic radiation with intensity-modulated radiotherapy for gynecologic cancer? Int J Radiat Oncol Biol Phys. 2003;57(1):230–8.
4. Mell LK, Tiryaki H, Ahn KH, Mundt AJ, Roeske JC, Aydogan B. Dosimetric comparison of bone marrow-sparing intensity-modulated radiotherapy versus conventional techniques for treatment of cervical cancer. Int J Radiat Oncol Biol Phys. 2008;71(5):1504–10.
5. Weiss E, Vorwerk H, Richter S, Hess CF. Interfractional and intrafractional accuracy during radiotherapy of gynaecologic carcinomas: a comprehensive evaluation using the ExacTrac system. Int J Radiat Oncol Biol Phys. 2003;56(1):69–79.
6. Cozzi L, Dinshaw KA, Shrivastava SK, Mahantshetty U, Engineer R, Deshpande DD, et al. A treatment planning study comparing volumetric arc modulation with RapidArc and fixed field IMRT for cervix uteri radiotherapy. Radiother Oncol. 2008;89(2):180–91.
7. Georg D, Georg P, Hillbrand M, Pötter R, Mock U. Assessment of improved organ at risk sparing for advanced cervix carcinoma utilizing precision radiotherapy techniques. Strahlenth Onkol. 2008;184(11):586–91.
8. Georg P, Georg P, Georg D, Hillbrand M, Kirisits C, Pötter R. Factors influencing bowel sparing in intensity modulated whole pelvic radiotherapy for gynaecological malignancies. Radiother Oncol. 2006;80(1):19–26.
9. van de Bunt L, van der Heide UA, Ketelaars M, de Kort GA, Jürgenliemk-Schulz IM. Conventional, conformal, and intensity-modulated radiation therapy treatment planning of external beam radiotherapy for cervical cancer: the impact of tumor regression. Int J Radiat Oncol Biol Phys. 2006;64(1):189–96.
10. Guerrero M, Li XA, Ma L, Linder J, Deyoung C, Erickson B. Simultaneous integrated intensity-modulated radiotherapy boost for locally advanced gynecological cancer: radiobiological and dosimetric considerations. Int J Radiat Oncol Biol Phys. 2005;62(3):933–9.
11. Mundt AJ, Lujan AE, Rotmensch J, et al. Intensity modulated whole pelvic radiotherapy in women with gynaecologic malignancies. Int J Rad Oncol Biol Phys. 2002;52:1330–7.
12. Portelance L, Chao KS, Grigsby PW, Bennet H, Low D. Intensity-modulated radiation therapy (IMRT) reduces small bowel, rectum, and bladder doses in patients with cervical cancer receiving pelvic and para-aortic irradiation. Int J Radiat Oncol Biol Phys. 2001;51(1):261–6.
13. Roeske JC, Lujan A, Rotmensch J, et al. Intensity modulated whole pelvic radiation therapy in patients with gynaecological malignancies. Int J Rad Oncol Biol Phys. 2000;48:1613–21.
14. Roeske JC, Bonta D, Mell LK, et al. A dosimetric analysis of acute gastrointestinal toxicity in women receiving intensity modulated whole pelvic radiation therapy. Radioth Oncol. 2003;69:201–7.
15. van de Bunt L, Jürgenliemk-Schulz IM, de Kort GA, Roesink JM, Tersteeg RJ, van der Heide UA. Motion and deformation of the target volumes during IMRT for cervical cancer: what margins do we need? Radiother Oncol. 2008;88(2):233–40.
16. Beadle BM, Jhingran A, Salehpour M, Sam M, Iyer RB, Eifel PJ. Cervix regression and motion during the course of external beam chemoradiation for cervical cancer. Int J Radiat Oncol Biol Phys. 2009;73:235–41.
17. Dimopoulos J, Schirl G, Baldinger A, Helbich T, Pötter R. MRI Assessment of Cervical Cancer for Adaptive Radiotherapy Strahlenth. Strahlenth Onkol. 2009;185:282–7.
18. Kerkhof EM, Raaymakers BW, van der Heide UA, van de Bunt L, Jürgenliemk-Schulz IM, Lagendijk JJ. Online MRI guidance for healthy tissue sparing in patients with cervical cancer: an IMRT planning study. Radiother Oncol. 2008;88(2):241–9.
19. Wo J, Viswanathan AN. Impact of radiotherapy on fertility, pregnancy, and neonatal outcomes in female cancer patients. Int J Radiat Oncol Biol Phys. 2009;73(5):1304–12.
20. Haie-Meder C, Mlika-Cabanne N, Michel G, Briot E, Gerbaulet A, Lhomme C, et al. Radiotherapy after ovarian transposition: ovarian function and fertility preservation. Int J Radiat Oncol Biol Phys. 1993;25(3):419–24.

21. Kry SF, Salehpour M, Followill DS, Stovall M, Kuban DA, White RA, et al. Out-of-field photon and neutron dose equivalents from step-and-shoot intensity-modulated radiation therapy. Int J Radiat Oncol Biol Phys. 2005;62(4):1204–16.
22. Olofsen-van Acht M, van den Berg H, Quint S, et al. Reduction of irradiated small bowel volume and accurate patient positioning by use of a bellyboard device in pelvic radiotherapy of gynecological cancer patients. Radioth Oncol. 2001;59:87–93.
23. Liu Y, Shiau C-Y, Lee M-L, et al. The role and strategy of IMRT in radiotherapy of pelvic tumors: dose escalation and critical organ sparing in prostate cancer. Int J Radiat Oncol Biol Phys. 2007;67:1113–23.
24. Mock U, Dieckmann K, Wolff U, Pötter R. Portal Imaging based definition of the planning target volume during pelvic irradiation for gynecologic malignancies. Int J Rad Oncol Biol Phys. 1999;45:227–32.
25. Stroom JC, Olofsen-van Acht MJ, Quint S, Seven M, de Hoog M, Creutzberg CL, et al. On-line set-up corrections during radiotherapy of patients with gynaecologic tumors. Int J Radiat Oncol Biol Phys. 2000;46(2):499–506.
26. White EA, Brock KK, Jaffray DA, Catton CN. Inter-observer variability of prostate delineation on cone beam computerised tomography images. Clin Oncol. 2009;21(1):32–8.
27. Huh SJ, Park W, Han Y. Interfractional variation in position of the uterus during radical radiotherapy for cervical cancer. Radiother Oncol. 2004;71(1):73–9.
28. Taylor A, Powell ME. An assessment of interfractional uterine and cervical motion: implications for radiotherapy target volume definition in gynaecological cancer. Radiother Oncol. 2008;88(2):250–7.
29. Lagendijk JJ, Raaymakers BW, Raaijmakers AJ, Overweg J, Brown KJ, Kerkhof EM, et al. MRI/linac integration. Radiother Oncol. 2008;86(1):25–9.
30. Aydogan B, Mundt AJ, Smith BD, et al. A dosimetric analysis of intensity-modulated radiation therapy (IMRT) as an alternative to adjuvant high-dose-rate (HDR) brachytherapy in early endometrial cancer patients. Int J Radiat Oncol Biol Phys. 2006;65:266–73.
31. Low DA, Grigsby PW, Dempsey JF, Mutic S, Williamson JF, Markman J, et al. Applicator-guided intensity-modulated radiation therapy. Int J Radiat Oncol Biol Phys. 2002; 52(5):1400–6.
32. Molla M, Escude L, Nouet P, et al. Fractionated stereotactic radiotherapy boost for gynecologic tumors: an alternative to brachytherapy? Int J Radiat Oncol Biol Phys. 2005;62:118–24.
33. Wahab SH, Malyapa RS, Mutic S, et al. A treatment planning study comparing HDR and AGIMRT for cervical cancer. Med Phys. 2004;31:734–43.
34. Dimopoulos JC, Kirisits C, Petric P, Georg P, Lang S, Berger D, et al. The Vienna applicator for combined intracavitary and interstitial brachytherapy of cervical cancer: clinical feasibility and preliminary results. Int J Radiat Oncol Biol Phys. 2006;66(1):83–90.
35. Pötter R, Dimopoulos J, Georg P, Lang S, Waldhäusl C, Wachter-Gerstner N, et al. Clinical impact of MRI assisted dose volume adaptation and dose escalation in brachytherapy of locally advanced cervix cancer. Radiother Oncol. 2007;83(2):148–55.
36. Assenholt MS, Petersen JB, Nielsen SK, Lindegaard JC, Tanderup K. A dose planning study on applicator guided stereotactic IMRT boost in combination with 3D MRI based brachytherapy in locally advanced cervical cancer. Acta Oncol. 2008;47(7):1337–43.
37. Georg D, Kirisits Ch, Hillbrand M, Dimopoulos J, Pötter R. Image-guided radiotherapy for cervix cancer: high-tech external beam therapy vs. High-tech brachytherapy. Int J Rad Onc Biol Phys. 2008;71:1272–8.
38. ICRU Report 50. Prescribing, recording, and reporting photon beam therapy. International Commission on Radiation Units and Meausrments, Bethesda.
39. Lang S, Kirisits C, Dimopoulos J, Georg D, Pötter R. Treatment planning for MRI assisted brachytherapy of gynecologic malignancies based on total dose constraints. Int J Radiat Oncol Biol Phys. 2007;69(2):619–27.

40. Kagei K, Tokuuye K, Okumura T, Ohara K, Shioyama Y, Sugahara S, et al. Long-term results of proton beam therapy for carcinoma of the uterine cervix. Int J Radiat Oncol Biol Phys. 2003;55(5):1265–71.
41. Kato S, Ohno T, Tsujii H, Nakano T, Mizoe JE, Kamada T, et al. Dose escalation study of carbon ion radiotherapy for locally advanced carcinoma of the uterine cervix. Int J Radiat Oncol Biol Phys. 2006;65(2):388–97.

Image-Guided Treatment Planning and Therapy in Postoperative Gynecologic Malignancies

7

Eric D. Donnelly, Tamer M. Refaat, and William Small, Jr

7.1 Conventional Two-Dimensional (2D) Treatment Regimen

Traditionally, radiation therapy has played a prominent role in the treatment of patients with gynecologic malignancies. The majority of endometrial and early-stage cervical carcinomas are treated upfront with hysterectomy with appropriate concurrent surgical staging. Based on the pathologic findings, patients at risk of local recurrence may be considered for radiation therapy, either in the form of external beam radiation therapy (EBRT) and/or brachytherapy. Large randomized trials have demonstrated that adjuvant radiation therapy significantly reduces the rate of local recurrences in postoperative endometrial and cervical cancer patients, most notably in those with positive nodes and/or high-grade disease [1, 4–6].

The target volume for pelvic radiation in postoperative gynecologic malignancies includes the parametrium, the upper vagina, and pelvic lymph nodes. Conventional radiation techniques used to treat the pelvic target volume for carcinoma of the uterine cervix or corpus post-hysterectomy involve either two (anteroposterior–posteroanterior [AP–PA]) or four (AP, PA, right, and left laterals) portal fields. Historically, radiation portals have been designed by means of plain radiographs, utilizing bony landmarks for borders based on the knowledge of anatomical landmarks from surgical trials [12]. Based on these studies, the superior border of the pelvis in gynecologic malignancies has traditionally been placed at the level of the L4–L5 or L5–S1 interspace, with upward extension if additional common

E.D. Donnelly (✉) and W. Small, Jr
Department of Radiation Oncology, Feinberg School of Medicine, Robert H. Lurie Comprehensive Cancer Center, Northwestern University, 251 E. Huron St., Galter LC-178, Chicago, IL, 60611 USA
e-mail: eric.d.donnelly@gmail.com; wsmall@nmff.org

T.M. Refaat
Clinical Oncology and Nuclear Medicine Department, University of Alexandria, Alexandria, Egypt

A.N. Viswanathan et al. (eds.), *Gynecologic Radiation Therapy*,
DOI: 978-3-540-68958-4_7, © Springer-Verlag Berlin Heidelberg 2011

iliac or para-aortic nodal coverage is indicated. The lateral borders of the anteroposterior treatment field should extend 1.5–2.0 cm beyond the widest portion of the bony pelvis to include the pelvic lymph nodes. When there is no vaginal extension, the inferior border is placed at the lower edge of the obturator foramen at least 3 cm below the lowest extent of disease. For patients with mid to distal vaginal extension, the entire vagina down to the level of the introitus should be included extend posteriorly the portal field. In addition, coverage of the inguinal nodes should be included in patients with distal vaginal involvement based on the increased incidence of metastatic spread in patients with vaginal involvement. The borders of the lateral fields extend to include the anterior most portion of the pubic symphysis. Posteriorly, the lateral field should extend posteriorly to include the sacral hollow [13].

The utilization of these techniques exposes the majority of the true pelvis to the total prescribed dose, often 45–50 Gy in 25–28 fractions. Frequently a considerable amount of small bowel is located within the treatment volume that can be associated with both short- and long-term morbidities. Reported acute gastrointestinal (GI) symptoms typically involve varying degrees of diarrhea, urgency, and abdominal cramping [14]. In addition to the small bowel, inclusion of the bladder and rectum in the conventional radiation fields tends to increase the incidence of radiation-induced toxicities within these organs [15]. Acute radiation-associated toxicity in the postoperative setting has been reported to occur in 65% of patients [16]. For gynecologic malignancies, late toxicities may arise months to years after radiation therapy, ranging from intermittent diarrhea and malabsorption to more severe toxicities including obstruction and fistulas. Grade 1 and 2 late toxicities have been reported in 18% of patients [14]; severe grade 3 and 4 toxicities in 2–11% of patients have also been reported [15, 16].

7.2 Delineation of Nodal Location and Clinical Volumes

Draining lymph node regions are included in the radiation target volume when tumor characteristics are such that there is significant risk of involvement. Anatomic studies have demonstrated that pelvic lymph nodes are positioned in close proximity to major blood vessels [17]. Conventional portals have not utilized techniques to more precisely delineate clinical nodal volumes based on individual anatomic variances. Thus, traditional fields risk insufficiently treating the pelvis if the entire extent of the clinical nodal volume does not fall within the historically established bony landmark boundaries. Several studies have evaluated the location of pelvic lymph nodes for patients based on radiographic surrogates of lymph node location, (e.g., lymphangiograms, CT, and MRI) [17–20].

A lymphangiogram (LAG) has been shown to be an accurate method for the delineation of lymph nodes within patients [17]. Using LAG studies in patients, Chao et al. [17] evaluated the location of lymph nodes relative to the pelvic vasculature. The average distance from the vessel wall to the LAG-avid lymph nodes was 22.2 ± 12.2 mm within the para-aortic region. Utilizing expansions on the vessels of 15 and 20 mm around the common iliac and external iliac vessels, respectively, yielded 82.3% ± 7.3% coverage of LAG-avid lymph nodes. Nodal volumes that fell outside of the expansion volume included nodes greater than 2 cm, nodes in the lateral external iliac region, and nodes in the obturator area. Because lymph nodes generally follow the path of the major blood vessels, contouring the vessels followed by a radial expansion may be a feasible technique to demarcate the nodal volume [21]. Shih et al. [22] noted that nodal metastases within the pelvis mapped much more tightly relative to the vasculature when examined utilizing LAG. A proposed 2-cm margin around vessels to delineate a nodal target volume was found to encompass 94.5% of the pelvic lymph nodes at risk. Taylor et al. [23] noted the percentage of lymph node contours covered by 7 and 10 mm margins to be 94% and 99%, respectively. These guidelines resulted in smaller volumes than those previously reported, secondary to the fact that LAG can increase the apparent size of the nodes [24]. The recommendations resulted in reducing the volume of bowel, bladder, and rectum by 23%, 24%, and 31%, respectively. Based on the data noting metastatic disease typically is found near the vessels and the decrease in normal tissue treated, the smaller margins are typically utilized for treatment planning.

Inadequate margins around CT-defined gross tumor volume results in decreased local control [25]. Accordingly, it is important to determine the ability of traditional fields to cover radiographically defined nodal volumes. Evaluating the ability of standard pelvic fields, based on bony anatomy within the pelvis, to cover nodal volumes obtained using LAG and CT-simulated nodal delineation show traditional fields do not provide optimal coverage in a significant portion of patients. A study performed at Fox Chase Cancer Center utilizing LAG demonstrated that 45% of patients would have had inadequate nodal irradiation based on standard field borders [26]. Utilizing CT simulation to delineate pelvic vessels and thus nodal volumes yields similar results. Finlay et al. [18] revealed that conventional pelvic fields did not provide adequate coverage in 95.4% of patients, the majority having inadequate margins located superiorly (79.1%). Additionally, within the same study, 55.8% of patients had margins that were deemed too generous, including an excessive volume of normal tissue. These studies demonstrate the clinical target volume can be missed when traditional radiation portals are based on bony anatomy. Based on

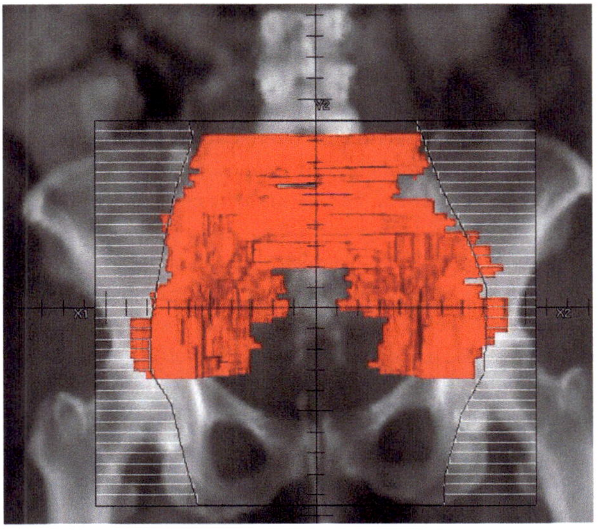

Fig. 7.1 Nodal clinical tumor volume (*red*) falling laterally outside a traditional field

individual anatomy, a significant portion of patients' volumes can fall outside traditional fields, most commonly the external iliac vessels (Fig. 7.1). Compared with conventional four-field techniques, IMRT plans have been shown to result in improved local control with similar late toxicity. In a study by Bouchard et al. [27] comparing IMRT to conventional fields, no relapses were noted in patients treated with IMRT. However, five relapses were noted in the control group at a median follow-up of 30.4 months. In addition to conventional fields missing the target, large areas of normal tissue volume can be located within the treatment design causing certain areas to receive treatment that could have been avoided. Therefore, it is imperative to radiographically assess the anatomy of each individual patient to outline contours of the clinical target volumes for the proper demarcation of unique treatment fields.

7.3 Image-Guided Three-Dimensional (3D) Treatment Planning

Imaging developments have enabled radiation oncologists to avoid the pitfalls associated with traditional 2D planning and to develop plans based on the unique anatomy inherent to each patient. CT simulators have revolutionized treatment planning for radiation oncology, allowing 3D visualization of the clinical target volume and organs at risk. The first and perhaps most important step in the planning process for image-guided planning involves patient positioning and immobilization. The goal is to place the position in a reproducible, yet comfortable, position in which the patient will be treated on a daily basis. Immobilization for gynecologic malignancies is typically accomplished with the use of devices that secure the part of the body that is being treated, including the mobile joints associated, in the case of gynecologic malignancies, the pelvis, and femur. The most common systems used to accomplish this goal are the Alpha Cradle (Smithers Medical Products, Akron, OH) and Vac-Lok (Med-Tec, Orange City, IA) systems [28]. Both systems form rigid geometric representations of the patients in the treatment position to aid in daily positioning and decrease intrafraction movement. It can be advantageous to place patients in the prone position, especially obese patients and patients with significant amounts of small bowel located low in the pelvis in an attempt to displace tissue folds and small bowel out of the pelvis [29].

Prior to the acquisition of images, patients should have a radiopaque marker placed spanning the extent of the vagina to the cervix/vaginal cuff to allow accurate visualization. Care must be taken to ensure the marker does not displace the anatomy; large obturators should not be utilized. Contrast material should be infused intravenously to delineate the vasculature anatomy and orally to delineate the small bowel. A rectal tube can also be inserted into the rectum and infused with contrast to help visualize the rectum. Radiopaque markers can be placed at the introitus as well as the anal verge. Patients should be instructed to maintain full bladders during simulation and later during treatment to help keep the small bowel away from the treatment volumes.

After proper patient positioning, immobilization, and placement of simulation markers, the acquirement of images is undertaken in preparation for volumetric definition. With the advent of image-guided treatment planning, comes the difficult task of delineating the targets and areas that need to be irradiated. Small et al. [10] developed an atlas of the clinical

Table 7.1 Consensus clinical target volume for adjuvant (postoperative) radiotherapy for cervical and endometrial cancer

Target site	Definition
Common iliac lymph nodes	From 7 mm below L4–L5 interspace to level of bifurcation of common iliac arteries into external and internal iliac arteries
External iliac lymph nodes	From level of bifurcation of common iliac artery into external artery to level of superior aspect of femoral head where it becomes femoral artery
Internal iliac lymph nodes	From level of bifurcation of common iliac artery into internal artery, along its branches (obturator, hypogastric) terminating in paravaginal tissues at level of vaginal cuff
Upper vagina	Vaginal cuff and 3 cm of vagina inferior to cuff
Parametrial/paravaginal tissue	From vaginal cuff to medial edge of internal obturator muscle/ischial ramus on each side
Presacral lymph nodes[a]	Lymph node region anterior to S1and S2 region

[a]If patient has cervical cancer or endometrial cancer with cervical stromal invasion
Adapted from Small et al. [10].

target volume definitions for postoperative radiotherapy of both endometrial and cervical cancer to be used for planning pelvic radiotherapy (Table 7.1). The researchers noted that the clinical target volume should include the common, external, and internal iliac lymph node regions, as well as the upper 3.0 cm of the vagina and paravaginal soft tissue lateral to the vagina. For patients with cervical cancer or those with endometrial cancer with cervical stromal invasion, the presacral lymph node region should be included. The clinical target volume was defined by adding a 7-mm margin around the vasculature, based on research by Taylor et al. [23] and extending it to include any adjacent visible or suspicious lymph nodes, lymphoceles, or surgical clips. The clinical target volume was modified to exclude vertebral bodies and muscle and to limit the dose to the bowel. In patients requiring presacral treatment, the coverage was discontinued when the piriformis muscle was clearly visualized. Generally, within the inferior portion of the clinical tumor volume, the vagina and adjacent lymph nodes were conjoined and the rectum, bladder, bone, and muscle were avoided (Fig. 7.2). The volume guidelines serve as a useful tool to both delineate volumes that need to be included and to produce a means of contouring similar volumes to enable future comparisons and evaluations across treatment centers.

7.4 Image Guidance–Based Intensity-Modulated Radiation Therapy in Gynecologic Cancer

Image-guided radiation therapy allows the at-risk pelvic nodal regions to be assessed based on vasculature anatomy during CT simulation to demarcate nodal regions for patients on an individualized basis. Utilization of contouring guidelines to delineate the clinical target

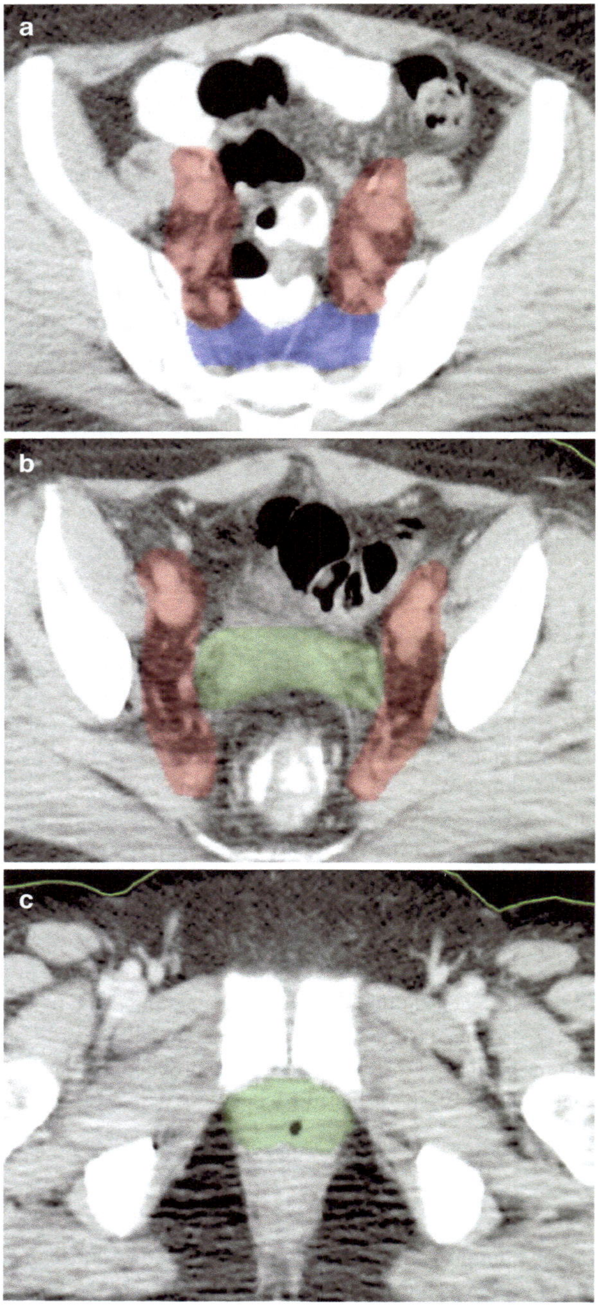

Fig. 7.2 (**a**) Superior clinical target volume – upper external and internal iliac (*red*) and presacral (*blue*). (**b**) Middle clinical target volume – external and internal iliac (*red*) and parametrial/vaginal (*green*). (**c**) Inferior clinical target volume – parametrial and vaginal

volumes assures the areas at risk for recurrence are included within the treatment field. Intensity-modulated radiotherapy has evolved as a technique that enables the treatment of tumors and areas at risk of recurrence while sparing adjacent normal tissues from high-dose irradiation [30]. IMRT is an advanced form of 3D-conforming radiotherapy that produces a high-dose optimized, nonuniform beam allowing the use of irregular shapes to conform to the clinical target volume. IMRT has the ability to utilize the information obtained using image guidance to treat complex shapes and/or concave regions. By conforming more closely to the target volume based on the individual's anatomy, image guidance treatment planning can help normal pelvic tissues to be relatively spared. IMRT is currently being used in the treatment of the head and neck, prostate, and other body sites to achieve more conformal treatment of irregular treatment volumes and to spare normal tissue. The use of image guidance, in particular IMRT, enables significantly better target coverage when compared to conventional field techniques. Bouchard et al. noted that IMRT allowed 93% of the primary tumor volume to be covered by the 45-Gy isodose curve versus only 76% coverage found with conventional four-field technique [27].

The major potential advantage of image-guided radiation therapy and IMRT in the treatment of postoperative gynecological carcinomas is not only the ability to more adequately cover the target volume but also the capability to shape a dose distribution that delivers a lower dose to intraperitoneal pelvic contents (i.e., small and large bowel) than to the surrounding pelvic lymph nodes and other areas at risk [30, 31]. IMRT has been shown to reduce normal tissue dose and is associated with decreased acute and chronic toxicity compared with conventional treatment [32, 33]. Studies have shown that IMRT reduces the volume of small bowel receiving radiation of 45 Gy or greater during whole pelvic radiation therapy (WPRT) for both cervical and uterine cancer. Portelance et al. [34] compared four-, seven,- and nine-field plans delivered by dynamic multileaf collimation (DMLC) with four-field box technique and showed a 58–67% reduction in the volume of small bowel irradiated to more than 45 Gy with IMRT. Roeske et al. [35] reported similar results in their study using radiation doses up to 45 Gy in 25 fractions to treat the proximal vagina, parametrial tissues, uterus, and pelvic nodes of ten patients with cervical or uterine carcinoma. The study noted a 50% reduction in the volume of small bowel receiving more than 45 Gy with a nine-field Corvus (Nomos Corporation, Cranberry Township, PA) plan when compared with four-field 3D conformal plan.

In 2002 and 2003, Mundt et al. published reports studying acute and chronic GI toxicity as well as hematologic toxicity in patients with cervical and endometrial carcinoma treated with IMRT compared with those treated with conventional WPRT [29, 33]. The researchers found that patients treated with IMRT had a lower rate of acute grade 2 GI toxicity than the WPRT-treated patients (60% vs. 91%; $P = 0.002$) [29]. The percentage of patients requiring no or only infrequent antidiarrheal medications was 75% in patients treated with IMRT compared to 34% in patients treated with conventional WPRT. In this same group, patients treated with IMRT had a lower rate of chronic GI toxicity compared to patients treated with conventional WPRT (11.1% vs. 54%, respectively; $P = 0.02$) [34]. A reduction in hematological toxicity (grade 2 or greater white blood cell toxicity) was also observed in patients treated with a combination of chemotherapy and IMRT when compared with standard WPRT (31% vs. 60%) [32]. This observation was attributed to a significant reduction in irradiated bone marrow, particularly within the iliac crests. While the results from Mundt and colleagues are very promising, the use of IMRT for gynecological malignancies still needs to be tested in a multi-institutional setting.

7.5 Challenges Associated with Image-Guided Planning and Treatment

Although image-guided results may seem promising, there are several issues of concern and caution. In a study by Ahamad et al. [36] a variety of clinical tumor volume parameters were used to generate IMRT plans. The investigators found that the volume of the normal tissue spared by IMRT relative to conventional techniques was very sensitive to small increases of the margin size used to generate the planning target volume. For example, with a 5 mm increase in margin size around the clinical tumor volume, the volume of small bowel spared 30 Gy or more was reduced by as much as 40%. The researchers also noted the effects of internal organ motion on IMRT. The vaginal vault and central pelvic tissues can move during treatment either due to random internal organ motion, or due to changes in filling of the rectum and bladder. Simulating patients with a full and empty bladder and fusing the images to obtain an internal target volume should be routinely accomplished as well as strong consideration for accommodating changes in rectal volume When compared to standard techniques, the very tight and conformal isodose curves around the outlined target volumes in IMRT increase the risk of missing areas containing subclinical disease when the volumes are not accurately drawn. As a result, there is an increased risk of marginal or out-of-field recurrence.

The margins utilized for delineation of target volumes for intensity-modulated pelvic radiotherapy in postoperative gynecologic malignancies have been an area of debate. As noted, Taylor et al. noted a 7 mm margin around the vessels encompassed >95% of the common iliac, internal iliac, medial and anterior external iliac, and obturator lymph node contours [24]. However, Chao and Lin, recommend larger margins of 15–20 mm based on data obtained with lymphangiograms [17]. The consensus guidelines by Small et al. developed an atlas of the clinical target volumes for postoperative radiotherapy of endometrial and cervical patients recommending a 7-mm margin around vessels, because lymphangiography might overestimate lymph node size [10]. This continues to be a controversial subject and an area where active research into patterns of recurrence is needed.

7.6 Conclusion

The use of radiotherapy after surgery for cervical and endometrial cancer reduces the risk of recurrence. Traditional radiotherapy based on bony landmarks is inadequate in terms of target volume coverage. All patients treated with radiotherapy should have image guidance utilized to help determine proper radiotherapy fields. Image guidance also makes the use of IMRT possible, although challenges remain and continued research is needed to confirm target volumes, organ motions, and techniques.

References

1. Keys HM, Roberts JA, Brunetto VL, et al. A phase III trial of surgery with or without adjunctive external pelvic radiation therapy in intermediate risk endometrial adenocarcinoma: a Gynecologic Oncology Group study. Gynecol Oncol. 2004;92:744–51.
2. Barillot I, Horiot JC, Pigneux J, et al. Carcinoma of the intact uterine cervix treated with radiotherapy alone: a French Cooperative Study: update and multivariate analysis of prognostic factors. Int J Radiat Oncol Biol Phys. 1997;38:969–78.
3. Keys HM, Bundy BN, Stehman FB, et al. Radiation therapy with and without extrafascial hysterectomy for bulky stage IB cervical carcinoma: a randomized trial of the Gynecologic Oncology Group. Gynecol Oncol. 2003;89:343–53.
4. Sedlis A, Bundy BN, Rotman MZ, et al. A randomized trial of pelvic radiation therapy versus no further therapy in selected patients with stage IB carcinoma of the cervix after radical hysterectomy and pelvic lymphadenectomy: a Gynecologic Oncology Group study. Gynecol Oncol. 1999;73:177–83.
5. Creutzberg CL, Van Putten WL, Koper PC, et al. Surgery and postoperative radiotherapy versus surgery alone for patients with stage 1 endometrial carcinoma: multicenter randomized trial. PORTEC Study Group. Lancet. 2000;355:1404–11.
6. ASTEC/EN.5 writing committee on behalf of the ASTEC/EN.5 Study Group. Adjuvant external beam radiotherapy in the treatment of endometrial cancer: Pooled trial results, systemic review and meta-analysis. Lancet. 2009;373:137–46.
7. Rose PG, Bundy BN, Watkins EB, et al. Concurrent cisplatin-radiotherapy and chemotherapy for locally advanced cervical cancer. N Engl J Med. 1999;340:1144–53.
8. Greven K, Winter K, Underhill K, et al. Preliminary analysis of RTOG 9708: adjuvant postoperative radiotherapy combined with cisplatin/paclitaxel chemotherapy after surgery for patients with high-risk endometrial cancer. Int J Radiat Oncol Biol Phys. 2004; 59:168–73.
9. Mell LK, Mundt AJ. Intensity-modulated radiation therapy in gynecologic cancers: growing support, growing acceptance. Cancer. 2008;14:198–9.
10. Small Jr W, Mell LK, Anderson P, et al. Consensus guidelines for delineation of clinical target volume for intensity-modulated pelvic radiotherapy in postoperative treatment of endometrial and cervical cancer. Int J Radiat Oncol Biol Phys. 2008;71:428–34.
11. Taylor A, Powell ME. An assessment of interfractional uterine and cervical motion: Implications for radiotherapy target volume definition in gynaecological cancer. Radiother Oncol. 2008;88:250–7.
12. Greer BE, Koh W-J, Figge DC, et al. Gynecologic radiotherapy fields defined by intraoperative measurements. Gynecol Oncol. 1990;38:421–4.
13. Perez CA. Uterine Cervix. In: Perez CA, Brady LW, editors. Principles and practice of radiation oncology. 3rd ed. Philadelphia: Lippincott-Raven; 1997. p. 1733–834.
14. Letschert JG, Lebesque JV, Aleman BM, et al. The volume effect in radiation-related late small bowel complications: results of a clinical study of the EORTC Radiotherapy Cooperative Group in patients treated for rectal carcinoma. Radiother Oncol. 1994;32: 116–23.
15. Jereczek-Fossa B, Jassem J, Nowak R, Badzio A. Late complications after postoperative radiotherapy in endometrial cancer: analysis of 317 consecutive cases with application of linear-quadratic model. Int J Radiat Oncol Biol Phys. 1998;41:329–38.

16. Weiss E, Hirnle P, Arnold-Bofinger H, et al. Therapeutic outcome and relation of acute and late side effects in the adjuvant radiotherapy of endometrial carcinoma stage I and II. Radiother Oncol. 1999;53:37–44.
17. Chao KS, Lin M. Lymphangiogram-assisted lymph node target delineation for patients with gynecologic malignancies. Int J Radiat Oncol Biol Phys. 2002;54:1147–52.
18. Finlay MH, Ackerman I, Tirona RG, et al. Use of CT simulation for treatment of cervical cancer to assess the adequacy of lymph node coverage of conventional pelvic fields based on bony landmarks. Int J Radiat Oncol Biol Phys. 2006;64:205–9.
19. Vilarino-Varela MJ, Taylor A, Rockall AG, et al. A verification study of proposed pelvic lymph node localisation guidelines using nanoparticle-enhanced magnetic resonance imaging. Radiother Oncol. 2008;89:192–6.
20. Dinniwell R, Chan P, Czarnota G, et al. Pelvic lymph node topography for Radiotherapy Treatment Planning From Ferumoxtran-10 Contrast-Enhanced Magnetic Resonance Imaging. Int J Radiat Oncol Biol Phys, 2009;74(3):844-51.
21. Heller PB, Malfetano JH, Bundy BN, et al. Clinical-pathologic study of stage IIB, III and IVA carcinoma of the cervix: Extended diagnostic evaluation for paraaortic node metastasis – A Gynecology Oncology Group study. Gynecol Oncol. 1990;38:425–30.
22. Shih HA, Harisinghani M, Zietman AL, et al. Mapping of nodal disease in locally advance prostate cancer: rethinking the clinical target volume for pelvic nodal irradiation based on vascular rather than bony anatomy. Int J Radiat Oncol Biol Phys. 2005;63:1262–9.
23. Taylor A, Rockall AG, Reznek RH, et al. Mapping pelvic lymph nodes: guidelines for delineation in intensity-modulated radiotherapy. Int J Radiat Oncol Biol Phys. 2005;63:1604–12.
24. McIvor J. Changes in lymph node size induced by lymphography. Clin Radiol. 1980;31:541–4.
25. Kim RY, McGinnis S, Spencer SA, et al. Conventional four-field pelvic radiotherapy technique without computer tomography-treatment planning in cancer of the cervix: Potential geographic miss and its impact on pelvic control. Int J Radiat Oncol Biol Phys. 1995;31:109–12.
26. Bonin SR, Lanciano RM, Corn BW, et al. Bony landmarks are not an adequate substitute for lymphangiography in defining pelvic lymph node location for the treatment of cervical cancer with radiotherapy. Int J Radiat Oncol Biol Phys. 1996;34:167–72.
27. Bouchard M, Nadeau S, Gingras L, et al. Clinical outcome of adjuvant treatment of endometrial cancer using aperture-based intensity-modulated radiotherapy. Int J Radiat Oncol Biol Phys. 2008;71:1343–50.
28. Bentel GC. Treatment Planning Pelvis. In: Radiation Therapy Planning. 2nd ed. New York: McGraw-Hill; 1992. p. 439–89.
29. Gallagher MJ, Brereton HD, Rostock RA, et al. A prospective study of treatment techniques to minimize the volume of pelvic small bowel with reduction of acute and late effects associated with pelvic irradiation. Int J Radiat Oncol Biol Phys. 1986;12:1565.
30. Mundt AJ, Lujan AE, Rotmensch J, et al. Intensity-modulated whole pelvic radiotherapy in women with gynecologic malignancies. Int J Radiat Oncol Biol Phys. 2002;52:1330–7.
31. Georg P, Georg D, Hillbrand M, et al. Factors influencing bowel sparing in intensity modulated whole pelvic radiotherapy for gynaecologic malignancies. Radiother Oncol. 2006;80:19–26.
32. Brixey CJ, Roeske JC, Lujan AE, et al. Impact of intensity-modulated radiotherapy on acute hematologic toxicity in women with gynecologic malignancies. Int J Radiat Oncol Biol Phys. 2002;54:1388–96.
33. Mundt AJ, Mell LK, Roeske JC. Preliminary analysis of chronic gastrointestinal toxicity in gynaecologic patients treated with intensity-modulated whole pelvic radiation therapy. Int J Radiat Oncol Biol Phys. 2003;56:1354–60.
34. Portelance L, Chao KS, Grigsby PW, et al. Intensity-modulated radiation therapy (IMRT) reduces small bowel, rectum, and bladder doses in patients with cervical cancer receiving pelvic and para-aortic irradiation. Int J Radiat Oncol Biol Phys. 2001;51:261–6.

35. Roeske JC, Lujan A, Rotmensch J, et al. Intensity-modulated whole pelvic radiation therapy in patients with gynecologic malignancies. Int J Radiat Oncol Biol Phys. 2000;48:1613–21.
36. Ahamad A, D'Souza W, Salehpour M, et al. Intensity-modulated radiation therapy after hysterectomy: comparison with conventional treatment and sensitivity of the normal-tissue-sparing effect to margin size. Int J Radiat Oncol Biol Phys. 2005;62:1117–24.

The Integration of 3D Imaging with Conformal Radiotherapy for Vulvar and Vaginal Cancer

8

Simul Parikh and Sushil Beriwal

8.1 Introduction

Vulva and vaginal cancers are ideal anatomic sites to exploit the advantages of conformal radiation therapy because of the proximity of the tumor volumes to critical structures. In addition to permitting dose escalation, these techniques can decrease the dose to normal structures such as the small bowel, rectum, bladder, and femoral heads [1, 2]. Despite the advantages of these techniques, there are pitfalls to be considered. There is an increase in integral dose and a decrease in dose homogeneity because of the usage of multiple fields. There is also risk of geographic miss because of target motion, difficulty with daily reproducibility, and anatomic changes due to tumor regression.

To utilize three-dimensional conformal radiotherapy (3D-CRT) or intensity-modulated radiation therapy (IMRT) effectively requires accurate staging, precise localization of gross tumor and critical structures, and precise information about intra-abdominal and intrapelvic motion. This chapter will discuss 3D imaging modalities and their use in staging, treatment planning, and the utility of imaging during and after therapy.

8.2 The Role of 3D Imaging in Staging Vulvar and Vaginal Cancer

8.2.1 Vulvar Cancer

Staging of the primary tumor in vulvar cancer is typically performed clinically utilizing physical exam findings; however there may be a role for imaging techniques. In a study by Sohaib et al. [3], the utility of preoperative magnetic resonance (MR) was utilized in

S. Parikh and S. Beriwal (✉)
Department of Radiation Oncology, Magee-Womens Hospital of UPMC,
300 Halket Street, 0725, Pittsburgh, PA15213, USA
e-mail: parikhs@upmc.edu; beriwals@upmc.edu

A.N. Viswanathan et al. (eds.), *Gynecologic Radiation Therapy*,
DOI: 10.1007/978-3-540-68958-4_8, © Springer-Verlag Berlin Heidelberg 2011

22 patients with vulvar cancer who were then surgically managed. MR was found to have an accuracy of 70%, with only moderate correlation with clinicopathologic findings. The authors conclude that magnetic resonance imaging (MRI) would be of limited value in patients with small lesions, but MRI may play a role in detecting extension into adjacent structures in patients with advanced disease. There is scanty data on computed tomography (CT) and positron emission tomography-computed tomography (PET-CT) imaging of vulvar carcinoma primary lesions.

The single most important prognostic factor in patients with vulvar cancer is the presence of lymph node metastases [4]. Physical examination is neither sensitive nor specific since 25% of patients with enlarged nodes are found to have no evidence of disease, while nearly 25% of patients with a normal exam are found to have occult metastatic disease [4]. Radiation has been found to be a viable technique to locally control the inguinal node region, comparable to lymphadenectomy; however, if conventional two-dimensional (2D) treatment planning is used there is a significant risk of underdosing the area at risk [2, 5]. Because of this risk, 3D imaging has been explored to improve the staging of vulvar cancer.

CT scanning of the pelvis and US with fine needle aspiration (FNA) of suspicious appearing nodes were assessed in a retrospective study of 44 patients who underwent imaging prior to unilateral or bilateral lymph node dissection [6]. The results indicated that CT had calculated sensitivity, specificity, negative predictive value (NPV), and positive predictive value (PPV) of 58%, 75%, 75%, and 58%, respectively. The ultrasound scanning with FNA cytology had calculated sensitivity, specificity, NPV, and PPV of 80%, 100%, 93%, and 100%. The authors concluded that because of low sensitivity and specificity, CT did not affect surgical management. However, in patients with clinically diseased groin nodes, CT is useful to assess the pelvic lymph nodes as well as the proximity of the groin nodes to the femoral vessels, specifically if patients would be treated with radiation therapy.

There have been multiple studies assessing the role of pelvic MRI in staging the groin in patients with vulvar carcinoma. In the largest study, 60 patients with vulvar carcinoma underwent preoperative MRI for staging [7]. Using size, presence or absence of fatty center, margin, and shape of the lymph node, each groin was classified as malignant or benign by two radiologists. The sensitivity, specificity, PPV, and NPV were 52%, 85–89%, 46–52%, and 87–89%, respectively, and these authors concluded that MRI had no role in evaluating lymph node involvement. In a second study, 59 women who underwent preoperative MRI were assessed [8]. Size, shape, and STIR (short tau inversion recovery)/T2 signal abnormality were used to determine whether a lymph node appeared to be pathologic on MRI. The sensitivity, specificity, PPV, and NPV were 85.7%, 82.1%, 64.3%, and 93.9%. The authors concluded that MRI was useful in determining which patients could be spared inguinofemoral lymphadenectomy, and this could lead to a reduction in surgical-related patient morbidity.

The role of PET and PET/CT remain undefined for vulvar cancer; however, there is one prospective assessment of PET for evaluation of groin metastases [9]. Fifteen patients with a total of 29 groins were assessed by PET prior to dissection. The sensitivity, specificity, PPV, and NPV were 67%, 95%, 86%, and 86%. The authors concluded that although PET was relatively insensitive and also not reliable as a surrogate for a pathologically negative groin, the high specificity makes it useful for radiation therapy planning (Fig. 8.1). All of

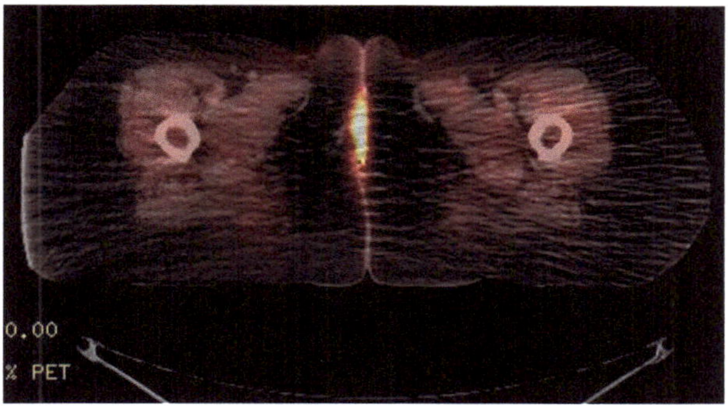

Fig. 8.1 Fluorodeoxyglucose positron emission tomography-computed tomography (FDG PET-CT) diagnostic and simulation scan of pelvis. This is an axial view showing an FDG avid area of uptake seen in the vulva, with no uptake seen in the inguinal nodes. Note the anterior and posterior markers delineating tumoral extent

these imaging modalities have high specificity but low sensitivity and thus cannot replace surgery in detecting microscopic disease. The high specificity may aid in deciding whether to dose escalate non-surgically managed involved nodes.

8.2.2 Vaginal Cancer

In a report on 25 patients with primary vaginal cancer, a study was undertaken to determine the imaging and staging features of this disease using MRI, as well as to suggest a role for MRI in the management of the disease [10]. The results indicate that MRI can be used to determine tumor dimensions, volume, and local extent (Fig. 8.3). The authors concluded that the use of MRI allows oncologists to assist in determining whether the patient can afford a more limited surgery, needs an exenterative surgery, or is a candidate for definitive radiation.

A prospective study of 23 patients compares the results of CT with PET in detecting the primary tumor and lymph node metastases in carcinoma of the vagina [11]. The PET scan identified abnormal uptake in all 21 patients with intact tumors, while the CT scan visualized it in 9/21 (43%). PET identified abnormal uptake in the groin and pelvis in 8/23 patients, while CT identified abnormalities in the groin and pelvis in 4/23 patients. The PET findings led to a modification of treatment planning in 14% of patients. Because all patients were treated with combined external beam radiation therapy and brachytherapy, there was no surgical "gold standard," and the sensitivity and specificity of either study could not be determined. The authors concluded that PET detected the primary tumor and abnormal lymph nodes more often than CT, that CT gleaned no further information than could be detected from exam alone and that PET/CT should be the standard for initial assessment and treatment planning for radiation therapy (Fig. 8.2).

The rationale for the use of CT, MRI, and PET for these diseases is based on the few studies described above and extrapolation from other gynecological malignancies. Therefore, clinical judgment is important in interpreting imaging results based on limited data and the low sensitivity of these tests.

8.3 Simulation for Image-Guided External Beam Radiation Therapy for Vulvar and Vaginal Cancer

Conventional radiation therapy treatment planning fields rely on bony anatomy and use wide margins to target tumor and nodal basins to specific doses with reasonable certainty. These large treatment fields lead to increased dose to critical tissues and can cause increased toxicities. Patient anatomy may vary and there may be a risk of geographical misses of the pelvic lymph nodes. For example, prescribing to a 3-cm depth may lead to significant under dosing of inguinal lymph nodes and using vertebral bodies as vascular landmarks a geographic miss [12]. The introduction of CT-based planning has allowed greater flexibility in designing treatment fields that are tailored to a patient's specific anatomy.

For both vaginal carcinoma and vulvar carcinoma, the patient should undergo CT or PET-CT simulation while positioned supine. Immobilization should include a knee sponge or other device to immobilize the lower extremities. For vulvar cancer, the maximal possible abduction that allows the patient to go through the scanner should be done to expose the groin folds. The distal extent of vaginal tumors may be demarcated by the placement of a radiopaque seed at the initial consultation. Vulvar tumoral extent can be delineated radiographically with radiopaque wiring, placed immediately before the simulation scan (Fig. 8.1). Unless contraindicated, simulation should include both oral and intravenous (IV) contrast. This will allow the rectum, bladder, and small bowel to be easily contoured, while also delineating the vascular structures that are surrogates for the lymph nodes. If possible, the diagnostic pelvic MRI can be fused to the CT/PET-CT scans or a workstation displaying the MRI should be available nearby (Figs. 8.2, 8.3 and 8.4). If the vulvar cancer is to be treated definitively or the tumor bed is to receive a boost postoperatively, the boost phase of the treatment may need to be re-simulated in "frog-leg" position so the patient can be treated with a direct electron boost.

8.4 Image-Guided Treatment Planning for Vulvar Cancer

Contouring may take place on the CT or PET-CT images obtained during simulation. For vulvar cancer, gross tumor volume (GTV) is defined as the extent of gross primary disease found on examination, palpable lymph nodes, lymph nodes >1.5 cm seen on CT, and FDG (fluorodeoxyglucose)-positive areas seen on the PET-CT. The clinical target volume (CTV) includes the GTV with a 1–2-cm expansion, the entire vulva or tumor bed if treating postoperatively, bilateral inguinal lymph nodes, and bilateral pelvic lymph nodes (including the external iliac, internal iliac, obturator, presacral lymph node regions and lower common iliac nodes). Care must be taken to contour the vulva generously since it is not well defined on CT, and bolus may be necessary to obtain the goal dose to the vulvar surface (Figs. 8.5 and 8.6). The bolus is integrated in the IMRT plan.

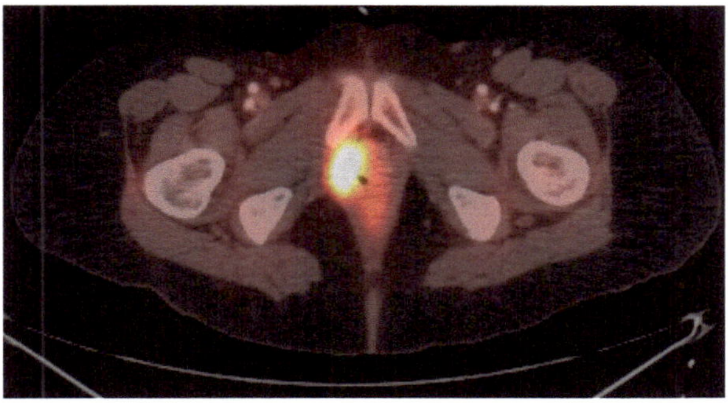

Fig. 8.2 FDG PET-CT diagnostic scan of pelvis. This is an axial view corresponding to the magnetic resonance imaging (MRI) described in Fig. 8.1. There is a heterogenous, irregular, FDG avid mass seen predominantly on the right side of the vagina, extending to the right pelvic sidewall and pelvic sling

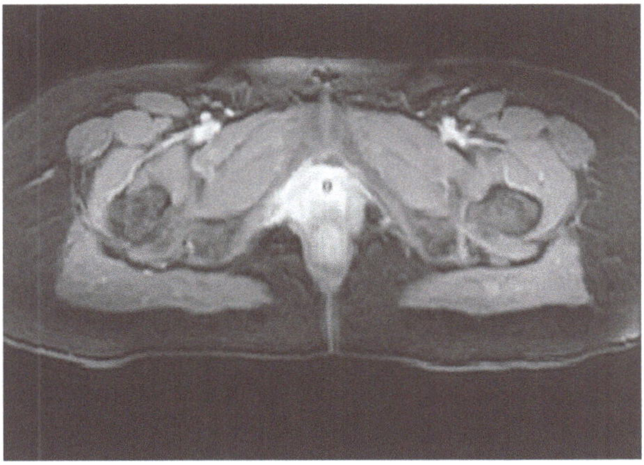

Fig. 8.3 MRI diagnostic scan of pelvis, T1 series with contrast. This is an axial view revealing an enhancing mass extending from the lower vagina measuring 4.2 × 3.4 × 3.8 cm representing a vaginal cancer. It extends laterally to right pelvic sidewall and anteriorly completely encases the urethra

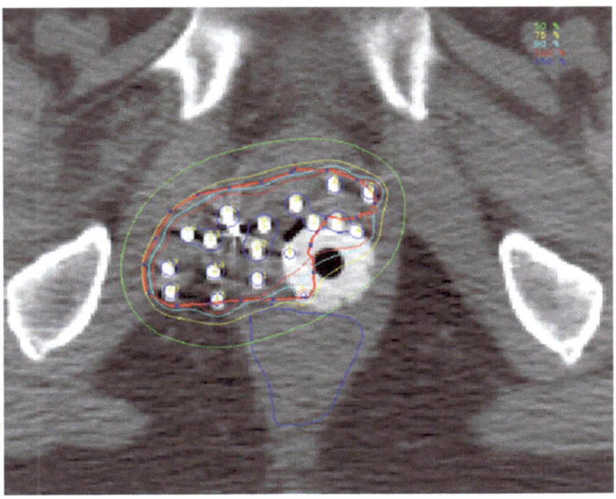

Fig. 8.4 Brachytherapy treatment planning non-contrast CT of pelvis showing interstitial needles covering the target volume in vagina and paravaginal area as seen in Figs. 8.2 and 8.3 while avoiding the rectum and bladder

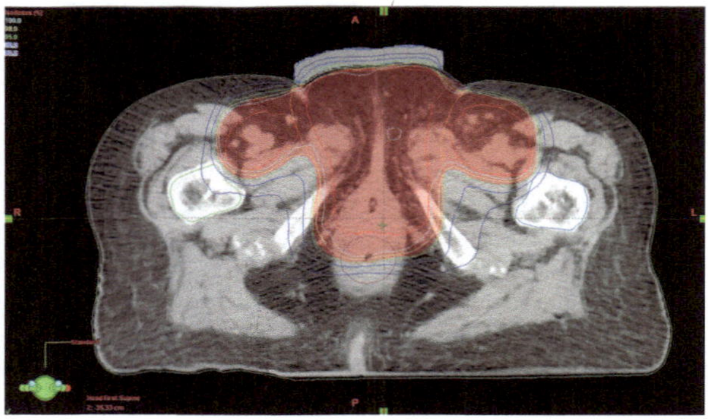

Fig. 8.5 External beam treatment planning CT scan of pelvis showing vulva and inguinal nodal region planning target volume (PTV) (*red*) covered by prescription 95% isodose line (*green*). Note the bolus that has been placed on the skin of the vulva and may be used as needed based on the three-dimensional (3D) plan

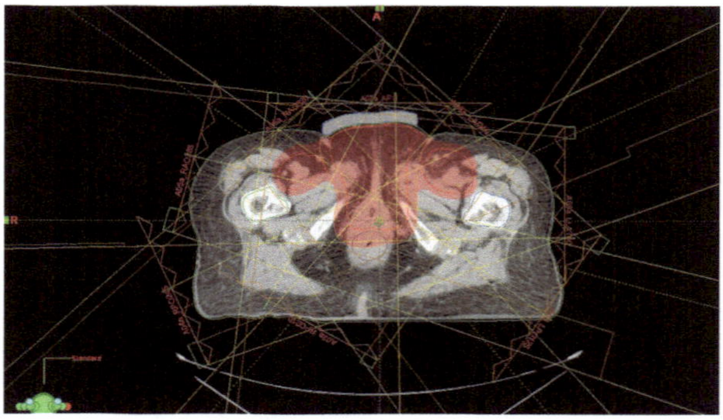

Fig. 8.6 External beam treatment planning CT scan of pelvis showing intensity-modulated radiation therapy (IMRT) beam arrangements covering PTV (*red*)

To define the pelvic nodal CTV, a 1-cm margin around the blood vessels edited for muscles and bones is used, while 2 cm with editing is used for inguinofemoral nodes. The inguinofemoral nodes are contoured inferiorly to the lowest aspect of the ischial tuberosity or to the lesser trochanter (Fig. 8.5). The planning target volume (PTV) includes the CTV with a 1-cm expansion, accounting for setup error and motion.

With 2D treatment planning, in order to treat the groin nodes, high-energy electrons are often used and this can result in severe skin reactions. With IMRT, 6 MV photons are used, which will significantly reduce the dose to the skin, potentially decreasing the need for a treatment break, and surgical complications in the preoperative setting. It is valuable to keep in mind during CT-based treatment planning, the patient's legs are not fully abducted, and a portion of the medial thigh may receive an increased dose.

At the University of Pittsburgh, the normal structures contoured are the small bowel, bladder, and rectum. Typical input parameters for IMRT planning of the PTV are as follows: ≤35% of small bowel to receive ≤35 Gy, with a dose maximum of 50 Gy; ≤40% of bladder to receive ≤40 Gy, with a dose maximum of 50 Gy; and ≤40% of the rectum to receive ≤40 Gy, with a dose maximum of 50 Gy. Quantec restrictions may be followed.

Table 8.1 Vulvar carcinoma radiation doses

	Volume	Dose (Gy)
Pre-operative	Primary tumor and lymph nodes	45–50.4
Definitive	No gross disease primary and regional lymph nodes	45–50.4
	Gross disease including primary and/or nodes	65–70[a]
Post-operative	Tumor bed and lymph nodes	45–50.4
	High-risk areas (ECE, positive margin)	60–65
	Undissected inguinal nodal region treated prophylactically	45–50.4

[a]May consider interstitial boost for significant vaginal or periurethral extension

Although the PTV overlaps the small bowel, daily variation of its position ensures that it does not receive full dose. These parameters were developed independently at our institution by comparing various 3D and IMRT plans with the desired goal of reducing dose to critical organs without compromising coverage of the PTV. The thought was that this reduction in dose to critical organs would lead to decreased toxicities. The IMRT plans are optimized to minimize the volume of PTV that receives less than 95% of the prescribed dose and the volume that receives more than 110% of the prescribed dose. TLDs (theromoluminescent dosimeters) are recommended for verification of dose to the primary vulvar site.

The dose for preoperative chemoradiation treatment for vulvar cancer is usually 45–50.4 Gy (Table 8.1) in either conventional fractionation or hybrid hyperfractionation [13, 14]. The patient may get an additional boost from 55 to 65 Gy to the site of involvement, if the plan is to treat definitively. In patients with significant extension of disease to the vagina or periurethral area, where surgery would confer significant morbidity, interstitial brachytherapy can be used to deliver higher doses to sites of gross disease, and this is further described in Chap. 24. In the postoperative setting, the dose is usually around 45–50.4 Gy with an additional boost to areas of positive margin or extracapsular extension to 55–60 Gy.

One series reports the experience of a single institution use treating locally advanced vulvar carcinoma with IMRT [13]. Eighteen patients were treated with chemoradiation therapy using a hybrid fractionation scheme delivering a dose of 46.4 Gy concurrent with cisplatin and 5 fluorouracil (5FU). A complete clinical response was seen in 72% of the patients and 14 of 18 underwent surgery (local excision +/− groin dissection). Nine of 14 patients had a pathological complete response while 5 of 14 had residual disease in the specimen. The 2-year disease specific and overall survival was 75% and 70% respectively. The patients tolerated the treatment well and none had confluent moist desquamation of the groin.

Prior to their outcome data, the same group reported dosimetric advantages as compared to 3D-CRT by reducing dose to bladder, rectum, and small bowel by 26%, 41%, and 27%, respectively [15]. They also noted that the conventional electron energies needed to treat the inguinal nodes could result in severe skin reactions. With 6 MV photon IMRT, the skin dose can be greatly reduced. The results of the treatment appear to confirm the theoretical dosimetric advantages.

Another group of investigators presented their experience with IMRT planning in patients with vulvar cancer undergoing pelvic inguinal radiotherapy [16]. They were able to reduce the dose to the small bowel, bladder, and rectum by 47%, 78%, and 35%, respectively, compared to conventional treatment planning. They also were able to spare the femoral heads, confirming the dosimetric advantages of IMRT.

8.5 Image-Guided Treatment Planning for Vaginal Cancer

8.5.1 Treatment Planning

For vaginal cancer, we define the GTV as the extent of gross disease found on examination, palpable lymph nodes, enlarged lymph nodes seen on CT, areas of abnormality seen on the MRI, and FDG-positive areas seen on the PET-CT. The CTV includes the GTV with a 1–2-cm expansion, the entire vagina, paravaginal area up to the sidewall, and bilateral pelvic lymph nodes (including the common iliac, external iliac, internal iliac, obturator, perirectal and presacral lymph node regions) (Fig. 8.7). If the distal vagina is involved, the inguinal lymph nodes should be included. The nodal CTV, PTV, and IMRT parameters are as defined above for vulvar cancer. For vaginal cancer, the dose prescription is to treat the initial PTV to 45–50.4 Gy with or without chemotherapy. The enlarged/involved nodes can be given an additional boost with either a sequential or concomitant technique to 55–65 Gy [17, 18].

After external beam radiation therapy, clinical examination should be obtained to determine whether the patient will be suited for treatment with intracavitary or interstitial brachytherapy, as it is an integral part of treatment in many cases of vaginal and vulvar cancer [19]. The superficial residual disease ≤5 mm in thickness can be treated with intracavitary brachytherapy, while thicker lesions are usually treated with interstitial brachytherapy. For apical lesions, real-time imaging or laparoscopic guidance is recommended for interstitial brachytherapy in order to ensure that bowel penetration of interstitial catheters is minimized. The total dose to the primary disease is usually around 75–85 Gy. A 2D point-based system has been the standard method of prescribing the dose [20]; however, there is evidence that this may lead to overestimation of dose to the tumor and underestimation of dose to the normal tissues [21, 22]. Because of this inference, image-guided techniques may be used for brachytherapy [23, 24].

If patients are unable to be treated with brachytherapy, they will need to complete treatment with an external beam boost. Patients with diffuse vaginal disease or thick posterior vaginal wall disease are usually not suitable for brachytherapy and can be treated with IMRT to a total dose of 70–75 Gy, with the parameters described in the above section on vulvar cancer.

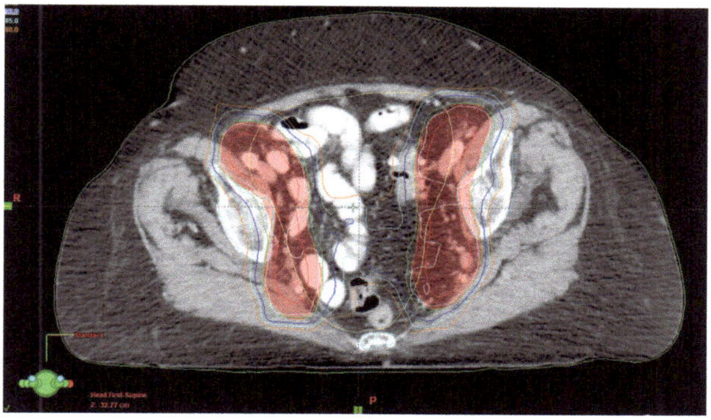

Fig. 8.7 External beam treatment planning CT scan of pelvis showing iliac nodal region PTV (*red*) covered by prescription 97.5% isodose line (*green*)

8.5.2 Vaginal Tolerance to Radiation

The tolerance dose of the vaginal mucosa is ill defined. There is a general assumption that the vagina is very radioresistant. Based on retrospective data from treatment of vaginal and cervical cancer, dose limits of 150 Gy (direct summation of EBRT and brachytherapy doses) to the anterior proximal vagina and 90–100 Gy to the distal vagina have resulted in minimal, manageable toxicity [25]. In an analysis by Grigsby et al., even this traditional tolerance level of 150 Gy was shown to be overly conservative and they reported based on their data with low-dose-rate brachytherapy that the tolerance dose for the proximal vagina for grade 3 morbidity is approximately 175 Gy [26]. However, as the therapeutic window is narrower for high-dose-rate brachytherapy compared with low-dose-rate brachytherapy, optimizing the dose to the vaginal surface may be of interest when using high-dose-rate brachytherapy. A prospective assessment of vaginal morbidity using objective criteria, such as fibrosis, vaginal atrophy, thinning, telangiectasia, and elasticity are needed to assess the true tolerance of vaginal mucosa with radiation.

8.6 Image Guidance During Treatment

The bladder filling position can cause significant motion of the vaginal apex. One way to account for this is to perform CT scans with a full and empty bladder, thus creating an internal target volume (ITV) for the vaginal region. The patient would then be treated with a full bladder. It is difficult to ensure reproducibility of the full bladder position. Use of daily ultrasound for localization of bladder may be another method of doing so. When using IMRT for vaginal cancer boost, daily catheterization to put a fixed amount of fluid in bladder may be another option to reduce internal motion. OBI (on-board imaging) with kilovoltage (KV) imaging can be also be used daily to reduce interfractional motion. A radiopaque marker can be placed at the apex of the vagina and daily AP and lateral images can be taken to confirm the position of the vagina. Cone-beam CT can also be used, and with this modality, both soft tissue and bone can be used as anatomic landmarks to assure that the patient is in the correct position. All of these techniques are evolving and are important when treating with conformal radiation therapy, particularly with IMRT.

8.7 Post-Therapy Imaging

The role for post-therapy imaging for vulvar and vaginal cancer remains undefined. There is evidence in the cervical and anal cancer literature indicating that posttreatment PET-CT response predicts outcome [27, 28]. In vaginal–vulvar cancers, in addition to a complete history and physical exam, obtaining follow-up CT, PET-CT, or MRI scans every 6 months during the first 3 years and annually thereafter may be considered for a follow-up regime.

8.8 Conclusion

In conclusion, 3D imaging plays an important role in the management of vulvar and vaginal cancers. Staging, simulation, treatment planning, and post-therapy evaluation may involve various modalities of imaging including CT, PET/CT and MRI. Judicious use of these modalities may allow for greater accuracy of staging, higher efficacy of treatment, lower morbidity, and overall better outcomes; further research in this area is well justified.

References

1. Leibel SA, Fuks Z, Zelefsky MJ, et al. Intensity modulated radiation therapy. Cancer J. 2007;8:164–76.
2. Nutting C, Dearnaley DP, Webb S. Intensity-modulated radiation therapy: a clinical review. Br J Radiol. 2000;73:459–69.
3. Sohaib SA, Richards PS, Ind T, et al. MR imaging of carcinoma of the vulva. AJR Am J Roentgenol. 2002;178:373–7.
4. Montana GS, Kang SK. Carcinoma of the vulva. In: Perez CA, Brady LW, Halperin EW, et al., editors. Principles and practice of radiation oncology. 4th ed. Philadelphia: Lippincott; 2004.
5. Petereit DG, Mehta MP, Buchler DA, et al. Inguinofemoral radiation of N0, N1 vulvar cancer may be equivalent to lymphadenectomy if proper technique is used. Int J Radiat Biol Phys. 1993;27:969–74.
6. Land R, Herod J, Moskovic E, et al. Routine computerized tomography scanning, groin ultrasound with or without fine needle aspiration cytology in the surgical management of primary squamous cell carcinoma. Int J Gynecol Cancer. 2006;16:312–7.
7. Bipat S, Fransen GA, Spijkerboer AM, et al. Is there a role for magnetic resonance imaging in the evaluation of inguinal lymph node metastases in patients with vulva carcinoma? Gynecol Oncol. 2006;103:1001–6.

8. Singh K, Orakwue CO, Honest H, et al. Accuracy of magnetic resonance imaging of inguinofemoral lymph nodes in vulval cancer. Int J Gynecol Cancer. 2006;16:1179–83.
9. Cohn D, Dehdashti GR, et al. Prospective evaluation of positron emission tomography for detection of groin node metastases from vulvar cancer. Gynecol Oncol. 2002;72:179–84.
10. Taylor MB, Dugar N, Davidson SE, et al. Magnetic resonance imaging of primary vaginal carcinoma. Clin Radiol. 2007;62:549–55.
11. Lamoreaux W, Grigsby PW, Dehdashti F, et al. FDG-PET evaluation of vaginal carcinoma. Int J Radiat Biol Phys. 2005;62:733–7.
12. Koh WJ, Chiu M, Stelzer KJ, et al. Femoral vessel depth and the implications for groin node radiation. Int J Radiat Oncol Biol Phys. 1993;27:969–74.
13. Beriwal S, Coon D, Heron DE, et al. Preoperative intensity-modulated radiotherapy and chemotherapy for locally advanced vulvar carcinoma. Gynecol Oncol. 2008;109:291–5.
14. Moore DH, Thomas GM, Montana GS, et al. Preoperative chemoradiation for advanced vulvar cancer: a phase II study of the Gynecologic Oncology Group. Int J Radiat Biol Phys. 1998; 42:79–85.
15. Beriwal S, Heron DE, Kim H, et al. Intensity-modulated radiotherapy for the treatment of vulvar carcinoma: A comparative dosimetric study with early clinical outcome. Int J Radiat Oncol Biol Phys. 2006;64:1395–400.
16. Garofalo M, Lujan A, Mundt A. (2002) Intensity-modulated radiation therapy in the treatment of vulvar carcinoma: a feasibility study. Paper presented at the 88th annual meeting of the radiologic society of North America. Chicago, IL, December 5, RSNA 2002 Archive.
17. Beriwal S, Gan G, Heron D, et al. Early clinical outcome with concurrent chemotherapy and extended field, intensity-modulated radiotherapy for cervical cancer. Int J Radiat Oncol Biol Phys. 2007;68:166–71.
18. Esthappan J, Chaudri S, Santanam L, et al. Prospective clinical trial of positron emission tomography/computed tomography image-guided intensity-modulated radiation therapy for cervical carcinoma with positive para-aortic lymph nodes. Int J Radiat Oncol Biol Phys. 2008;72:1134–9.
19. Frank SJ, Jhingran A, Levenback C, et al. Definitive radiation therapy for squamous cell carcinoma of the vagina. Int J Radiat Oncol Biol Phys. 2005;62:138–47.
20. International Commission of Radiation Units and Measurements (1985) Dose and volume specification for reporting intracavitary therapy in gynecology. ICRU Report, 38. Bethesda: ICRU.
21. Datta NR, Srivastava A, Maria Das KJ, et al. Comparative assessment of doses to tumor, rectum, and bladder as evaluated by orthogonal radiographs vs. computer enhanced computed tomography-based intracavitary brachytherapy in cervical cancer. Brachytherapy. 2006;5:223–9.
22. Kim RY, Pareek P. Radiography-based treatment planning compared with computed tomography (CT)-based treatment planning for intracavitary brachytherapy in cancer of the cervix: analysis of dose-volume histograms. Brachytherapy. 2003;2:200–6.
23. Beriwal S, Heron DE, Mogus R, et al. High-dose rate brachytherapy (HDRB) for primary or recurrent cancer in the vagina. Radiat Oncol. 2008;3:166–71.
24. Viswanathan AN, Cormack R, Holloway C, et al. Magnetic resonance-guided interstitial therapy for vaginal recurrence of endometrial cancer. Int J Radiat Oncol Biol Phys. 2006;66:91–9.
25. Hintz BL, Kagan AR, Chan P, et al. Radiation tolerance of the vaginal mucosa. Int J Radiat Oncol Biol Phys. 1980;6:711–6.
26. Au SP, Grigsby PW. The irradiation tolerance dose of the proximal vagina. Radiother Oncol. 2003;67:77–85.
27. Schwarz JK, Siegel BA, Dehdashti F, et al. Association of posttherapy positron emission tomography with tumor response and survival in cervical carcinoma. JAMA. 2007;298:2289–95.
28. Schwarz JK, Siegel BA, Dehdashti F, et al. Tumor response and survival predicted by posttherapy FDG-PET/CT in anal cancer. Int J Radiat Biol Phys. 2008;71:180–6.

Part III

Image-Guided Brachytherapy

Adaptive Contouring of the Target Volume and Organs at Risk

9

Primož Petrič, Richard Pötter, Erik Van Limbergen, and Christine Haie-Meder

9.1 Introduction

The most common method of brachytherapy (BT) treatment planning is based on different systems of points, defined on two orthogonal pelvic radiographs with the applicator in place. In cervical cancer BT, this approach refers mainly to dose prescription to point A [1, 2]. In definitive radiotherapy for endometrial cancer, several reference points (My-point, S-point, A-line) have been used for dose specification [3]. Dose to the organs at risk (OAR) has been often reported at points suggested by the International Commission on Radiation Units and Measurements (ICRU) Report 38 [1]. These point-based systems, however, have nonstandard correlations with the true pathoanatomical situation, which differs from organ to organ, patient to patient, application to application, and even within the same application. Due to the lack of visual information on spatial relationships between the tumor, applicator, and OAR, the capability for clinically meaningful and reproducible dose adaptation in X-ray-based BT is limited.

In patients with gross residual disease at the time of BT that extends beyond the standard isodose distribution, parts of the tumor are not covered with the prescribed dose, leading to

P. Petrič (✉)
Department of Brachytherapy, Institute of Oncology Ljubljana,
Zaloška c. 2 1000, Ljubljana, Slovenia
e-mail: ppetric@onko-i.si

R. Pötter
Department of Radiotherapy, Vienna General Hospital,
Medical University of Vienna, Währinger Gürtel 18-20, 1090 Vienna, Austria

E. Van Limbergen
Department of Radiation Oncology, University Hospital Gasthuisberg,
Herestraat, 49 3000, Leuven, Belgium

C. Haie-Meder
Brachytherapy Service, Institut Gustave Roussy, Rue Camille Desmoulins 94800,
Villejuif, France

A.N. Viswanathan et al. (eds.), *Gynecologic Radiation Therapy*,
DOI: 10.1007/978-3-540-68958-4_9, © Springer-Verlag Berlin Heidelberg 2011

"cold spots" that predispose to treatment failure. Mock et al. performed computed tomography (CT)–assisted treatment planning for endometrial cancer BT and demonstrated that the standard treatment planning strategy resulted in inclusion of 66% of uterine volume inside the treated volume [4]. For cervical cancer BT, it has been shown that the dose to point A may overestimate the tumor dose, with the prescribed pear-shaped volume encompassing 80–99% and 60–80% of computed tomography (CT)–defined tumor volume in Fédération Internationale de Gynécologie et d'Obstétrique (FIGO) stages IB and IIB–IIIB, respectively [5]. In a study by Datta et al., the percentage of tumor volume encompassed within the prescribed dose to point A ranged from 61% to 100% [6]. The tumor coverage in these studies and in general depends on tumor volume at the time of BT, with larger tumors less likely to be encompassed by the prescribed isodose [5–10]. These dosimetric results are in line with clinical outcomes of conventional BT, with reported local control rates of 75–95% and 40–75% for FIGO stages I–II and III–IV cervical cancer, respectively [11–18].

Regarding the OAR, the definition of point-related normal tissue dose constraints is also controversial, due to the steep dose gradient, dose inhomogeneity, and noncontiguous high-dose regions over the irradiated volume [18, 19]. In addition, the conventional approach using ICRU point doses may underestimate maximum doses to the OAR, in particular for the bladder [6, 20–22]. Nevertheless, numerous published results support a correlation between the ICRU point dose and probability of late complications for bladder and rectum [23–29]. However, the doses to sigmoid colon, the small bowel, the vagina, the ureters, and some other pelvic tissues at risk from radiation toxicity have not been systematically reported using the conventional radiography-based approach. It is more reliable to correlate the effects of radiation on tissues with doses absorbed in certain volumes, rather than at specific points. The incorporation of three dimensional (3D) imaging into radiotherapy treatment planning allows a comprehensive assessment of correlations between dose-volume parameters and effects in the target volume and in irradiated normal tissues.

9.2 The Role of Clinical Examination and Sectional Imaging in Brachytherapy for Gynecological Malignancies

The clinical gynecological examination plays a critical role in the evaluation of disease extent at time of diagnosis, remission during external-beam radiotherapy, and residual tumor at time of BT. Inspection and palpation are critical for assessment of vaginal involvement, where sectional imaging plays a less important role [30]. Lateral (and to a lesser extent anteroposterior) dimensions of the target volume are readily accessible to bimanual palpation, whereas the height of the tumor, particularly in cases of endocervical growth or uterine involvement, may be clinically inaccessible. While sectional imaging, especially MRI, can detect tumor invasion of the bladder or rectal wall, cystoscopy and rectoscopy are standard methods for verification of mucosal involvement [30].

Therefore, clinical examination remains an essential component of an appropriate BT planning procedure. Accurate description of clinical findings, including written documentation and schematic drawings of initial tumor extension, pattern of regression during external beam radiotherapy (EBRT), and situation at time of BT, should be created and made available for appropriate adaptation of application technique and target volume determination. Systematic incorporation of these findings during sectional imaging-based Gross Tumor Volume (GTV) and Clinical Target Volume (CTV) delineation is highly valuable and recommended (Figs. 9.1, 9.2, and 9.4) [31, 32].

Nevertheless, compared with clinical examination, sectional imaging offers a more reproducible estimation of dimensions, shape, and topography of the target volume and OAR at diagnosis, during the course of EBRT, and at the time of BT [30, 33–39].

While image-based conformal treatment planning has been widely adopted for EBRT of gynecological malignancies, it has been implemented in BT only recently. Over the last decade, we have witnessed its systematic incorporation at a growing number of institutions. Combined with utilization of remote afterloading technologies and advances in computer-based dosimetry, this approach allows for an individualized, anatomy-based dose adaptation and escalation in the target volume, while respecting normal tissue dose constraints [7, 9, 40–44]. In fact, repetitive 3D image–based evaluation of target extent in relation to the applicator and OAR during the course of treatment allowed the evolution of 3D into a four dimensional image-guided adaptive brachytherapy approach (4D IGABT) approach: while an optimized dose distribution of the first BT application is adapted to instantaneous topographic relations in the pelvis at that time, successive applications, accompanied by repetitive imaging, allow for dose adaptation/escalation to a shrinking target.

The ability to perform accurate and reproducible delineations of target volumes and OAR is a precondition for reliable dose delivery and reporting, and is influenced by the choice of the most appropriate sectional imaging modality. While ultrasound (US) is currently used for guidance during applicator insertion in a large number of institutions, further research is required before its systematic implementation into conformal BT planning for gynecological malignancies. Currently, CT and magnetic resonance imaging (MRI) are the basis of IGABT planning in these tumors. The relatively limited availability of CT and especially of MRI, however, prevented early widespread adoption of these promising techniques. Nevertheless, based on encouraging dosimetric and clinical outcome data [7–9, 40–45], we anticipate that 4D IGABT will become more widespread. Information obtained from positron emission tomography (PET) may eventually enable individualized dose escalation to areas of residual metabolic activity at the time of BT.

9.2.1 Ultrasound

Ultrasound (US), in particular endosonography, plays an important role in detection of gynecological malignancies and assessment of tumor dimensions and topography at the time of diagnosis. It enables accurate evaluation of the local spread of the tumor, depiction of intracervical and intrauterine disease extent, parametrial and vaginal infiltration, and involvement of bladder and rectal wall [46]. In addition, US is relatively inexpensive, portable, and may be more readily available in clinical practice than CT or MRI. These characteristics make US a promising and attractive imaging modality in the field of gynecological BT planning.

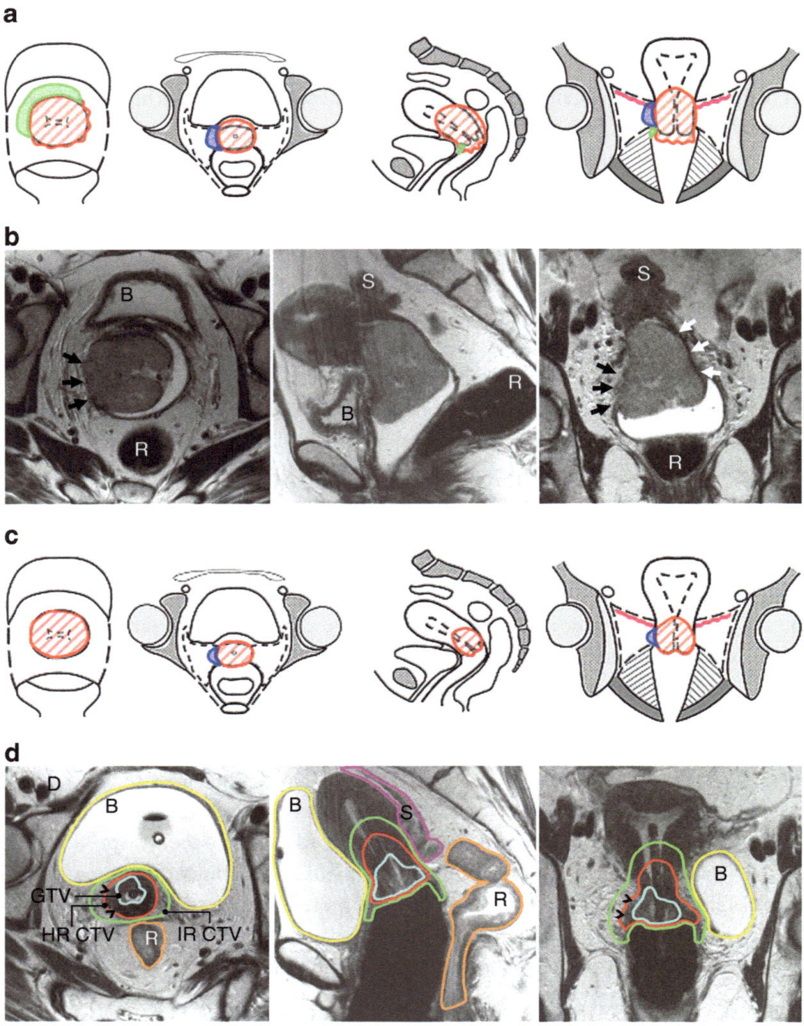

Fig. 9.1 Gross tumor volume (GTV), clinical target volume (CTV), and organs at risk delineation at time of brachytherapy in a FIGO stage IIB cervical tumor with good response to combined chemoirradiation. (**a**) Initial clinical examination. Exophytic tumor, extending to anterior and right fornix. Proximal invasion of right parametrium. (**b**) Magnetic resonance imaging (MRI) in transverse, sagittal, and coronal plane. Hyperintensity-signal lesion in the cervix. Proximal infiltration of right parametrium (*black arrows*). No signs of parametrial invasion on the left, with partially preserved hypointense rim of cervical stroma (*white arrows*). (**c**) Clinical findings at time of brachytherapy. Good partial remission with minimal residual infiltration of right parametrium. (**d**) MRI at time of brachytherapy in paratransverse, parasagittal, and paracoronal orientation. Tandem–ring applicator in place. Small high-signal intensity tumor residuum in the cervix. Gray zones in the proximal third of right parametrium (*black arrow-heads*). Intermediate-risk CTV (IR CTV) encompasses the high-risk CTV (HR CTV) and initial macroscopic tumor extension, superimposed on pelvic topography at time of brachytherapy. Bladder (B), rectum (R), and sigmoid colon (S)

The rationale behind US guidance in BT is twofold: (1) to ensure optimal positioning of BT catheters within the target volume by controlling their insertion; and (2) to assist in detection and contouring of the target volume and OAR. Post-insertion or real-time intraoperative US-guided placement of intracavitary and interstitial applicators has been used in gynecological BT at many centers for decades. In challenging clinical situations, including retroverted uterus or tumor-related distortion or obliteration of the cervical canal, US-guided insertion of an intrauterine tandem has proved helpful in achieving optimal applicator position and preventing inadvertent uterine perforation and its complications [47–50]. US-guided placement of interstitial needles in primary and recurrent vaginal, cervical, and endometrial cancer is a feasible, safe, and relatively inexpensive method for achieving an optimal implant geometry [51, 52].

While systematic US-assisted delineation of target volume and OAR has become a standard approach in the field of prostate cancer BT, it is currently used only to a limited extent for gynecological BT planning. In BT of primary or recurrent vaginal cancer and postoperative vaginal vault irradiation, endosonography adds very useful information to clinical and pathological findings with regard to definition of the target volume and OAR dimensions and topography [3]. In definitive irradiation of uterine cancer, endosonography allows for identification of tumor location, estimation of its volume, and depth of infiltration across the uterine wall, assisting in the definition of BT target volumes [3, 53]. Van Dyk et al. recently reported the use of US guidance for applicator insertion and conformal planning in cervical cancer BT. They suggested that, compared with a 2D X-ray image-based approach, US-assisted BT planning can substantially reduce doses to OAR without compromising the target dose and is associated with a dosimetric outcome comparable to the MRI-guided method [54]. Nevertheless, before systematic implementation of US into conformal gynecological BT planning, further developments in this field are required. Technological adaptations of current sonographic devices to meet the specific demands of gynecological BT may eventually be needed. In addition, systematic evaluation of sonographic findings at the time of diagnosis and BT in the context of traditional clinical experience and current gold standards in gynecological IGABT are required to arrive at a reproducible target concept before this approach can be fully exploited in the clinic.

9.2.2
Computed Tomography

Ling et al. were the first to compare conventional X-ray-based cervical cancer BT planning with a sectional imaging approach using CT. They reported the inaccuracy of the conventional method when estimating maximum OAR doses and emphasized the importance of CT-assisted evaluation [21]. The role of CT in BT treatment planning was later evaluated by a number of groups. Appreciating individual topographic relations between pathoanatomical structures, CT-based generation of dose-volume histograms (DVH) allows for a more reliable estimation of doses to OAR [6, 21, 22, 55–59] than traditional X-rays and is superior to conventional point A planning in terms of conformal target volume coverage [6, 60–63]. To date, there have been only a few reports on the use of CT in

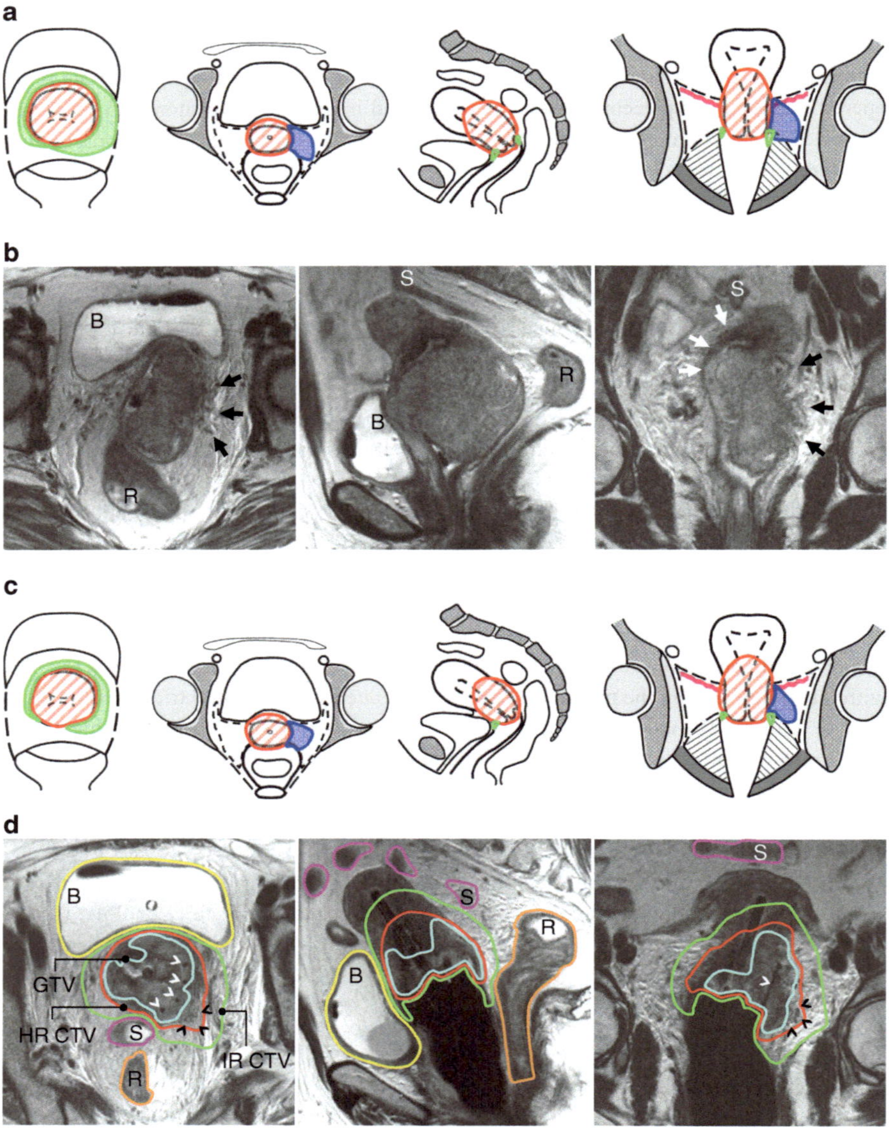

Fig. 9.2 Delineation of gross tumor volume (GTV), Clinical target volume (CTV) and at time of brachytherapy in a large, FIGO stage IIIB cervical tumor with poor remission after combined chemoirradiation. (**a**) Initial clinical findings. Infiltrative tumor, replacing the portio and extending to fornices. Invasion of left parametrium up to the pelvic sidewall. (**b**) MRI in transverse, sagittal, and coronal plane. Hyperintensity-signal lesion, replacing the cervix. Gross infiltration of left parametrium up to its distal third (*black arrows*). No signs of parametrial invasion on the right, with partially preserved hypointense rim of cervical stroma (*white arrows*). No infiltration of

BT for inoperable endometrial cancer. By superimposing the isodose distributions on CT sections of the uterus in inoperable endometrial cancer patients, Bond et al. calculated the dose at several points on the uterine serosa and surrounding normal tissues [64], whereas Mock et al. utilized CT-based dose optimization to increase the proportion of uterine volume included inside the treated volume [4]. In a series by Weitmann et al., CT alone was used for target delineation and dose optimization in 8 out of 16 endometrial cancer patients treated with definitive irradiation [45]. CT has been used in postoperative vaginal cylinder (VC) brachytherapy (Chap. 10). However, CT may have limited soft tissue contrast between the tumor and surrounding normal tissues.

9.2.3 Magnetic Resonance Imaging

Because differences in magnetic resonance (MR) characteristics of soft tissues are more pronounced than variations in X-ray attenuation coefficients, MRI is better than CT in depicting soft tissues. Its capability for non-reconstructed multiplanar imaging further enhances the discrimination of tumor from surrounding structures and assessment of its three-dimensional extent and topography. No ionizing radiation is used, and no intravenous contrast agents are needed for adequate visualization of the pathoanatomical structures during diagnostic imaging and BT planning [30, 33, 36]. Results of clinical–pathological studies in operable cervical cancer demonstrate superior assessment of tumor size, detection of parametrial and uterine invasion, and inter-reader agreement for MRI compared with CT [30, 36, 37, 65–67].

The first reports on the value of MRI in BT planning, illustrating the specific advantages of MRI-based approaches, date back to the 1990s. This early work demonstrated that multiplanar MRI allows adequate depiction of size, location, and paracervical involvement of the tumor and its relations to the applicator, while CT may fail to distinguish cervical tumor from surrounding normal tissues such as small bowel [68–74].

Applying specific protocols for image acquisition, Dimopoulos et al. recently analyzed the potential of MRI to identify the regions of interest in cervical cancer BT

bladder or rectum. (**c**) Clinical findings at time of brachytherapy. Persistent tumor at the portio and fornices. Residual distal infiltration of left parametrium. (**d**) MRI at time of brachytherapy in paratransverse, parasagittal and paracoronal orientation. Tandem–ring applicator and four interstitial needles (*white arrow-heads*) in place. Residual high-signal intensity tumor in the cervix and left parametrium. Gray zones in the dorsolateral region of left parametrium up to its distal third (*black arrow-heads*). Intermediate risk CTV (IR CTV) encompasses the high risk CTV (HR CTV) and initial macroscopic tumor extension, superimposed on pelvic topography at time of brachytherapy. A margin of 1 cm is added to the HR CTV on the left side where remission of less than 1 cm was achieved. Bladder (B), rectum (R), and sigmoid colon (S)

planning. They demonstrated that MRI provides the necessary information for accurate definition of pathoanatomical structures and the applicator. The ability to visualize OAR was also excellent [33]. In a study directly comparing CT- and MRI-based contouring, Viswanathan et al. concluded that either modality is adequate for delineation of OAR. However, tumor contours outlined on CT can overestimate the tumor width compared with MRI [43].

The value of MRI in assessment of GTV and CTV in definitive BT of endometrial cancer has been addressed systematically [3]. Weitmann et al. reported on 16 endometrial cancer patients treated with modified Heyman packing and sectional imaging-based treatment planning. CT alone was used in eight patients, MRI alone in five, and alternating imaging in three patients. The dosimetric and clinical outcomes were encouraging, and MRI was identified as a superior modality for delineation of GTV and CTV [45].

Regarding IGABT of primary and recurrent vaginal cancer, there are a growing number of publications on the advantages of MRI-assisted treatment planning [43, 53, 75–77].

Overall, MRI is the imaging modality of choice for GTV and CTV definition in IGABT of gynecological malignancies. CT seems adequate for delineation of OAR, but its potential for GTV and CTV contouring is limited. T2-weighted MRI has been recommended for target volume and OAR delineation in image-based cervical cancer BT both by the American Brachytherapy Society (ABS) and by the Groupe Européen de Curiethérapie of the European Society for Therapeutic Radiology and Oncology (GEC-ESTRO) [31, 32, 78].

9.2.4 Positron Emission Tomography

18F-fluorodeoxyglucose (FDG) PET is routinely used as an important diagnostic procedure for staging of patients with gynecological tumors at a growing number of institutions worldwide. Furthermore, the level of pre- and postirradiation metabolic activity, as assessed by FDG uptake, may be used as an indicator of prognosis in cervical cancer patients. In a study by Grigsby et al., persistent or new abnormal FDG uptake following irradiation has been identified on multivariate analysis as the most significant prognostic factor for developing metastases and death from cervical cancer [79]. Another study demonstrates that the level of FDG uptake within primary tumor, as measured by standardized uptake value (SUV) prior to initiation of radiotherapy, may identify cervical cancer patients who require more intensive treatment [80].

FDG-PET-assisted delineation of metabolically active tumor volume has been used also for conformal cervical cancer BT planning with encouraging results, indicating the potential for improved target volume coverage while sparing surrounding normal tissues [81, 82]. Incorporation of information from PET imaging using FDG and new tracers as radiopharmaceutical agents (for angiogenesis, hypoxia, etc.) may therefore represent an important opportunity for improvement of conformal BT planning, including individualized definition of tumor subvolumes that require higher doses. However, due to a lack of clinical data in this field, PET-based IGABT currently remains an experimental approach.

9.3 Target Volume Definition with an Emphasis on MRI Assessment of GTV and CTV

Individualized adaptation of dose distribution in 4D IGABT is based on specific topographical relationships between the delineated regions of interest. Applying a common set of rules for volume definition is essential for standardization of the BT procedure. In the field of cervical cancer BT, the concepts and terms for 3D image-based treatment planning were systematically developed over the last few years and published by both the ABS and GEC-ESTRO [31, 32, 78]. In order to facilitate inter-institutional standardization of recording and reporting, the GEC-ESTRO nomenclature has been accepted by both organizations for future clinical work and research [83].

The GEC-ESTRO target concept at the time of BT includes the GTV and two categories of CTV: high-risk and intermediate-risk CTV (HR CTV and IR CTV). These entities are defined at each BT application, taking into account the changes in tumor and true pelvis topography and dimensions during treatment. Assuming a fixed relation between the applicator and the target, no safety margins are applied, and planning target volume (PTV) equals CTV [31].

GTV at time of BT represents the macroscopic tumor as visible and palpable on clinical examination and detectable on T2-weighted MRI as high signal intensity mass(es) (Figs. 9.1 and 9.2).

The HR CTV is assumed to carry a high density of tumor cells and is characterized by a high risk of recurrence. It includes at least the whole cervix, as well as eventual intra- and extra-cervical extension of GTV. In addition, any high- to intermediate-signal intensity areas in the parametria, uterus, or vagina, indicating residual macroscopic disease and areas of low-signal intensity (gray zones) in the parametria corresponding to the topography of initial tumor spread, should be regarded as regions at high risk of developing residual macroscopic disease. As such, they should be included in the HR CTV (Figs. 9.1 and 9.2). The HR CTV is a purely biological concept, and no geometric safety margins are added during its delineation. It requires delivery of a correspondingly high dose, appropriate for eradication of macroscopic residual disease and areas at high risk of recurrence (>80–90 Gy).

The IR CTV is assumed to carry a significant microscopic tumor load. It is characterized by an intermediate risk of local recurrence and requires delivery of a dose appropriate for eradicating microscopic disease (60 Gy). In principle, the IR CTV surrounds the HR CTV like a shell and should therefore be delineated on each slice as a ring, encircling the HR CTV contour. For practical reasons, however, it is recommended to outline it as a volume, encompassing the HR CTV with a margin. In extensive disease, treated with a combination of EBRT and BT, the amount of margin around the HR CTV depends on the size and topography of initial tumor extent and on pattern and degree of regression. At a minimum, the IR CTV encompasses the HR CTV and initial macroscopic tumor extension superimposed on the pelvic topography at the time of BT (Fig. 9.1). In cases of partial or no remission with extra-cervical residual disease, a margin of at least 10 mm needs to be added to the HR CTV (Fig. 9.2). In tumors, smaller than 4 cm, the treatment may consist of BT alone or upfront BT followed by surgery or EBRT. In these clinical situations, IR CTV is delineated by adding a safety margin around HR CTV of up to 5 mm in an anterior–posterior direction, and 10 mm in cranio-caudal and lateral directions. An additional margin of 5 mm is applied in the direction of potential spread in case of laterally growing or endocervical tumors. As they are dependent on initial tumor extension, regression, and treatment strategy, the margins around HR CTV are typically asymmetrical. In addition, during the process of IR CTV delineation, natural anatomical borders (bladder, rectum, sigmoid colon, parametria, and pelvic sidewalls) have to be respected. By definition, organ walls (not lumen) are included in the IR CTV only in case of tumor invasion at time of diagnosis [31]. It can therefore be concluded that utilization of treatment planning system (TPS) tools for automatic creation of margins around the HR CTV will introduce inconsistencies in the IR CTV delineation, which has been demonstrated in one study [84].

One report on sectional imaging-based BT planning in endometrial cancer treated with modified Heyman packing included a systematic delineation of GTV and CTV with DVH analysis. In this series, published in 2005 by Weitmann et al., the GTV was defined as visible tumor on T2-weighted MRI, whereas in patients with CT-based treatment planning, GTV was contoured according to the findings of transvaginal US or hysteroscopy. The entire uterus and proximal vagina were included in the CTV, following the traditional approach to definitive irradiation. Although only 68% of the CTV could be covered with the prescribed dose, the treatment outcome was excellent, and the authors stressed that total enclosure of the CTV with prescribed dose does not seem to be required [45]. This concept was systematically described in the GEC-ESTRO Handbook of Brachytherapy in 2002, referring to the MRI-based definition of GTV and the classical description of the CTV, including the whole uterus [3]. Based on these reports and on earlier data [4], it can be concluded that the GTV and adjacent layers of uterine wall, with a large tumor load and high risk of recurrence (HR CTV), need a sufficiently high dose to eradicate tumor cells

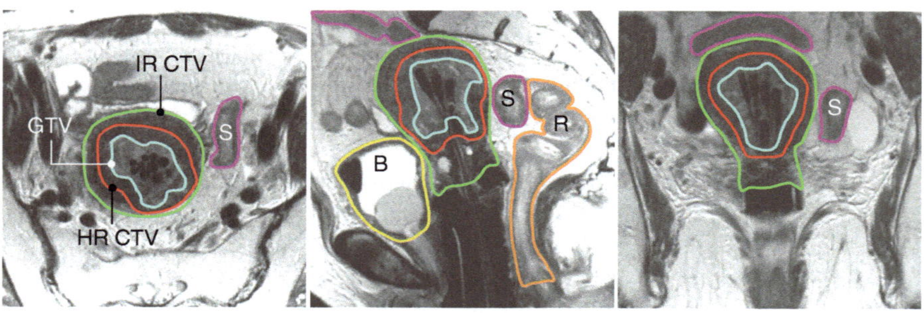

Fig. 9.3 Delineation of gross tumor volume (GTV), Clinical target volume (CTV) and organs at risk in a FIGO stage IB, grade 2, medically inoperable endometrial adenocarcinoma, treated with upfront brachytherapy, followed by external beam irradiation. MRI in paratransverse, parasagittal, and paracoronal plane with applicators in place. Modified Heyman packing technique, combined with a ring applicator in the vagina. High-signal intensity endometrial tumor (GTV) in the uterine cavity with varying depths of infiltration at different parts of the muscular wall. Modified GEC-ESTRO recommendations for cervix cancer BT have been applied in this case to delineate the CTV. High risk CTV (HR CTV) encompassed the GTV and adjacent muscular wall. In regions of superficial tumor growth, internal half of uterine wall was included, whereas in regions with infiltration into outer half, HR CTV was extended up to serosa. Intermediate risk CTV (IR CTV) encompassed the entire uterus. Bladder (B), rectum (R), and sigmoid colon (S)

(>80–90 Gy). In other parts of the CTV carrying a significant microscopic tumor load and an intermediate risk of recurrence (IR CTV), a lower dose may be sufficient (60 Gy). It seems reasonable to apply an adapted GEC-ESTRO nomenclature, as introduced for cervical cancer, for BT of endometrial cancer (Fig. 9.3), taking into account its specific pattern of spread of uterine endometrial cancer.

In the absence of formal contouring guidelines for vaginal and vulvar cancer, the GEC-ESTRO recommendations for cervical cancer BT may also be applied in clinical practice

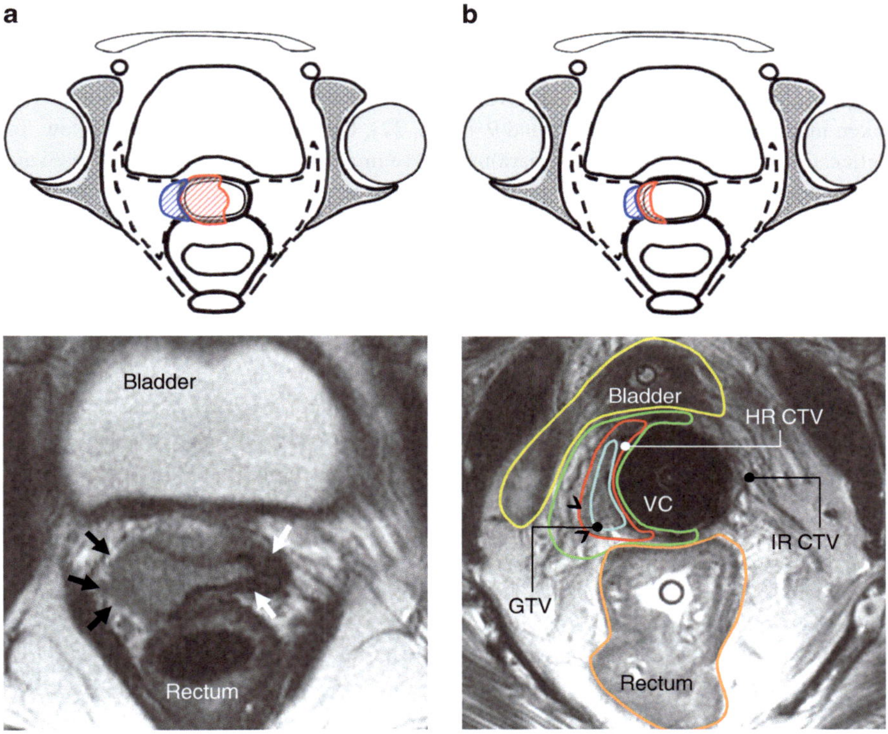

Fig. 9.4 Delineation of gross tumor volume (GTV), Clinical target volume (CTV) and organs at risk in a FIGO stage IIB vaginal cancer. (**a**) Initial clinical and MRI findings in transverse orientation. On clinical examination, an exophytic tumor, involving right, anterior, and posterior vaginal walls with proximal infiltration of the right paracolpium was found. MRI in transverse orientation reveals a hyperintensity-signal exophytic tumor of the right, anterior and posterior vaginal walls with distal infiltration of the right paracolpium (*black arrows*). No invasion on the left aspect of vagina with preserved hypointense muscular wall (*white arrows*). (**b**) Clinical and MRI findings at time of brachytherapy with the applicator in place in paratransverse orientation. Individualized intracavitary vaginal cylinder (VC) with a central channel and peripheral channels on the right side. Small hyperintensive tumor residuum (GTV) on the right with gray zones extending less than 1 cm into the right paracolpium (*black arrow-heads*). Adapted GEC-ESTRO recommendations for cervix cancer BT have been applied to delineate the high risk CTV (HR CTV) and intermediate risk CTV (IR CTV) in this case. HR CTV includes the GTV and the residual gray zones in the right paracolpium. The IR CTV corresponds to the initial tumor extension, superimposed on the MRI at time of brachytherapy

for these tumor sites, where BT also plays a major role (Fig. 9.4). The MRI-based target concept for IGABT of primary and recurrent vaginal and vulvar tumors was first indicated in the GEC-ESTRO Handbook of Brachytherapy [53] and was developed more comprehensively in [77] and in recent work by Dimopoulos et al. [75, 76]. The first clinical results on systematic implementation of this concept in clinical practice were presented recently, demonstrating the feasibility and an encouraging clinical outcome [76]. Viswanathan et al. reported on real-time MRI-guided needle insertion and MRI-assisted delineation of the GTV, CTV, and OAR for BT of vaginal recurrence in endometrial cancer. High accuracy of needle placement and limited toxicity of the approach were demonstrated. Highly homogeneous dose distributions around clearly visualized target volumes were achieved [43].

During the delineation process, detailed information on clinical findings at time of diagnosis and BT, including detailed written documentation and tumor drawings, must be taken into account (Figs. 9.1, 9.2, and 9.4) [31, 32]. Currently available TPSs allow for delineation in a reference, usually (para)transverse image orientation, and enable viewing the contouring result in multiple reconstructed planes. However, due to the finite slice thickness of 4–5 mm, these reconstructed images are characterized by poor quality and do not allow for a meaningful assessment of pathoanatomical structures. Therefore, it is essential that, in addition to the MR images in the (para)transverse plane, non-reconstructed MR images in paracoronal and parasagittal orientation at time of diagnosis and BT are available during delineation. In this way, all imaging information on tumor response and spatial relations between the pathoanatomical structures and the applicator can be integrated into treatment planning. Utilization of T2-weighted fast recovery fast spin echo MRI with 1-mm isotropic voxel size for BT planning has been proposed as an alternative in one study [85]. Using this approach, due to the small voxel size, high-quality image reconstruction in any orientation was possible in the TPS environment, providing a basis for simultaneous and interactive delineation in multiple image planes. When compared with the standard approach using T2-weighted fast spin echo MRI with 4-mm slice thickness, there were only minor volumetric, topographic, and DVH deviations [85].

Accurate and reproducible delineation of GTV and CTV is a precondition for accurate treatment delivery and consistent recording and reporting. It can be achieved only through adequate training and strict adherence to a common set of rules for contouring [31, 32].

9.4 Delineation of Organs at Risk

The tolerance of normal pelvic structures to irradiation is a major limiting factor when applying high doses to the target volume, in particular when using brachytherapy. The most important critical normal structures in gynecological BT are the hollow visceral organs of the true pelvis: urinary bladder, rectum, and sigmoid colon. Although there is a lack of reliable data on dose-response relationships for other parts of the bowel, the vagina, and the ureters, these regions also need to be considered, since they may receive a significant dose [32, 86].

Regarding the imaging modality for OAR delineation, CT was shown to be as accurate for delineation of outer OAR contours as MRI in one study [87]. MRI may enable superior discrimination of organ walls from their contents and from surrounding tissues. In a study by Dimopoulos et al., the overall ability to visualize bladder, rectum, sigmoid colon, and vaginal wall on MRI was excellent, exceeding 98% [33]. On T2-weighted MRI, the muscular wall of OAR can be depicted as a band of low-signal intensity with thickness ranging from 2–8 mm, depending on the filling status. OAR can be contoured by outlining the whole organ, including its contents, or just the organ wall. When outlining the whole organ, parts of delineated volumes that receive the highest dose may not be located entirely within the organ wall, especially if the wall is very thin. Therefore, it is more appropriate to delineate organ walls instead of whole organs for recording and reporting the dose to OAR. However, given the lack of capability for automatic contour generation in the majority of TPSs, this approach requires a time-consuming slice-by-slice delineation. In addition, due to the varying thicknesses of organ walls, inaccuracies introduced during manual or automatic delineation may lead to major variations in the reported dose [88]. Wachter-Gerstner et al. have analyzed the correlation between dose-volume histograms for bladder and rectum, based on whole-organ and organ-wall volumes. They demonstrated that when volumes of 2 cm^3 (D_{2cc}) were considered, the doses computed for the whole organ served as a good estimate for doses to the organ wall. In contrast, for volumes of 5 cm^3 (D_{5cc}) or larger, this correspondence was no longer evident [89]. The reliability of whole-organ DVH parameters for estimating the dose to the organ wall is also dependent on the wall thickness and therefore the filling status. If the organ wall is thick, it is probable that the high-dose-volume is situated inside the wall. In such cases, the whole-organ DVH parameters therefore serve as a good estimate for organ-wall values. However, for fully filled organs with thin walls, there will be greater differences between DVH parameters for organ wall and whole organ. In a study by Olzsewska et al., it was shown that rectal wall thickness had only a minor impact on the D_{2cc} value, whereas it became more critical when the D_{5cc} for whole organ and organ wall were compared [90]. Therefore, when recording and reporting the dose to organ wall volumes of up to 2–3 cm^3, whole-organ contouring is advisable. However, when doses to larger volumes are considered, organ walls should be delineated [32].

9.5 Interobserver Variability in Contouring

Target and OAR delineation inconsistencies can reduce the accuracy of any conformal radiotherapy approach. The degree of dose conformity and capability for local dose escalation afforded by modern 4D IGABT exceed any other radiotherapy modality [91]. Due to inhomogeneous dose distributions and sharp dose fall-off, even minimal delineation inaccuracies may therefore be reflected in significant uncertainties regarding the optimized dose distribution in the tissues. These may have clinical implications and can compromise the reproducibility of treatment recording and reporting, undermining the overall efficacy of IGABT. Accurate and reproducible definition and delineation of GTV, CTV, and OAR is therefore a precondition for translation of conformal dose escalation into favorable clinical results and for researchers and clinicians in this area to speak a common language.

Common sources of systematic contouring variability include the choice of imaging modality and observer-specific subjectivity of image interpretation. This inference points to the need for standardization and training in target and OAR delineation. Several recent studies have demonstrated an encouraging level of interobserver agreement when contouring is performed by experienced observers according to GEC-ESTRO recommendations [84, 85, 87, 92–94]. In two multi-institutional intercomparisons involving three centers with different historical backgrounds of BT delivery, there was good agreement in volumetric and DVH parameters [92, 93]. In a study analyzing the agreement between target volumes, as delineated by two observers on two different MR image planes, the interobserver and interplanar conformity indexes (CI – ratio between common and encompassing volume) were high, 0.7–0.8. Only minor topographic deviations in contour extent were found [94]. In a similar analysis involving two observers and two MRI approaches (fast recovery fast spin echo vs. fast spin echo MRI), the interobserver and inter-approach CIs were around 0.8. A thorough topographic analysis of delineation differences using a dedicated software tool revealed no observer- or imaging-specific deviations [85]. Dimopoulos et al. have analyzed the variation in GTV, HR CTV, and IR CTV contouring between two observers from different centers. A systematic application of contouring recommendations resulted in small volumetric and dosimetric variations, despite different traditions regarding application technique, CTV assessment, and dose prescription at the respective institutions [84]. Experience from two transatlantic contouring workshops, organized in 2006 in Washington and in 2007 in Milwaukee, is in line with results of these studies. In a setting with favorable teaching conditions and experienced observers, a satisfactory CI of 0.6–0.7 was demonstrated (unpublished results). In an early European contouring workshop in Dublin (2005), where inexperienced observers were evaluated, the CI for HR CTV and IR CTV only reached 0.3 [95]. Recently, a contouring workshop was carried out in Utrecht for the purpose of the international study on MRI-guided brachytherapy in locally advanced cervical cancer (EMBRACE) study with observers of varying degrees of experience in this field. Average CIs of 0.4, 0.6, and 0.7 for GTV, HR CTV, and IR CTV, respectively, were revealed when individual contours were compared with the reference delineations (unpublished results).

During gynecological BT, posterior and inferior bladder wall, anterior walls of rectum and sigmoid colon, and vaginal wall adjacent to the applicator are typically close to BT sources, within the region of high and inhomogeneous dose. Due to a steep dose gradient, minimal inaccuracies in delineation of these parts of OAR can result in large uncertainties in the reported dose. It seems prudent to pay special attention on contouring accuracy in these regions. Parts of the OAR that are typically located farther from BT sources (anterior and superior bladder wall, posterior walls of rectum and sigmoid, and usually the lower vagina) receive a lower and more homogeneous dose, which has only a minor impact on the commonly reported DVH parameters. The effect of delineation uncertainties on the reported dose in these regions is less pronounced and of less consequence.

In a study by Saarnak et al., the interobserver variation in delineation of bladder and rectum outer contour resulted in 10% and 11% (one average relative standard deviation) variation in the reported minimal dose to the 2 cm^3 of the most exposed OAR (D_{2cc}), respectively [96].

Overall, the published results of the interobserver studies in this field seem to indicate a high degree of agreement among experienced observers. However, larger studies with more observers and patients are needed to confirm these findings. Furthermore, major efforts in education and training need to be undertaken before appropriate knowledge and experience can be assumed to put the complex 4D IGABT approach into clinical practice.

9.6 Conclusion

4D gynaecological IGABT is becoming more widely implemented in clinical practice worldwide. Compared with a conventional X-ray-based approach, 4D IGABT enables a greater and more reproducible dose adaptation/escalation to the target volume while respecting OAR dose constraints. However, interobserver variability in the definition of GTV, CTV, and OAR is a major source of uncertainty in BT treatment planning. It can be reduced by systematic application of contouring recommendations and radiological training. In the absence of clinicopathologic studies in locally advanced cervical cancer, emerging favorable clinical results can be regarded as indirect evidence of the appropriateness of MRI-based definition of GTV, CTV, and OAR.

References

1. ICRU, International Commission of Radiation Units and Measurements. Dose and volume specification for reporting intracavitary therapy in gynaecology. ICRU report 38, Bethesda, MD; 1985.
2. Pötter R, Van Limbergen E, Wambersie A. Reporting in brachytherapy. In: Gerbaulet A, Pötter R, Mazeron JJ, Meertens H, Van Limbergen E, editors. The GEC ESTRO handbook of brachytherapy. Brussels: European Society of Therapeutic Radiology and Oncology; 2002. p. 153–215.
3. Pötter R, Gerbaulet A, Haie-Meder C. Endometrial cancer. In: Gerbaulet A, Pötter R, Mazeron JJ, Meertens H, Van Limbergen E, editors. The GEC ESTRO handbook of brachytherapy. Brussels: European Society of Therapeutic Radiology and Oncology; 2002. p. 365–401.
4. Mock U, Knocke TH, Fellner C, et al. Comparison of different application systems and CT-assisted treatment planning procedures in the treatment of primary endometrium carcinoma: Is it technically possible to include the whole uterus volume in the volume treated by brachytherapy? Strahlenther Onkol. 1998;174:320–8.
5. Kim RY, Pareek P. Radiography-based treatment planning compared with computed tomography (CT)-based treatment planning for intracavitary brachytherapy in cancer of the cervix: analysis of dose-volume histograms. Brachytherapy. 2003;2:200–6.
6. Datta NR, Srivastava A, Maria Das KJ, et al. Comparative assessment of doses to tumor, rectum, and bladder as evaluated by orthogonal radiographs vs. computer enhanced computed tomography-based intracavitary brachytherapy in cervical cancer. Brachytherapy. 2006;5:223–9.
7. De Brabandere M, Mousa AG, Nulens A, et al. Potential of dose optimisation in MRI-based PDR brachytherapy of cervix carcinoma. Radiother Oncol. 2008;88(2):217–26.
8. Hudej R, Petric P, Burger J. Standard versus 3D optimized MRI-based planning for uterine cervix cancer brachyradiotherapy-the Ljubljana experience. Zbornik predavanj, konferenca MEDICON, Ljubljana; 2007.

9. Lindegaard JC, Tanderup K, Nielsen SK, et al. MRI-guided 3D optimization significantly improves DVH parameters of pulsed-dose-rate brachytherapy in locally advanced cervical cancer. Int J Radiat Oncol Biol Phys. 2008;71(3):756–64.
10. Petric P, Hudej R, Rogelj P, et al. Frequency-distribution mapping of HR CTV in locally advanced cervix cancer: a new tool for development of novel brachytherapy techniques. Radiother Oncol. 2009;91 Suppl 1:18–9.
11. Fletcher GH, Hamburger AD. Female pelvis. Squamous cell carcinoma of the uterine cervix. In: Fletcher GH, editor. Textbook of radiotherapy. 3rd ed. Philadelphia: Lea & Febiger; 1980. p. 720–89.
12. Gerbaulet A, Pötter R, Haie-Meder C. Cervix cancer. In: Gerbaulet A, Pötter R, Mazeron JJ, Meertens H, Van Limbergen E, editors. The GEC ESTRO handbook of brachytherapy. Brussels: European Society of Therapeutic Radiology and Oncology; 2002. p. 301–63.
13. Horiot JC, Pigneux J, Pourquier H. Radiotherapy alone in carcinoma of intact uterine cervix according to Fletcher guidelines: A French cooperative study of 1383 cases. Int J Radiat Oncol Biol Phys. 1988;14(4):605–11.
14. Ito H, Kutuki S, Nishiguchi I, et al. Radiotherapy for cervical cancer with high dose rate brachytherapy-correlation between tumour size, dose and failure. Radiother Oncol. 1994;31:240–7.
15. Perez CA, Breaux S, Bedwinek JM, et al. Effect of tumor size on the prognosis of carcinoma of the uterine cervix treated with irradiation alone. Cancer. 1992;69:2796–806.
16. Pernot M, Hoffstetter S, Peiffert D, et al. Statistical study of a series of 672 cases of carcinoma of the uterine cervix. Results and complications according to age and modalities of treatment. Bull Cancer. 1995;82(7):568–81.
17. Petereit DG, Pearcey R. Literature analysis of high dose rate brachytherapy fractionation schedules in the treatment of cervical cancer: Is there an optimal fractionation schedule? Int J Radiat Oncol Biol Phys. 1999;43:359–66.
18. Pötter R, Knocke TH, Fellner C, et al. Definitive radiotherapy based on HDR brachytherapy with Iridium – 192 in cervix cancer – report on the recent Vienna university hospital experience (1993–1997) compared to the preceding period, referring to ICRU 38 recommendations. Bull Cancer Radiother. 2000;4:159–72.
19. Visser AG, Symonds RP. Dose and volume specification for reporting gynaecological brachytherapy: time for a change. Radiother Oncol. 2001;58:1–4.
20. Barillot I, Horiot JC, Maingon P, et al. Maximum and mean bladder dose defined from ultrasonography. Comparison with the ICRU reference in gynaecological brachytherapy. Radiother Oncol. 1994;30(3):231–8.
21. Ling CC, Schell MC, Working KR, et al. CT-assisted assessment of bladder and rectum dose in gynecological implants. Int J Radiat Oncol Biol Phys. 1987;13(10):1577–82.
22. LaVigne SSL, ML MMK, et al. Three-dimensional treatment planning of intracavitary gynaecologic implants: analysis of ten cases and implications for dose specification. Int J Radiat Oncol Biol Phys. 1994;28(1):277–83.
23. Barillot I, Horiot JC, Maingon P, et al. Impact on treatment outcome and late effects of customized treatment planning in cervix carcinomas: baseline results to compare new strategies. Int J Radiat Oncol Biol Phys. 2000;48(1):189–200.
24. Chen SW, Liang JA, Yeh LS, et al. Comparative study of reference points by dosimetric analyses for late complications after uniform external radiotherapy and high-dose-rate brachytherapy for cervical cancer. Int J Radiat Oncol Biol Phys. 2004;60(2):663–71.
25. Ferrigno R, dos Santos Novaes PE, Pelizzon AC, et al. High-dose-rate brachytherapy in the treatment of uterine cervix cancer. Analysis of dose effectiveness and late complications. Int J Radiat Oncol Biol Phys. 2001;50(5):1123–35.
26. Kim HJ, Kim S, Ha SW, et al. Are doses to ICRU reference points valuable for predicting late rectal and bladder morbidity after definitive radiotherapy in uterine cervix cancer? Tumori. 2008;94(3):327–32.

27. Ogino I, Kitamura T, Okamoto N, et al. Late rectal complication following high dose rate intracavitary brachytherapy in cancer of the cervix. Int J Radiat Oncol Biol Phys. 1995;31(4):725–34.
28. Perez CA, Grigsby PW, Lockett MA, et al. Radiation therapy morbidity in carcinoma of the uterine cervix: dosimetric and clinical correlation. Int J Radiat Oncol Biol Phys. 1999;44(4):855–66.
29. Roeske JC, Mundt AJ, Halpern H, et al. Late rectal sequelae following definitive radiation therapy for carcinoma of the uterine cervix: a dosimteric analysis. Int J Radiat Oncol Biol Phys. 1997;37(2):351–8.
30. Boss EA, Barentsz JO, Massuger LFAG, et al. The role of MR imaging in invasive cervical carcinoma (review). Eur Radiol. 2000; 10:256–70; Subak LL, Hricak H, Powell CB, et al. Cervical carcinoma: computed tomography and magnetic resonance imaging for preoperative staging. Obstet Gynecol 1995; 86:43–50.
31. Haie-Meder C, Pötter R, Van Limbergen E, et al. Recommendations from Gynaecological (GYN) GEC-ESTRO Working Group (I): concepts and terms in 3D image based 3D treatment planning in cervix cancer brachytherapy with emphasis on MRI assessment of GTV and CTV. Radiother Oncol. 2005;74:235–45.
32. Pötter R, Haie-Mader C, Van Limbergen E, et al. Recommendations from gynaecological (GYN) GEC-ESTRO Working Group: (II): concepts and terms of 3D imaging, radiation physics, radiobiology, and 3D dose volume parameters. Radiother Oncol. 2006;78:67–77.
33. Dimopoulos JCA, Schard G, Berger D, et al. Systematic evaluation of MRI findings in different stages of treatment of cervical cancer: potential of MRI on delineation of target, pathoanatomical structures and organs at risk. Int J Radiat Oncol Biol Phys. 2006;64:1380–8.
34. Dimopoulos JCA, Schirl G, Baldinger A, et al. MRI assessment of cervical cancer for adaptive radiotherapy. Strahlentherapie und Onkologie. 2009;185(5):282–7.
35. Kerkhof EM, Raaymakers BW, van der Heide UA, van de Bunt L, Jürgenliemk-Schulz IM, Lagendijk JJ. Online MRI guidance for healthy tissue sparing in patients with cervical cancer: an IMRT planning study. Radiother Oncol. 2008;88(2):241–9.
36. Mitchell DG, Snyder B, Coakley F, et al. Early invasive cervical cancer: tumor delineation by magnetic resonance imaging, computed tomography, and clinical examination, verified by pathologic results, in the ACRIN 6651/GOG 183 Intergroup Study. J Clin Oncol. 2006;24(36):5687–94.
37. Oszarlak O, Tjalma W, Scheppens E, et al. The correlation of preoperative CT, MR imaging, and clinical staging (FIGO) with histopathology findings in primary cervical carcinoma. Eur Radiol. 2003;13(10):2338–45.
38. van de Bunt L, Jurgenliemk-Schulz IM, de Kort GA, Roesink JM, Tersteeg RJ, van der Heide UA. Motion and deformation of the target volumes during IMRT for cervical cancer: what margins do we need? Radiother Oncol. 2008;88:233–40.
39. van de Bunt L, van der Heide UA, Ketelaars M, de Kort GA, Jurgenliemk-Schulz IM. Conventional, conformal, and intensity-modulated radiation therapy treatment planning of external beam radiotherapy for cervical cancer: The impact of tumor regression. Int J Radiat Oncol Biol Phys. 2006;64:189–96.
40. Haie-Meder C et al. MRI-based brachytherapy (BT) in the treatment of cervical cancer: experience of the Institut Gustave-Roussy. Radiother Oncol. 2007;83 Suppl 1:S11–2.
41. Kirisits C, Pötter R, Lang S, et al. Dose and volume parameters for MRI based treatment planning in intracavitary brachytherapy of cervix cancer. Int J Radiation Oncology Biol Phys. 2005;62(3):901–11.
42. Pötter R, Dimopoulos J, Georg P, et al. Clinical impact of MRI assisted dose volume adaptation and dose escalation in brachytherapy of locally advanced cervix cancer. Radiother Oncol. 2007;83:148–55.
43. Viswanathan AN, Cormack R, Holloway CL, et al. Magnetic resonance-guided interstitial therapy for vaginal recurrence of endometrial cancer. Int J Radiat Oncol Biol Phys. 2006;66(1):91–9.

44. Wachter-Gerstner N, Wachter S, Reinstadler E, et al. The impact of sectional imaging on dose escalation in endocavitary HDR-brachytherapy of cervical cancer: results of a prospective comparative trial. Radiother Oncol. 2003;68(1):51–9.
45. Weitmann HD, Pötter R, Waldhäusl C, et al. Pilot study in the treatment of endometrial carcinoma with 3D image-based high-dose-rate brachytherapy using modified Heyman Packing: clinical experience and dose-volume histogram analysis. Int J Radiat Oncol Biol Phys. 2005;62(2):468–78.
46. Bernaschek G, Deutinger J, Kratochwill A. Endosonographic diagnosis of carcinoma. In: Endosonography in obstetrics and gynecology. Berlin, Heidelberg: Springer; 1990. p. 97–121.
47. Davidson MT, Yuen J, D'Souza D, et al. Optimization of high-dose-rate cervix brachytherapy applicator placement: the benefits of intraoperative ultrasound guidance. Brachytherapy. 2008;7:248–53.
48. Granai CO, Allee P, Doherty F, et al. Ultrasound used for assessing the in situ position of intrauterine tandems. Gynecol Oncol. 1984;18(3):334–8.
49. Mayr NA, Montebello JF, Sorosky JI, et al. Brachytherapy management of the retroverted uterus using ultrasound-guided implant applicator placement. Brachytherapy. 2005;4:24–9.
50. Sahinler I, Cepni I, Colpan D, et al. Tandem application with transvaginal ultrasound guidance. Int J Radiat Oncol Biol Phys. 2004;59(1):190–6.
51. Stock RG, Chan K, Terk M, et al. A new technique for performing Syed–Neblett template interstitial implants for gynecologic malignancies using transrectal-ultrasound guidance. Int J Radiat Oncol Biol Phys. 1997;37:819–25.
52. Weitmann HD, Knocke TH, Waldhäusl C, et al. Ultrasound-guided interstitial Brachytherapy in the treatment of advanced vaginal recurrences from cervical and endometrial carcinoma. Strahlentherapie und Onkologie. 2006;182:86–95.
53. Gerbaulet A, Pötter R, Haie-Meder C. Primary vaginal cancer. In: Gerbaulet A, Pötter R, Mazeron JJ, Meertens H, Van Limbergen E, editors. The GEC ESTRO handbook of brachytherapy. Brussels: European Society of Therapeutic Radiology and Oncology; 2002. p. 153–215.
54. Van Dyk S, Narayan K, Fisher R, Bernshaw D. Conformal brachytherapy planning for cervical cancer using transabdominal ultrasound. Int J Radiat Oncol Biol Phys. 2009; 75(1):64–70.
55. Kapp KS, Stuecklschweiger GF, Kapp DS, et al. Dosimetry of intracavitary placements for uterine and cervical carcinoma: results of orthogonal film, TLD, and CT-assisted techniques. Radiother Oncol. 1992;24(3):137–46.
56. Kim RY, Shen S, Duan J. Image-based three-dimensional treatment planning of intracavitary brachytherapy for cancer of the cervix: dose-volume histograms of the bladder, rectum, sigmoid colon, and small bowel. Brachytherapy. 2007;6(3):187–94.
57. Pelloski CE, Palmer M, Chronowski GM, et al. Comparison between CT-based volumetric calculations and ICRU reference-point estimates of radiation doses delivered to bladder and rectum during intracavitary radiotherapy for cervical cancer. Int J Radiat Oncol Biol Phys. 2005;62(1):131–7.
58. Sun LM, Huang EY, Ko SF, et al. Computer-tomography-assisted three-dimensional technique to assess rectal and bladder wall dose in intracavitary brachytherapy for uterine cervical cancer. Radiother Oncol. 2004;71(3):333–7.
59. van den Bergh F, Mertens H, Moonen LMF, et al. The use of a transverse CT image for the estimation of the dose given to the rectum in intracavitary brachytherapy for carcinoma of the cervix. Radiother Oncol. 1998;47:85–90.
60. Eisbruch A, Johnston CM, Martel MK, et al. Customized gynecologic interstitial implants: CT-based planning, dose evaluation and optimization aided by laparotomy. Int J Radiat Oncol Biol Phys. 1998;40(5):1087–93.

61. Fellner C, Pötter R, Knocke T, et al. A comparison of radiography and computed-tomography-based treatment planning in cervix cancer brachytherapy with specific attention to some quality assurance aspects. Radiother Oncol. 2001;58:53–62.
62. Mai J, Rownd J, Erickson B. CT-guided high-dose-rate dose prescription for cervical carcinoma: the importance of uterine wall thickness. Brachytherapy. 2002;1(1):27–35.
63. Shin KH, Kim TH, Cho JK, et al. CT-guided intracavitary radiotherapy for cervical cancer: comparison of conventional point A plan with clinical target volume-based three-dimensional plan using dose volume parameters. Int J Radiat Oncol Biol Phys. 2006;64(1):197–204.
64. Bond MG, Workman G, Martland J, et al. Dosimetric considerations in the treatment of inoperable endometrial carcinoma by a high dose rate afterloading packing technique. Clin Oncol. 1997;9(1):41–7.
65. Bipat S, Glas AS, van der Velden J, et al. Computed tomography and magnetic resonance imaging in staging of uterine cervical carcinoma: a systematic review. Gynecol Oncol. 2003;91(1):59–66.
66. Hricak H, Gatsonis C, Coakley FV, et al. Early invasive cervical cancer: CT and MR imaging in preoperative evaluation – ACRIN/GOG comparative study of diagnostic performance and interobserver variability. Radiology. 2007;245(2):491–8.
67. Jung DC, Ju W, Choi HJ, et al. The validity of tumour diameter assessed by magnetic resonance imaging and gross specimen with regard to tumour volume in cervical cancer patients. Eur J Cancer. 2008;44(11):1524–8.
68. Lukas P, Heuck A. The use of magnetic resonance tomography in cancer of the cervix and uterus. Rontgenpraxis. 1990;43(12):439–44.
69. Pötter R, Kovacs G, Haverkamp U. 3D Conformal Therapy in Brachytherapy. 8th International Brachytherapy Conference, Nice 1995. Nucletron-Oldelft, Veenendaal. p. 34–39.
70. Pötter R, Kovacs G, Lenzen B, et al. Technique of MRI assisted brachytherapy treatment planning. Activity. Selectr Brachyther J. 1991;5(3):145–8.
71. Pötter R. Modern imaging methods used for treatment planning and quality assurance for combined irradiation of cervix cancer, Workshop Integration of external beam therapy and brachytherapy in the treatment of cervix cancer: clinical, physical and biological aspects. Annual Brachytherapy Meeting GEC-ESTRO Stockholm, 5–7 May 1997; European Society for Therapeutic Radiology and Oncology, Groupe Européen de Curiethérapie 1997; p. 27–39.
72. Schmidt BF, Hirnle P, Kaulich TW, et al. The value of NMR tomography in the planning of HDR-afterloading brachytherapy in cervical carcinomas: The experience with 41 patients. Rofo. 1991;155(2):109–16.
73. Schoeppel SL, Ellis JH, LaVigne ML, et al. Magnetic resonance imaging during intracavitary gynecologic brachytherapy. Int J Radiat Oncol Biol Phys. 1992;23(1):169–74.
74. Tardivon AA, Kinkel K, Lartigau E, et al. MR imaging during intracavitary brachytherapy of vaginal and cervical cancer: preliminary results. Radiographics. 1996;16(6):1363–70.
75. Dimopoulos J, Fidarova E, Pötter R. Definitive radiotherapie und radiochemotherapie der vulva und vagina. Onkologe. 2009;15:54–63.
76. Dimopoulos J, Schmid M, Berger D et al. MRI-guided BT with EBRT plus chemotherapy for the treatment of locally advanced vaginal cancer. Radiother Oncol. 2009;91 (Suppl.1): S18–19.
77. Pötter R. Vaginalkarzinom. In: Strnad V, Pötter R, Kovacs G, editors. Stand und Perspektiven der klinischen Brachytherapie. Bremen: UNI-MED; 2004. p. 114–21.
78. Nag S, Cardenes H, Chang S, et al. Proposed guidelines for image-based intracavitary brachytherapy for cervical carcinoma: report from image-guided brachytherapy working group. Int J radiat Oncol Biol Phys. 2004;60(4):1160–72.
79. Grigsby PW, Siegel BA, Dehdashti F, et al. Posttherapy [^{18}F] fluorodeoxyglucose positron emission tomography in carcinoma of the cervix: response and outcome. J Clin Oncol. 2004;22:2167–71.

80. Xue F, Lin LL, Dehdashti F, et al. F-18 fluorodeoxyglucose uptake in primary cervical cancer as an indicator of prognosis after radiation therapy. Gynecol Oncol. 2006;101:147–51.
81. Malyapa RS, Mutic S, Low DA, et al. Physiologic FDG-PET three dimensional brachytherapy treatment planning for cervical cancer. Int J Radiat Oncol Biol Phys. 2002;54(4):1140–6.
82. Mutic S, Grigsby PW, Low DA, et al. PET-guided three-dimensional treatment planning of intracavitary gynecologic implants. Int J Radiat Oncol Biol Phys. 2002;52(4):1104–10.
83. Nag S. Controversies and new developments in gynecologic brachytherapy: image-based intracavitary brachytherapy for cervical carcinoma. Semin Radiat Oncol. 2006;16(3):164–7.
84. Dimopoulos JC, De Vos V, Berger D, et al. Inter-observer comparison of target delineation for MRI-assisted cervical cancer brachytherapy: application of the GYN GEC-ESTRO recommendations. Radiother Oncol. 2009;91(2):166–72.
85. Petric P, Hudej R, Rogelj P, et al. 3D T2-weighted fast recovery fast spin echo sequence MRI for target contouring in cervix cancer brachytherapy. Brachytherapy. 2008;7(2):109.
86. Berger D, Dimopoulos J, Georg P, et al. Uncertainties in assessment of the vaginal dose for intracavitary brachytherapy of cervical cancer using a tandem-ring applicator. Int J Radiat Oncol Biol Phys. 2007;67(5):1451–9.
87. Viswanathan AN, Dimopoulos JCA, Kirisits C, et al. CT versus MRI-based contouring in cervical cancer brachytherapy: results of a prospective trial and preliminary guidelines for standardized Contours. Int J Radiat Oncol Biol Phys. 2007;68:491–8.
88. Shenfield CB, Berger D, Dimopoulos JCA, et al. Systematic comparison of two methods of bladder contouring in cervix cancer brachytherapy: 'Direct' vs. 'indirect'. Brachytherapy. 2009;8(2):141–2.
89. Wachter-Gerstner N, Wachter S, Reinstadler E, et al. Bladder and rectum dose defined from MRI based treatment planning for cervix cancer brachytherapy: comparison of dose-volume histograms for organ contours and organ wall, comparison with ICRU rectum and bladder reference point. Radiother Oncol. 2003;68(3):269–76.
90. Olszewska AM, Saarnak AE, De Boer RW, et al. Comparison of dose-volume histograms and dose-wall histograms of the rectum of patients treated with intracavitary brachytherapy. Radiother Oncol. 2001;61(1):83–5.
91. Georg D, Kirisits C, Hillbrand M, et al. Image-guided radiotherapy for cervix cancer: high-tech external beam therapy versus high-tech brachytherapy. Int J Radiat Oncol Biol Phys. 2008;71(4):1272–8.
92. Lang S, Nulens A, Briot E, et al. Intercomparison of treatment concepts for MR image assisted brachytherapy of cervical carcinoma based on GYN GEC-ESTRO recommendations. Radiother Oncol. 2006;78:185–93.
93. Nulens A, Lang S, Briot E, et al. Evaluation of contouring concepts and dose volume parameters of MR based brachytherapy treatment plans for cervix cancer: results and conclusions of the GEC-ESTRO, GYN working group delineation workshops GEC-ESTRO Meeting, Budapest 2005. Radiother Oncol. 2005;75(1):S9.
94. Petric P, Dimopoulos J, Kirisits C, et al. Inter- and intraobserver variation in HR CTV contouring: Intercomparison of transverse and paratransverse image orientation in 3D-MRI assisted cervix cancer brachytherapy. Radiother Oncol. 2008;89(2):164–71.
95. Kelly C, Thirion P, Grimley J, et al. Quantification of interobserver variation in delineation of target volumes using the GEC-ESTRO recommendations for MRI based brachytherapy of the cervix. Radiother Oncol. 2006;81 suppl 1:663.
96. Saarnak AE, Boersma M, van Bunningen BN, et al. Inter-observer variation in delineation of bladder and rectum contours for brachytherapy of cervical cancer. Radiother Oncol. 2000;56(1):37–42.

Clinical Aspects of Treatment Planning 10

Jacob C. Lindegaard, Richard Pötter, Eric Van Limbergen,
and Christine Haie-Meder

10.1 Introduction

The goal of treatment planning in image-guided brachytherapy (BT) is to widen the therapeutic window, i.e., to obtain the best possible chance for an uncomplicated cure of the patient [1] by optimizing the organization and delivery of the treatment. If a medical compromise has to be accepted it is vital to have maximal information about the consequences of any decisions taken during the treatment planning process. From quantitative radiobiology [2] and clinical experience [3, 4] we know that the dose-response curves for many organs at risk (OAR) in the pelvis are almost as steep as the dose fall-off curve of BT, implying that we may often balance on the knife's edge between success and failure in our attempt to selectively deliver a high curative dose to the tumor.

Over decades of traditional X-ray–based two-dimensional BT for gynecological cancer, invaluable experience has been gained in treatment planning [4–8]. With the advent of image-based BT, new volumetric (3D) and temporal (4D) information has deepened our understanding of BT thus far [9–18] but also presents us with new medical challenges and concepts that must be understood and interpreted correctly to reap the potential benefit of image-based BT treatment planning [19].

J.C. Lindegaard (✉)
Department of Oncology, Aarhus University Hospital,
Nörrebrogade 44, 8000 Aarhus C, Denmark
e-mail: jacolind@rm.dk

R. Pötter
Department of Radiotherapy, Vienna General Hospital,
Medical University of Vienna, Währinger Gürtel 18-20, 1090 Vienna, Austria

E.Van Limbergen
Department of Radiotherapy, University Hospital Gasthuisberg, Herestraat 49,
3000 Leuven, Belgium

C. Haie-Meder
Department of Radiotherapy, Brachytherapy Unit, Institut Gustave Roussy,
39 Rue Camille Desmoulins, 94800 Villejuif, France

A.N. Viswanathan et al. (eds.), *Gynecologic Radiation Therapy*,
DOI: 10.1007/978-3-540-68958-4_10,

The aim of this chapter is to focus on the general medical aspect of the treatment planning process in image-guided BT in gynecology, not only at the overall strategic level but also for optimization of the individual BT implant and BT fraction. Inevitably, this chapter will reflect the fact that most of our experience with image guidance so far has been accumulated in the treatment of locally advanced cervical cancer.

10.2 Implant and Fractionation Strategies for Image-Guided BT in Gynecology

For gynecological malignancies in general and cervical cancer in particular, BT is most often used in combination with external-beam radiotherapy (EBRT) [20]. Typically, the elective pelvic nodes are treated with EBRT to a dose level of 45–50 Gy given in 1.7–2.0 Gy/fraction. From this dose, level BT is used to boost the primary tumor to much higher doses, e.g., 75–95 Gy [20–22]. The fundamental rules and principles for applying traditional X-ray–based BT with EBRT are similar for image-guided BT, but are likely more important to respect, since the dose delivered by BT is now tailored closely to the tumor extension as presented on imaging at the time of BT, using a plan-of-the-day approach [19].

Tumor regression during EBRT evaluated in 3D is often significant and may amount to 70–80% of the pre-therapeutic tumor volume [23–27]. The majority of the tumor regression occurs during the first 3–4 weeks of treatment with little further effect observed during the final 2–3 weeks of treatment. To take maximal advantage of this regression pattern, which in fact is the very essence of the 4D image-guided adaptive BT concept [18, 19], and also to avoid the detrimental effect of prolonging the overall treatment time beyond 7 weeks [28–30], it is recommended to deliver BT during the last 2–3 weeks of the 6–7 week overall treatment period. For small or radiosensitive tumors, BT may be delivered early (i.e., weeks 4–6), whereas the full time frame of 7 weeks is needed for large tumors with poor response.

Treatment planning for image-guided BT is more demanding upon both patient and staff than traditional X-ray–based BT [31]. The possible advantages of more complex applicators used with 3D imaging (e.g., combined intracavitary/interstitial techniques [32] or custom-made vaginal molds [33]) may require a rethinking of the overall implant and fractionation strategy when switching from X-ray–based to 3D image-guided BT. Thus, the more complex the implant, the more important it is to deliver the entire BT dose in one or two implants with ideal geometry. For pulsed dose rate (PDR) the optimal schedule may involve fewer implants and larger fraction sizes with the dose delivered by an increasing number of pulses [13, 15, 16]. For high dose rate (HDR) a hybrid strategy has been developed in which more than one fraction of BT is delivered through the same implant over a few days [14, 34].

With fewer implants, the demand for a perfect implant from day 1 increases, especially with large and inaccessible tumors. 3D image-guided BT is therefore not an appropriate tool for improving the capabilities of a suboptimal implant. On the contrary, to confirm the choice of applicator and to determine the need for "add-ons" such as needles or cylinders [13, 35], or to produce an individualized vaginal applicator such as a mold [33], several institutions hold a preplanning session, especially for difficult cases. One approach is to

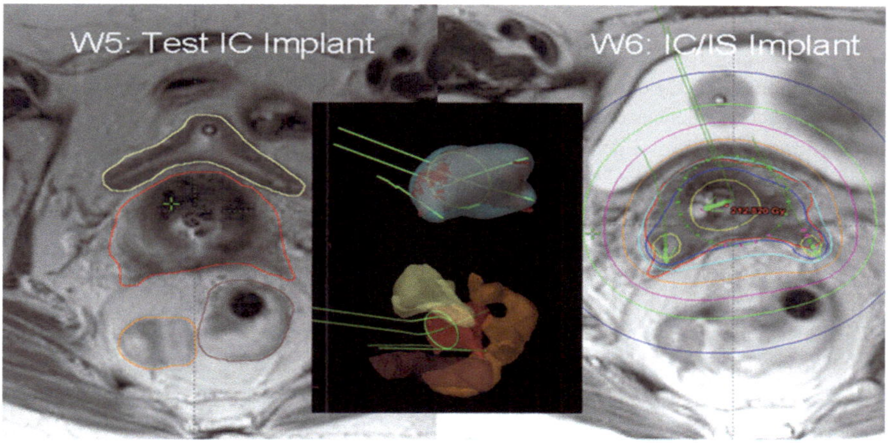

Fig. 10.1 An example of image-guidance used for planning of a combined intracavitary/interstitial (IC/IS) implant in a locally advanced cervical cancer with poor response to initial EBRT and concomitant Cisplatin. In week 5 (W5) of the treatment, a test implant was performed with the basic IC applicator (tandem–ring). Magnetic resonance imaging (MRI) was performed and a virtual treatment plan using two free titanium needles was generated. The actual IC/IS implant was performed in week 6 (W6): the titanium needles were inserted at specific positions and to a predetermined depth. The first brachytherapy (BT) fraction was then delivered on the W6 IC/IS implant. A second and similar IC/IS implant was performed in week 7

perform a magnetic resonance imaging (MRI) with the basic intracavitary element of the BT applicator in situ a few days before the actual implant to work out an individualized MRI-based implantation plan (Fig. 10.1).

There are no firm data on how to optimize the fractionation of image-guided BT. However, it is well known that acute and late radiation morbidity may be correlated with each other [36], which argues against combining concomitant chemotherapy involving multiple drug regimens [37] with high-dose-rate brachytherapy or accelerated radiotherapy regimens requiring a high weekly cumulative dose [38, 39]. Most institutions using HDR would therefore not give more than 2 BT fractions per week for a cumulative prescribed BT dose of 15–18 Gy (EQD2). For PDR with protracted dose delivery over 40–60 h (average dose rate <0.6 Gy/h), this issue is less relevant; but for higher dose rates (i.e., around 1 Gy/h) it may be important.

10.3 Evaluating the Combined Treatment Plan of EBRT and BT

A fundamental prerequisite for image-based BT treatment planning is the ability to evaluate the cumulative dose delivered by EBRT and BT in 3D [22]. Currently a simplistic approach is generally accepted: it assumes mono-exponential repair with repair half time of 1.5 h and the linear–quadratic model with values for α/β of 10 for tumor and 3 for organs at risk [13, 15–17, 40]. By applying this model and summing the equivalent dose in 2 Gy fractions (EQD2) derived from EBRT and BT, a total dose can be calculated. The validity and consequences of the radiobiological uncertainties of these assumptions for the calculation of cumulative dose are discussed in Chap. 7. Obviously, the radiobiological calculations are most critical for comparison of DVH parameters between institutions and when major changes are made within an institution; for instance, changing from PDR to HDR or vice versa. For a commonly employed fractionation schedule of EBRT and BT, less emphasis is given to radiobiological uncertainties, as these calculations mainly will reflect relative changes in DVH parameters [13].

Another important issue is the sensitivity of the calculation method to a heterogeneous EBRT dose distribution, especially for the central pelvis, where a significant dose from BT will also be delivered [19]. For EBRT delivered with a conformal box technique, dose homogeneity should not be an issue, and the dose delivered by EBRT to the International Commission on Radiation Units and Measurements (ICRU) reference point can readily be used for further calculations. However, when several EBRT dose levels are used (for instance, to boost the parametria or metastatic pelvic nodes in close proximity to the BT target), a tail of EBRT dose spillage may incur on the critical volumes receiving a high dose from BT. In this situation a complex evaluation is needed to establish the maximal dose the most irradiated volumes of the organs at risk (OAR) are likely to receive from EBRT. In contrast, the minimal dose received from EBRT should be used for the tumor targets (High Risk Clinical Target Volume [HR CTV] and Intermediate Risk Clinical Target Volume [IR CTV]). Therefore, from the outset of BT treatment plan optimization, the use of multiple dose levels of EBRT may call for extremely careful selection of the BT dose distribution.

Adding doses from EBRT and BT implies a conservative approach in assuming a stable geometry between the most exposed parts of the OAR and the BT sources, both during BT fractions and between BT implants, i.e., confirming that the same part of the OAR receives the high dose from BT for each fraction and/or implant. While geometric stability may be a reasonable assumption for rectum and vagina, the often large changes in the 3D shapes of the sigmoid, bowel, and bladder in relation to the BT sources may lead to overestimation of the total dose to these organs. Before reducing the dose to the tumor target, it is therefore important to carefully evaluate the mobility of these organs from implant to implant.

10.4 Dose Prescription and DVH Constraints for Image-Guided BT

Point A and the 60 Gy ICRU38 reference volume have been the dominating concepts in traditional X-ray–based treatment planning and reporting in gynecological BT for decades [42, 43]. Like traditional X-ray–based EBRT, in which the target and the treatment technique are determined in one step (for instance four-field box), there is no clear distinction between target and treatment planning for 2D BT – point A representing the point for both dose prescription and dose reporting. With 3D BT, a conceptual change has occurred by which target definition, treatment planning, and dose reporting now are performed in

Table 10.1 Dose volume parameters from five institutions for the high risk clinical target volume (HR CTV) and organs at risk using MRI-guided brachytherapy in locally advanced cervix cancer treated and reported according to the Groupe Européen de Curiethérapie - European Society for Therapeutic Radiology and Oncology (GEC ESTRO) guidelines

Department	Dose rate & applicator	No. of pts.	HR CTV D90 (EQD2)	Bladder D_{2cc} (EQD2)	Rectum D_{2cc} (EQD2)	Sigmoid D_{2cc} (EQD2)
Vienna	HDR/ring	141	86	95	65	62
Leuven	PDR/ovoids	56	82	85	63	66
Paris	PDR/mould	45	75	72	61	61
Utrecht	PDR/ovoids	29	88	83	67	61
Aarhus	PDR/ring	100	91	72	65	67

independent steps. The HR CTV and IR CTV used in image-based 3D BT have nevertheless emerged from the traditions of 2D BT [21].

Since the HR CTV includes remaining tumor at the time of BT, a high dose (similar to the dose previously prescribed for point A) is recommended [21, 44]. As the dose is prescribed to a volume, the Dose Volume Histogram (DVH) parameters D100 and D90 are used. However, the D100 is sensitive to small uncertainties in contouring and dose calculations in the treatment planning system. The D90 is a much more robust and representative DVH parameter for the dose to the HR CTV and is therefore used in most institutions. Now there is insufficient knowledge on the impact of different prognostic factors on the relation between dose to the HR CTV and local control (see Chap. 12). Most institutions are currently aiming for a D90 of at least 85 Gy (EQD2) for optimization of the dose to the HR CTV (Table 10.1), which is supported by a recent analysis showing a clear dose-response relationship with less than 4% risk of local recurrence if a D90 of more than 87 Gy (EQD2) is reached [45, 46]. For the D100 a somewhat smaller dose (65–75 Gy) (EQD2) is usually reported. When the D100 is small it is important to visually inspect the BT plan to avoid a contiguous volume of underdosage that would be large enough (1–2 cc) to potentially harbor the origin of a recurrence.

For the IR CTV, this concept is linked to the extension of the primary tumor at diagnosis [21]. The purpose of the IR CTV is primarily to ensure that a sufficient dose is delivered to positions from which the macroscopic tumor has withdrawn but where a significant risk of microscopic disease remains. In most situations the contour of the IR CTV will be situated sufficiently close to the HR CTV such that the intended dose level (i.e., 60 Gy EQD2) will be reached in the IR CTV even when dose optimization is performed for the HR CTV only. However, for specific topographic situations such as distal vaginal involvement at diagnosis with marked regression at time of BT, sufficient coverage of IR CTV is not guaranteed and merits special attention, for instance by additional loading in the vagina.

Due to the steep gradient involved in gynecological BT, for instance, as compared to intensity modulated radiotherapy (IMRT), an accurate evaluation of the dose to the most exposed part of the OAR requires a DVH analysis based on doses to absolute volumes [22]. Currently it is recommended to evaluate the minimal dose to the most exposed $D_{0.1cc}$ and D_{2cc} of the OAR. Providing that the thickness of the OAR wall is in the range 2–4 mm

[47, 48], the diameter of the most exposed surface of the organ at the D_{2cc} level will be in the region of 25–35 mm and at the $D_{0.1cc}$ level, 6–8 mm. Thus, taking, e.g., the rectum as the model, the dose at the $D_{0.1cc}$ level may be relevant for the development of ulceration, necrosis, and fistula and at the D_{2cc} level for telangiectasia.

Current DVH constraints for both PDR [13, 15–17] and HDR [14, 40] are 90 Gy (EQD2) for bladder and 70–75 Gy (EQD2) for both rectum and sigmoid as minimal doses to the most exposed D_{2cc} of the OAR. The clinical relevance of using a 70–75 Gy constraint for rectum has recently been proven [49], whereas clinical dose-effect relationships for sigmoid, bowel, and bladder still need to be defined. There are no generally accepted constraints for the $D_{0.1cc}$ level. However, the $D_{0.1cc}$ and the D_{2cc} doses are inherently linked (Fig. 10.2). By analyzing the DVH data from the Aarhus series [13, 41], DVH constraints at the D_{2cc} level of 70–75 and 90 Gy would reflect dose constraints of about 80–85 and 110–115 Gy at the $D_{0.1cc}$ level, respectively. However, as shown in Fig. 10.2, the deviations from the tendency line may amount to 5–10 Gy in individual patients, meaning that the $D_{0.1cc}$ dose should always be reviewed individually by DVH analysis.

It is important to remember that current DVH constraints are recommended only for BT combined with homogenous whole-pelvic EBRT given to a dose level of 45–50 Gy. If

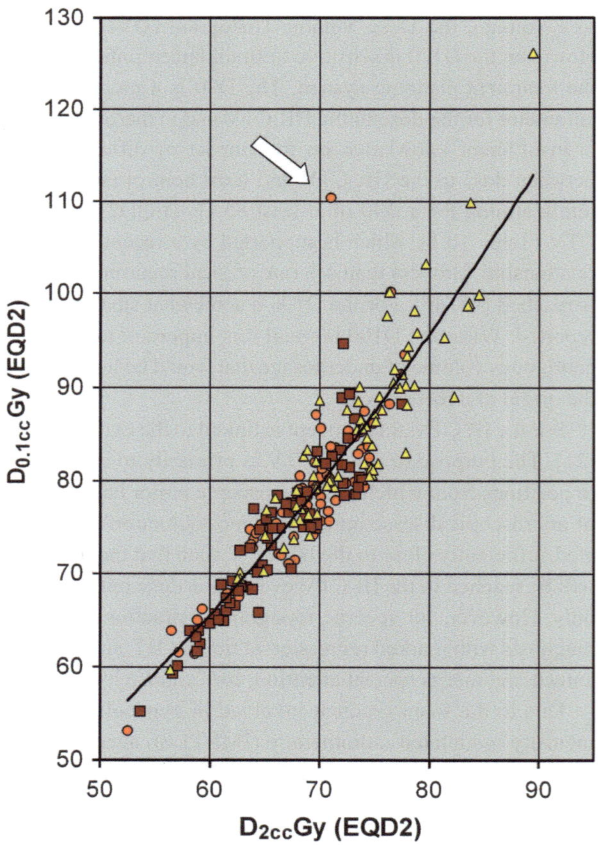

Fig. 10.2 Relationship between minimal dose (EQD2) to the most exposed D_{2cc} and $D_{0.1cc}$ of organs at risk (OAR) (yellow = bladder; brown= rectum, orange = sigmoid) in 72 patients treated at Aarhus University Hospital [41]. This figure demonstrates the relationship between the minimal doses to the most exposed $D_{0.1cc}$ and D_{2cc} of the OAR. However, the deviations from the tendency line may amount to 5–10 Gy on the level of the individual patients. The sigmoid outlier with a $D_{0.1cc}$ =110 Gy (*white arrow*) despite an acceptable D_{2cc} was caused by unintentional loading in a needle stopping position in the vicinity of the sigmoid. This example illustrates the importance of tracking the DVH parameters at both OAR volume levels as a quality assurance measure in adaptive BT dose planning

significant parts of the OAR are exposed to higher EBRT doses, these constraints should be used with caution, and it may also be necessary to evaluate the dose to D_{5cc} and even D_{10cc}. However, there are not yet any recommended DVH constraints for this situation. Representative mean DVH values reported for bladder, rectum, and sigmoid derived from image-guided 3D BT in cervical cancer are given in Table 10.1.

Due to difficulties in defining the vagina on images and the steep dose gradients with very close proximity to BT sources, a meaningful DVH analysis and correlation of dose to vaginal morbidity have so far been impossible [50]. A practical approach to this problem is to inspect the high dose volumes (200% and 400%) of the optimized plan intended for treatment to ensure that these very high doses are kept inside the applicator to the same degree as with a non-optimized standard plan. For bowel there are currently also no available constraints. Several institutions have chosen to tackle this problem by contouring bowel loops within 1–2 cm of the HR CTV and evaluating these by the same method used for the sigmoid.

In addition to dose, it is also necessary to know the position of the most exposed parts of the organ and whether they are positioned in continuous or separate volumes. For instance, the bladder neck is believed to be more sensitive than the posterior bladder wall, and even 90 Gy may affect voiding [19]. However, the bladder neck is normally positioned caudally to the vaginal source, probably explaining the lack of significant morbidity in many patients treated with doses even higher than 90 Gy [40]. For the rectum and sigmoid, special attention has to be directed toward the transition zone. If the volume of the most exposed part of rectum and sigmoid is confluent, the DVH parameters may be underestimating the D_{2cc} dose by as much as 4–5 Gy [51]. In this situation, a combined rectosigmoid reference structure should be contoured and evaluated by separate DVH analysis.

10.5 Quantitative Impact of Image-Based Dose Optimization

Image-based DVH analysis of standard point A prescription has shown highly variable tumor doses, resulting in target doses (D90 of HR CTV) ranging from 52–160% of the prescription dose [13]. This effect is mainly caused by the inverse square law [19, 41], such that only tumors with a HR CTV of less than 30–35 cm^3 are likely to receive a tumoricidal dose (Fig. 10.3). Treatment plan optimization makes it possible to expand the prescription isodose by 5 mm for an intracavitary implant [12] and by about 15 mm for a combined intracavitary/interstitial implant [11]. As shown in Fig. 10.3, the D90 of the HR CTV for image-based implants is much less depending on target volume making it possible to deliver sufficient dose also to poorly responding tumors with a HR CTV volume measuring 80–100 cm^3 [19, 41].

For the OAR, the ICRU reference points have been shown to underestimate the maximal dose to the bladder as evaluated by the minimal dose to the most exposed D_{2cc} [9, 10, 13, 16]. For the rectum there is a better correlation between the ICRU reference point and the D_{2cc} [9], but often the most exposed part of the rectum receives a higher point dose [52], and for the sigmoid no system for evaluation has been available. By evaluation of dose

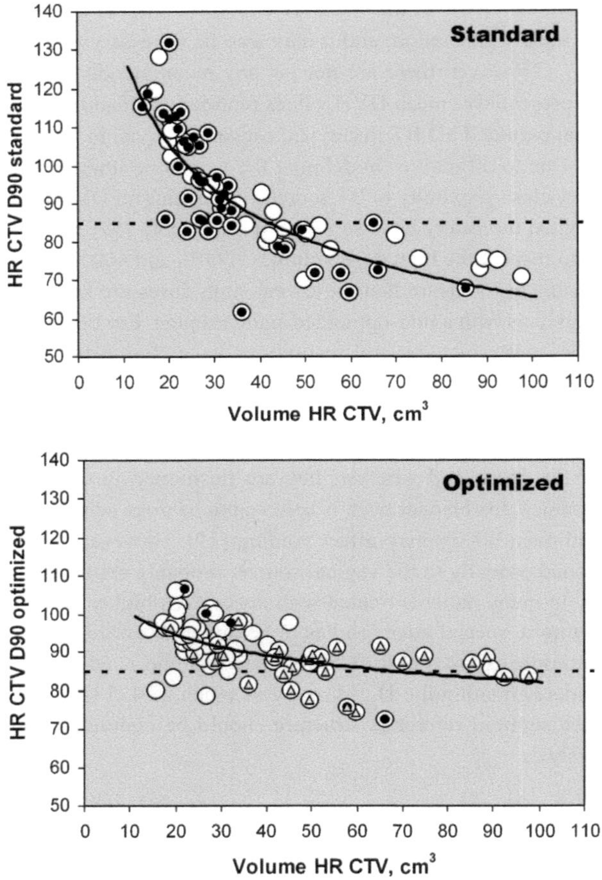

Fig. 10.3 D90 as a function of high risk clinical target volume (HR CTV) volume comparing standard 2D and optimized 3D treatment plans in a consecutive series of 72 locally advanced cervix cancer patients treated at Aarhus University Hospital with tandem and ring intracavitary brachytherapy plus additional interstitial needles in selected cases [41]. The black horizontal line indicates the desired D90 of 85 Gy for HR CTV. The OAR constraints were not respected in patients with a black dot. In patients with yellow triangles interstitial needles were applied (optimized plans). All constraints (HR CTV *and* OAR) were met in 14/72 patients for standard versus in 56/72 patients for optimized plans ($p < 0.0001$, two-tailed Fishers Exact Test)

distribution derived from 2D BT standard plans, both De Brabandere et al. [16] and Lindegaard et al. [13] found that DVH constraints were exceeded in the majority of patients. However, MRI-based dose optimization has made it possible to avoid this situation and even to increase the dose to the tumor [17, 41].

The benefit of optimization has been shown to depend on the tumor volume (Fig. 10.3). For small tumors, where the OAR may be in close proximity to the BT sources, the benefit of optimization is mainly the reduction of the treated volume, i.e., the prescription isodose is moving closer to the applicator, and overdosing of the OAR is avoided [17]. Comparing an optimized to a standard plan may demonstrate a 30–40% change in point A dose. For large tumors the OAR are often displaced by the tumor, and the primary objective is obtain better tumor coverage. In this situation the point A dose will increase and sometimes become meaningless if needles are loaded close by [11, 13]. However, it is recommended to still report the dose to point A to ensure consistent communication between centers [22].

10.6 Conclusion

3D imaging with the applicator in situ is a powerful tool for treatment planning of BT in gynecological cancer. Compared to X-ray–based BT, 3D imaging has been shown to provide a much more precise estimation of where the BT dose is actually placed in the patient. Equally important is the fact that 3D image-guided treatment planning also provides a channel for communication and research, including better dose-response data, which will enable us to fine-tune the currently used prescription doses and DVH constraints to further improve the therapeutic ratio in the individual patient.

References

1. Holthusen H. Erfahrungen über die Verträglichkeitsgrenze für Röntgenstrahlung and deren Nutzanwendung zur Verhütung von Schäden. Strahlentherapie. 1936;57:254–69.
2. Bentzen SM. Quantitative clinical radiobiology. Acta Oncol. 1993;32(3):259–75.
3. Petereit DG, Sarkaria JN, Potter DM, Schink JC. High-dose-rate versus low-dose-rate brachytherapy in the treatment of cervical cancer: analysis of tumor recurrence–the University of Wisconsin experience. Int J Radiat Oncol Biol Phys. 1999;45(5):1267–74.
4. Perez CA, Grigsby PW, Chao KS, Mutch DG, Lockett MA. Tumor size, irradiation dose, and long-term outcome of carcinoma of uterine cervix. Int J Radiat Oncol Biol Phys. 1998;41(2): 307–17.
5. Eifel PJ, Thoms Jr WW, Smith TL, Morris M, Oswald MJ. The relationship between brachytherapy dose and outcome in patients with bulky endocervical tumors treated with radiation alone. Int J Radiat Oncol Biol Phys. 1994;28(1):113–8.
6. Pernot M, Hoffstetter S, Peiffert D, Carolus JM, Guillemin F, Verhaeghe JL, et al. Statistical study of a series of 672 cases of carcinoma of the uterine cervix. Results and complications according to age and modalities of treatment. Bull Cancer. 1995;82(7):568–81.
7. Gerbaulet A, Michel G, Haie-Meder C, Castaigne D, Lartigau E, L'Homme C, et al. The role of low dose rate brachytherapy in the treatment of cervix carcinoma. Experience of the Gustave-Roussy Institute on 1245 patients. Eur J Gynaecol Oncol. 1995;16(6):461–75.
8. Horiot JC, Pigneux J, Pourquier H, Schraub S, Achille E, Keiling R, et al. Radiotherapy alone in carcinoma of the intact uterine cervix according to G. H. Fletcher guidelines: a French cooperative study of 1383 cases. Int J Radiat Oncol Biol Phys. 1988; 14(4):605–11.
9. Pelloski CE, Palmer M, Chronowski GM, Jhingran A, Horton J, Eifel PJ. Comparison between CT-based volumetric calculations and ICRU reference-point estimates of radiation doses delivered to bladder and rectum during intracavitary radiotherapy for cervical cancer. Int J Radiat Oncol Biol Phys. 2005;62(1):131–7.
10. Barillot I, Horiot JC, Maingon P, Bone-Lepinoy MC, Vaillant D, Feutray S. Maximum and mean bladder dose defined from ultrasonography. Comparison with the ICRU reference in gynaecological brachytherapy. Radiother Oncol. 1994;30(3):231–8.
11. Kirisits C, Lang S, Dimopoulos J, Berger D, Georg D, Potter R. The Vienna applicator for combined intracavitary and interstitial brachytherapy of cervical cancer: design, application, treatment planning, and dosimetric results. Int J Radiat Oncol Biol Phys. 2006; 65(2):624–30.

12. Kirisits C, Potter R, Lang S, Dimopoulos J, Wachter-Gerstner N, Georg D. Dose and volume parameters for MRI-based treatment planning in intracavitary brachytherapy for cervical cancer. Int J Radiat Oncol Biol Phys. 2005;62(3):901–11.
13. Lindegaard JC, Tanderup K, Nielsen SK, Haack S, Gelineck J. MRI-guided 3D optimization significantly improves DVH parameters of pulsed dose rate brachytherapy in locally advanced cervical cancer. Int J Radiat Oncol Biol Phys. 2008;71(3):756–64.
14. Viswanathan AN, Cormack R, Holloway CL, Tanaka C, O'Farrell D, Devlin PM, et al. Magnetic resonance-guided interstitial therapy for vaginal recurrence of endometrial cancer. Int J Radiat Oncol Biol Phys. 2006;66(1):91–9.
15. Chargari C, Magne N, Dumas I, Messai T, Vicenzi L, Gillion N, et al. Physics Contributions and Clinical Outcome with 3D-MRI-Based Pulsed-Dose-Rate Intracavitary Brachytherapy in Cervical Cancer Patients. Int J Radiat Oncol Biol Phys. 2008;74(1):133–9.
16. De Brabandere M, Mousa AG, Nulens A, Swinnen A, Van LE. Potential of dose optimisation in MRI-based PDR brachytherapy of cervix carcinoma. Radiother Oncol. 2008;88(2): 217–26.
17. Jurgenliemk-Schulz IM, Tersteeg RJ, Roesink JM, Bijmolt S, Nomden CN, Moerland MA, et al. MRI-guided treatment-planning optimisation in intracavitary or combined intracavitary/interstitial PDR brachytherapy using tandem ovoid applicators in locally advanced cervical cancer. Radiother Oncol. 2009;93(2):322–30.
18. Tanderup K, Georg D, Pötter R, Kirisits C, Grau C, Lindegaard JC. Adaptive management of cervical cancer radiotherapy. Sem Radiat Oncol. 2010; 20(2):121–9.
19. Pötter R, Kirisits C, Fidarova EF, Dimopoulos JC, Berger D, Tanderup K, et al. Present status and future of high-precision image-guided adaptive brachytherapy for cervix carcinoma. Acta Oncol. 2008;47(7):1325–36.
20. Gerbaulet A, Pötter R, Mazeron JJ, Meertens H, van Limbergen E. The GEC ESTRO Handbook of Brachytherapy. 1 ed. 2002. ESTRO, Brussels, www.estro-education.org
21. Haie-Meder C, Potter R, van Limbergen E, Briot E, De Brabandere M, Dimopoulos J, et al. Recommendations from Gynaecological (GYN) GEC-ESTRO Working Group (I): concepts and terms in 3D image based 3D treatment planning in cervix cancer brachytherapy with emphasis on MRI assessment of GTV and CTV. Radiother Oncol. 2005;74(3):235–45.
22. Pötter R, Haie-Meder C, Limbergen EV, Barillot I, Brabandere MD, Dimopoulos J, et al. Recommendations from gynaecological (GYN) GEC ESTRO working group (II): concepts and terms in 3D image-based treatment planning in cervix cancer brachytherapy-3D dose volume parameters and aspects of 3D image-based anatomy, radiation physics, radiobiology. Radiother Oncol. 2006;78(1):67–77.
23. Mayr NA, Yuh WT, Taoka T, Wang JZ, Wu DH, Montebello JF, et al. Serial therapy-induced changes in tumor shape in cervical cancer and their impact on assessing tumor volume and treatment response. AJR Am J Roentgenol. 2006;187(1):65–72.
24. Beadle BM, Jhingran A, Salehpour M, Sam M, Iyer RB, Eifel PJ. Cervix regression and motion during the course of external beam chemoradiation for cervical cancer. Int J Radiat Oncol Biol Phys. 2009;73:235–41.
25. Lim K, Chan P, Dinniwell R, Fyles A, Haider M, Cho YB, et al. Cervical cancer regression measured using weekly magnetic resonance imaging during fractionated radiotherapy: radiobiologic modeling and correlation with tumor hypoxia. Int J Radiat Oncol Biol Phys. 2008;70(1):126–33.
26. van de Bunt L, van der Heide UA, Ketelaars M, de Kort GA, Jurgenliemk-Schulz IM. Conventional, conformal, and intensity-modulated radiation therapy treatment planning of external beam radiotherapy for cervical cancer: the impact of tumor regression. Int J Radiat Oncol Biol Phys. 2006;64(1):189–96.
27. Dimopoulos JC, Schirl G, Baldinger A, Helbich TH, Potter R. MRI assessment of cervical cancer for adaptive radiotherapy. Strahlenther Onkol. 2009;185(5):282–7.

28. Fyles AW, Pintilie M, Kirkbride P, Levin W, Manchul LA, Rawlings GA. Prognostic factors in patients with cervix cancer treated by radiation therapy: results of a multiple regression analysis. Radiother Oncol. 1995;35(2):107–17.
29. Petereit DG, Sarkaria JN, Chappell R, Fowler JF, Hartmann TJ, Kinsella TJ, et al. The adverse effect of treatment prolongation in cervical carcinoma. Int J Radiat Oncol Biol Phys. 1995;32(5):1301–7.
30. Chen SW, Liang JA, Yang SN, Ko HL, Lin FJ. The adverse effect of treatment prolongation in cervical cancer by high-dose-rate intracavitary brachytherapy. Radiother Oncol. 2003;67(1): 69–76.
31. Pötter R, Kirisits C, Lievens Y. What kind of equipment do we need in gynaecological brachytherapy? Clinical, technical and econimical aspects for standard and new techniques. Radiother Oncol. 2005;75 Suppl 1:S1.
32. Dimopoulos JC, Kirisits C, Petric P, Georg P, Lang S, Berger D, et al. The Vienna applicator for combined intracavitary and interstitial brachytherapy of cervical cancer: clinical feasibility and preliminary results. Int J Radiat Oncol Biol Phys. 2006;66(1):83–90.
33. Albano M, Dumas I, Haie-Meder C. Brachytherapy at the Institut Gustave-Roussy: personalized vaginal mould applicator: technical modification and improvement. Cancer Radiother. 2008;12:822–6.
34. Kirisits C, Lang S, Dimopoulos J, Oechs K, Georg D, Pötter R. Uncertainties when using only one MRI-based treatment plan for subsequent high-dose-rate tandem and ring applications in brachytherapy of cervix cancer. Radiother Oncol. 2006;81(3):269–75.
35. Petric P, Hudej R, Music M. MRI assisted cervix cancer brachytherapy pre-planning, based on insertion of the applicator in para-cervical anaesthesia: preliminary results of a prospective study. J Contemp Brachytherapy. 2009;3:163–9.
36. Wang CJ, Leung SW, Chen HC, Sun LM, Fang FM, Huang EY, et al. The correlation of acute toxicity and late rectal injury in radiotherapy for cervical carcinoma: evidence suggestive of consequential late effect (CQLE). Int J Radiat Oncol Biol Phys. 1998;40(1):85–91.
37. Rose PG, Bundy BN, Watkins EB, Thigpen JT, Deppe G, Maiman MA, et al. Concurrent cisplatin-based radiotherapy and chemotherapy for locally advanced cervical cancer. New Engl J Med. 1999;340:1144–53.
38. Serkies K, Kobierska A, Konopa K, Sawicki T, Jassem J. The feasibility study on continuous 7-day-a-week external beam irradiation in locally advanced cervical cancer: a report on acute toxicity. Radiother Oncol. 2001;61(2):197–202.
39. Hellebust TP, Kristensen GB, Olsen DR. Late effects after radiotherapy for locally advanced cervical cancer: comparison of two brachytherapy schedules and effect of dose delivered weekly. Int J Radiat Oncol Biol Phys 2009;76(3):713–8.
40. Pötter R, Dimopoulos J, Georg P, Lang S, Waldhausl C, Wachter-Gerstner N, et al. Clinical impact of MRI assisted dose volume adaptation and dose escalation in brachytherapy of locally advanced cervix cancer. Radiother Oncol. 2007;83(2):148–55.
41. Tanderup K, Nielsen SK, Nyvang G, Pedersen EP, Røhl L, Fokdal L, et al. From point A to the sculpted pear: MR image guidance significantly improves tumour dose and sparing of organs at risk in brachytherapy of cervical cancer. Radiother Oncol. 2010;94(2):173–80.
42. International Commission on Radiation Units and Measurements, ICRU Report 38. Dose and volume specifications for reporting intracavitary therapy in gynaecology. Bethesda: ICRU; 1985.
43. Pötter R, van Limbergen E, Gerstner N, Wambersie A. Survey of the use of the ICRU 38 in recording and reporting cervical cancer brachytherapy. Radiother Oncol. 2001;58(1):11–8.
44. Pötter R, Dimopoulos J, Kirisits C, Lang S, Haie-Meder C, Briot E, et al. Recommendations for image-based intracavitary brachytherapy of cervix cancer: the GYN GEC ESTRO Working Group point of view: in regard to Nag et al. (Int J Radiat Oncol Biol Phys. 2004;60:1160–72). Int J Radiat Oncol Biol Phys. 2005 ;62(1):293–5.

45. Dimopoulos JC, Lang S, Kirisits C, Fidarova EF, Berger D, Georg P, et al. Dose-volume histogram parameters and local tumor control in magnetic resonance image-guided cervical cancer brachytherapy. Int J Radiat Oncol Biol Phys. 2009;75(1):56–63.
46. Dimopoulos JC, Potter R, Lang S, Fidarova E, Georg P, Dorr W, et al. Dose-effect relationship for local control of cervical cancer by magnetic resonance image-guided brachytherapy. Radiother Oncol. 2009;93(2):311–5.
47. van den Bergh F, Meertens H, Moonen L, van Bunningen B, Blom A. The use of a transverse CT image for the estimation of the dose given to the rectum in intracavitary brachytherapy for carcinoma of the cervix. Radiother Oncol. 1998;47(1):85–90.
48. Blatt AH, Titus J, Chan L. Ultrasound measurement of bladder wall thickness in the assessment of voiding dysfunction. J Urol. 2008;179(6):2275–8.
49. Georg P, Kirisits C, Goldner G, Dorr W, Hammer J, Potzi R, et al. Correlation of dose-volume parameters, endoscopic and clinical rectal side effects in cervix cancer patients treated with definitive radiotherapy including MRI-based brachytherapy. Radiother Oncol. 2009;91(2):173–80.
50. Berger D, Dimopoulos J, Georg P, Georg D, Potter R, Kirisits C. Uncertainties in assessment of the vaginal dose for intracavitary brachytherapy of cervical cancer using a tandem-ring applicator. Int J Radiat Oncol Biol Phys. 2007;67(5):1451–9.
51. Lang S, Trodella L, Kirisits C, Dimopoulos J, Georg D, Pötter R. Dose reporting for rectum and sigmoid colon in 3D image based brachytherapy for cervical cancer: the importance of the location of the rectosigmoid junction. Radiother Oncol. 2008;88:S91.
52. Cheng JC, Peng LC, Chen YH, Huang DY, Wu JK, Jian JJ. Unique role of proximal rectal dose in late rectal complications for patients with cervical cancer undergoing high-dose-rate intracavitary brachytherapy. Int J Radiat Oncol Biol Phys. 2003;57(4):1010–8.

Radiobiological Aspects of Brachytherapy in the Era of 3-Dimensional Imaging

11

Alexandra J. Stewart and Søren M. Bentzen

11.1 Introduction

Radiobiological principles are increasingly well understood for external beam radiotherapy (EBRT) for a variety of tumor histologies and the associated normal tissue effects. Application of this knowledge in the daily use of brachytherapy is much more challenging, although equally important. Brachytherapy was initially developed empirically with dose being determined predominantly by clinical effect. In the modern era, radiobiological modeling is used to predict the biological effect of varying dose prescriptions. The challenges involved in applying radiobiological principles within brachytherapy have been emphasized by the move from low dose rate (LDR) treatment to fractionated high dose rate (HDR) and pulsed brachytherapy (PB) treatment. Radiobiological thinking in the early era of HDR predicted a worse efficacy: toxicity ratio for HDR compared with LDR [1–3]. It is only relatively recently that the reasons why this was not seen in clinical trials have become clearer. Of course, it must be remembered that source placement remains the single most important factor in brachytherapy such that, in an implant with poor geometry, changing radiobiologic factors, such as fractionation or dose rate, may not ensure an acceptable clinical outcome.

A.J. Stewart (✉)
Consultant Clinical Oncologist, St Luke's Cancer Centre,
Royal Surrey County Hospital, Egerton Rd,
Guildford, GU2 7XX, England
e-mail: Alexandra.stewart@nhs.net

S.M. Bentzen
Department of Human Oncology, University of Wisconsin School of
Medicine and Public Health, K4/316 Clinical Science Center, 600 Highland Avenue,
Madison, WI 53792, USA

A.N. Viswanathan et al. (eds.), *Gynecologic Radiation Therapy*,
DOI: 10.1007/978-3-540-68958-4_11, © Springer-Verlag Berlin Heidelberg 2011

11.1.1 Dose Rates

Three ranges of brachytherapy dose rate were defined in the International Commission on Radiation Units and Measurements (ICRU) 38 report [4]:

- Low dose rate (LDR) – a range of 0.4–2 Gy/h.
- Medium dose rate (MDR) – a range of 2–12 Gy/h.
- High dose rate (HDR) – over 12 Gy/h.

Note, that dose-rate effects cannot be seen in isolation from total dose and overall treatment time. This is because sublethally damaged lesions (which govern the observed magnitude of the dose-rate effect) may repair during the ongoing treatment and the amount of such repair is time-dependent. Since the treatment time is in turn related to the prescribed dose it is clear that radiobiological characterization of LDR, MDR, and HDR cannot be achieved by consideration of dose rate alone [5].

Pulsed brachytherapy delivers radiation dose in short pulses in an attempt to achieve the dose optimization available with an HDR stepping source combined with the radiobiologic and toxicity profile associated with LDR brachytherapy. Generally, the same dose and overall time as an LDR implant are prescribed with the pulses delivered every 1 to 4 h. If PB is delivered at a pulse width of 10 min and a 1-h pulse interval, the dose is probably equivalent to LDR 60 cGy/h [6, 7] and has shown similar cell killing effects to LDR in vivo [8, 9]. If the dose per pulse is small (≤0.5 Gy) and the repair half time is over 30 min, the differential effect to LDR is less than 10% [10]. However, if the interval between pulses is longer, thus increasing the dose per pulse (over 2 Gy) or the tissue repair half time is under half an hour this is not the case and the PB effect becomes biologically closer to a highly fractionated HDR treatment, especially in close proximity to the source [11]. In this case, a similar biological effect will be achieved if a lower total dose than LDR is prescribed in the same overall time.

11.1.2 General Radiobiology Principles

The linear-quadratic (LQ) model is the most commonly used tool for estimating biologically equivalent dose (BED) adjusted for dose rate, dose per fraction, and overall treatment time [12, 13]. Historically the LQ model was introduced on the basis of hypothesized differences in the shape of the in vitro radiation cell survival curves for the putative target cells whose depletion was thought to cause early versus late side effects. With an increased appreciation of non-targeted effects of radiation as well as the importance of damage processing at the tissue level for the pathogenesis of many late side effects, the LQ model is now seen more as a heuristic formula for estimating equivalent dose for various time-dose-fractionation schemes [14]. For continuous irradiation the equivalent dose in 2-Gy fractions is estimated as

$$EQD_2 = D\cdot\frac{d\cdot g + \alpha/\beta}{2 + \alpha/\beta}$$

where D is the total dose, d is dose per fraction (i.e., the total dose in one brachytherapy application), and α/β is the endpoint-specific parameter quantifying the sensitivity to changes in dose per fraction or dose rate. Values of α/β estimated from human data for many normal tissue endpoints and tumors have been tabulated in Bentzen and Joiner [14]. For a single application d is equal to the total dose D. g is a function of the duration of delivery of dose d and the so-called recovery half time $T_{1/2}$:

$$g = \frac{2\left(\mu t - 1 + exp\left(-\mu t\right)\right)}{(\mu t)^2}$$

where $\mu = \log_e(2)/T_{1/2}$ For very short delivery time, i.e., $t << T_{1/2}$, g approaches 1. In this limit, the dose-rate effect disappears and the isoeffect formula becomes identical with the one that governs the effect of fractionated external beam (sometimes referred to as acute dose rate) radiotherapy. For very protracted delivery, i.e., very low dose rate, g tends to zero. The $T_{1/2}$ is also an endpoint-specific empirical parameter to be estimated from clinical data, a compilation of values are given in Bentzen and Joiner [14]. Some authors refer to $T_{1/2}$ as the repair half time. However, in a more general setting it may reflect other recovery processes in addition to sublethal damage repair. The $T_{1/2}$ of late normal tissue effects has been estimated to be in the range of anything from 1½ to 6 h or more [15, 16].

11.1.3 Validity of the LQ Model and the Precision of α/β Estimates

The α/β ratio is a measure of the fraction sensitivity of an endpoint, i.e., how much the BED will change in response to a change in fractionation or dose rate. Early endpoints have a high α/β ratio (10–20 Gy) and express damage from radiotherapy in the hours to days after exposure. Late endpoints have a low α/β ratio (0.5–6 Gy) and express damage in the months to years following exposure [17]. Typically in cervix cancer an α/β ratio of 10 Gy is used for tumor and 3 Gy for normal tissues [18]. In practice, this may be an underestimate for a squamous cell carcinoma and an overestimate for the rectum. However, use of an α/β ratio of 3 Gy for the rectum has been correlated with late rectal complications [19, 20] and thus can be considered a safe parameter to use. Similarly, a dose-response relationship can be seen in cervix cancer brachytherapy using an α/β ratio of 10 [21]. The α/β ratio for other late-responding normal tissues (small bowel, bladder, sigmoid) is again conventionally taken as 3 Gy and in these cases doses received have not been clearly correlated with late toxicity. Further follow-up and radiobiological modeling in the era of improved dosimetric analysis may allow a more accurate estimation of the true α/β ratio of these tissues.

There are concerns regarding the validity of the LQ model at very low or very high dose per fraction [14, 22]. Although no definite limits can be stated, it is felt that the LQ model is useful for dose per fraction ranging from around 1 Gy to 5–6 Gy. At the low dose per fraction, low dose hyper-radiosensitivity may mean that the LQ model will underestimate the actual biological effect. At high dose per fraction, there are data suggesting that the LQ model may overestimate the biological effect. This overestimation is likely to be more pronounced for endpoints characterized by low α/β values.

A second line of concern is the (lack of) precision of human estimates of α/β. For many human endpoints there are no estimates at all – but even where estimates are available, the relative precision of these limits our ability to extrapolate from standard doses to high dose per fraction.

11.1.4 Recovery Kinetics

There are experimental data showing fast and slow $T_{1/2}$ components for the same endpoint [23, 24]. However, multicomponent recovery kinetics has generally not been resolvable from clinical data sets. Consequently, most studies assume mono-exponential kinetics when trying to estimate recovery half times. As mentioned above, the recovery kinetics are a strong determinant of the dose-rate effect. For increasing recovery half times, the theoretical advantage of LDR over fractionated HDR brachytherapy will diminish [25].

It is generally assumed that the recovery taking place between fractionated HDR is mechanistically identical to the recovery taking place during continuous exposure. More specifically, it is assumed that the α/β and $T_{1/2}$ parameters characterizing the capacity for and the kinetics of recovery are the same in the two situations. Indeed, these parameters have been estimated from clinical data derived from both continuous LDR irradiation [26, 27] as well as from fractionated EBRT [16, 28]. Unfortunately, the $T_{1/2}$ estimates obtained under the two conditions are not very consistent. Roberts et al. analyzed tumor control and normal tissue complications in 517 patients who received brachytherapy for stage I or II cervix carcinoma at Christie Hospital in Manchester with over 5 years follow-up [27]. In four consecutive trials with a common control arm, patients were randomly allocated to treatment with radium (control group) or Cesium applicators (experimental group). Controls received 75 Gy to point A in two fractions at a dose rate of 0.53 Gy/h, in an overall time of 10–14 days. The experimental arm used dose rates of 1.5–1.7 Gy/h with total doses varying from 75 to 60 Gy. The authors fitted a series of models to the trial data, typically fixing one or more of the model parameters. No attempt was made to reduce the dose distribution to an equivalent dose: the prescribed dose to point A was used as the tumor dose and 60% of this dose was assumed to be the dose to organs at risk. The modeling concluded that high α/β ratios and short $T_{1/2}$ values provided the best fits for both tumor control and late effects. However, there were very large confidence limits associated with these estimates.

This leaves the $T_{1/2}$ estimates from fractionated EBRT as the main source of quantitative recovery kinetics. Estimates are available for head and neck mucositis [28] as well as for several late endpoints in humans [16], all of them pointing to considerably slower recovery kinetics than estimated from the above studies. For mucositis, a reanalysis of data from a number of trials of two or more fractions per day, provided estimates of $T_{1/2} > 2$ h or even longer. The data for late effects mainly originate from the CHART (continuous hyperfractionated accelerated radiotherapy) head and neck cancer trial where three fractions per day, with a minimum 6-h interval between fractions, were delivered on 12 consecutive days with estimated recovery half times of 3.8–4.9 h. The outcomes from several other altered fractionation trials are consistent with such long recovery half times, but unfortunately few independent estimates are available.

11.1.5 The Effect of Dose Distribution

The simple LQ formalism only applies to a uniform dose distribution or to the dose-time-fractionation at a specific reference point. This may be a fair approximation for EBRT where most delivery techniques aim for a uniform dose distribution in the target volume and where – at least historically – parallel opposing field and "box" techniques led to partial organ irradiation to a fairly uniform dose. With modern "conformal" delivery techniques such as intensity modulated radiotherapy (IMRT) and rotational delivery techniques, dose will vary as a function of location within most organs at risk. The same is generally true for brachytherapy dose distributions.

11.1.6 Concurrent or Sequential Chemoradiotherapy

The addition of cytotoxic chemotherapy or molecular targeted agents to a radiotherapy regime will result in a change in the biological effect on both tumors and normal tissues. Attempts to quantify these effects empirically [29] or through a modification of the LQ model [30, 31] have been made but there is still a lack of high-quality parameter estimates that allows quantification of these effects. Interactions between chemotherapy on one hand and dose-time-fractionation or dose-volume relationships on the other hand cannot be ruled out, although hard data on such effects are scarce.

11.2 The Application of Radiobiology in 3D Conformal Brachytherapy

With the advent of image-guided brachytherapy for gynecologic cancer we have moved from point-based to volume-based dose-prescribing. This has resulted in some differences in the application of radiobiology to clinical practice with an increased importance of the understanding of the role of radiobiology within brachytherapy prescribing. The main differences pertinent to radiobiology can be summarized as follows:

11.2.1 Moving from LDR to HDR

Image-based gynecologic brachytherapy requires the delivery of dose using a stepping source with an optimized dose distribution; this means that dose is optimally delivered using HDR or PB. Where LDR uses fixed source positions and strengths to calculate the dose at the prescription point, afterloading machines and computerized dosimetry systems allow optimization of source dwell times to customize dose delivery to the patient's individual anatomy and tumor volume. Optimization results in nonuniform source loadings that give greater dose uniformity and CTV coverage that is often similar to an idealized Manchester dosimetry system implant [32, 33]. Individual dwell times can be modified to alter the dose locally, allowing the dose to the tumor to vary without increasing dose to the organs at risk, e.g., in intracavitary cervix implants tapering of the dose at the uterine tube tip results in a lower dose to the small bowel and sigmoid and decreases the grade 3–5 late complications without affecting local control [34–36]. Now that computerized dose optimization is available, brachytherapists may be tempted to abandon knowledge of the previous LDR dosimetric systems [32, 37] and place sources as they see fit, using the computer to calculate dose distribution. This approach risks overdosing part of the volume. There is a steep dose gradient around each wire and wide-spaced sources may form large high-dose regions and increase the risk of necrosis. In the same way, an isodose that covers the volume but is at a large distance from the sources may also cause necrosis in the vicinity of the sources. In using interstitial needles, the maximum source separations and treatment thickness in the Paris system [37] are useful rules to remember to decrease this risk. The principle of extending the sources beyond the target or crossing at the ends should also be remembered, to overcome the inherent dose fall off at the end of the source, this can be achieved using optimization with PB or HDR brachytherapy.

The use of HDR as an alternative to LDR for cervical carcinoma has been reported in four randomized prospective trials [38–41] and in a number of retrospective series [42]. The randomized trials have shown comparable results for HDR and LDR in all stages of cervical cancer. No statistically significant difference in disease-free survival was detected for any stage of cervical cancer. One series showed a statistically significant decrease in overall survival for stage I patients with HDR (66% vs. 89%) [38]. However, this study used selective randomization allocating older, medically unfit patients to the HDR arm. A meta-analysis of five randomized trials (including one published to date in abstract form only [43]) has shown no differences between HDR and LDR for overall survival, local recurrence, or late complications [44]. Most series show comparable rates of grades 3 to 5 late complications with LDR and HDR therapy. Comparison between studies of HDR and LDR for cancer of the cervix may be difficult because of a lack of detailed information on the radiation administered and a wide range of external-beam and intracavitary dose and fractionation schedules. Not all of the prospective trials were blinded clinical trials and the retrospective series may suffer from the potential bias of historic controls, stage migration over time, and improvement in radiotherapy techniques and dosimetry with modern imaging. The use of PB has not yet been compared to LDR or HDR in a randomized setting.

The four "Rs" of fractionated radiotherapy, the four factors affecting normal tissue and tumor response to changes in time-dose-fractionation: repair, reoxygenation, repopulation, and reassortment, can be examined with reference to the change in brachytherapy dose rates from LDR to HDR or PB [45]. It would appear that the differing techniques each carry their own potential radiobiological advantages and disadvantages [45], which probably equal out in clinical practice, a finding reflected by the results of the prospective clinical trials for cervix HDR and LDR. For example in the area of reoxygenation, the length of administration of LDR allows time for transient acute hypoxia to correct within the tumor during treatment [46]. However, between HDR fractions time is allowed for tumor shrinkage, reducing the distance between capillary vessels in the tumor and increasing oxygen delivery to the cells reoxygenating areas of chronic hypoxia.

The effects of brachytherapy increase as the dose per fraction increases due to a decrease in repair; therefore, less total dose is needed. This effect is more marked in late-responding normal tissue giving a theoretical late repair advantage to LDR. However this does not account for volume effects and the improved immobilization and packing achieved by HDR, the dose to OAR is decreased not only physical dose sparing but also radiobiological dose sparing because of the decrease both in dose and in dose rate with distance. In HDR there is also a decrease in dose per fraction with distance. Only a small amount of physical dose sparing is needed with HDR to offset potential disadvantages to late tissue in comparison to LDR [47]. BED values for HDR will generally be higher than LDR closer to the sources and lower than LDR at distances further from the prescription point [48]. In LDR a dose-rate effect has been seen, with increased morbidity if the dose rate is 0.8 Gy/h rather than 0.4 Gy/h [49, 50]; thus, similarly to HDR if the dose rate in LDR or dose per pulse in PB is increased then the total brachytherapy dose must be decreased.

11.2.2 Different Applicators

The rise in 3D brachytherapy has seen a change in applicators used from the traditional tandem and ovoid in use virtually since the inception of cervix brachytherapy to the tandem and ring that allows greater flexibility of source dwell positions for more individualized dose prescribing. The ring is shown to be hotter at the surface than ovoids [34] when the standardized "Fletcher" loading is used, though since the radiation tolerance of the upper vagina is high [51] the impact on late toxicity may be minimal. The concept of dose gradient and source spacing has been continued with modifications of the tandem and ring to allow interstitial needle placement in a predictable and reproducible geometric fashion [52]. This procedure not only ensures that a greater volume of tissue can receive the higher dose delivered by the brachytherapy boost but also ensures that dose gradients in tissue are minimized. However, the use of interstitial catheters may alter the radiobiology of the surrounding tissue as interstitial implants have been shown to cause tissue hypoxia an hour after implantation in experimental models with recovery in some but not all tumors by 24 h [53]. Whether this would be an area for specific targeting with hypoxic sensitizers is an area for future research.

11.2.3 Physical Biological Treatment Planning

When the first standardized treatment planning for cervix cancer was conceived, point doses were defined, which would deliver an LDR boost to the majority of the cervix while minimizing dose to surrounding structures [32]. However, improved imaging has shown that these point doses may fail to cover the residual cancer [54], in fact its very definition as a determinant of the point where the ureter and the uterine artery cross may not be very accurate [55]. The point dose prescribing also failed to take into account the dose received by normal tissues, which became more important as the dose per fraction rose with the advent of fractionated HDR brachytherapy. Thus, the ICRU cervix cancer normal tissue reference dose points were defined [4]. These dose points correlated with late effects but in the era of 3D imaging it could often be seen that they may not accurately represent the actual dose received [56–58]. Thus 3D OAR dose reporting was developed. This uses volumetric dose received combined with radiobiologic principles to ensure that not only the individual dose per fraction is not exceeded but also that the cumulative doses are considered with respect for the dose delivered by EBRT and that the individual normal tissue tolerances were considered. One drawback is that α/β ratios are assumed as 10 for tumor and 3 for late-reacting normal tissue [18, 59]. These ratios may be over- or underestimates and may also vary from patient to patient, however, they are more representative of the patient population as a whole than nonbiological models. Individualization of dose prescription may allow dose escalation to the tumor, which is useful in cancers showing a dose dependence, more important in some tumors types such as squamous cell carcinoma of the cervix [60, 61] than others such as adenocarcinoma of the endometrium [62]. The effect of tissue movement in the time between treatment planning and delivery must not be ignored; volumetric dosimetry is a dynamic process, compared to static point dosimetry.

11.2.4 Dose Prescribing

Volume-based dose prescribing has allowed precise dose prescription to residual tumor. This may result in isoeffective increased dose to the traditional volume but as yet there is no evidence that these volumes should be decreased. For HDR to be equivalent to LDR, the dose per fraction should be kept as low as possible. This condition affects both normal tissue and tumor, e.g., in postoperative treatment of endometrial cancer when two fractionation schemes were compared, 2.5 Gy × 6 fractions versus 5 Gy × 6 fractions, similar locoregional recurrence rates were seen, but there were much lower rates of vaginal morbidity in the lower dose per fraction group [62]. However when comparing 6 Gy versus 7.5 Gy per fraction for the brachytherapy of cervix cancer no significant difference was seen in control rates or complications [63], though this was before the era of 3D planning and OAR avoidance.

Fractionation is dependent on $T_{1/2}$; if the tumor $T_{1/2}$ for cervix cancer is 1.5 h then an HDR dose of 2–3 Gy per fraction would be equivalent to LDR at 0.5 Gy/h. However, if the $T_{1/2}$ were 4 h an HDR dose of 5–12 Gy/h would be equivalent, which more closely follows current fractionation schedules [15, 25, 48]. Repair may slow with higher doses and dose rates [11]. It must be remembered when fractionating HDR that the benefits of a lower dose per fraction must not be outweighed by a prolongation of overall treatment time, shorter overall treatment times allow less time for cell repopulation or accelerated repopulation to occur. It can be seen that use of HDR could result in extended overall treatment time [64], which consequently can lead to a decrease in overall survival [65] without a corresponding improvement in morbidity. Thus, it is recommended to commence the HDR during the EBRT course [66] but equally it is important to allow adequate time for tumor shrinkage with EBRT. Hama et al. showed increased complications with an increased dose per fraction in retrospective review [67] but equally Patel et al. gave a large dose per fraction in the prospective randomized setting and did not show an increase in complications [39]. The importance of good fractionation of the EBRT must also be remembered.

The use of more precise target definition and volume-based biologic OAR dose reporting gives the opportunity for dose escalation with a low predicted late morbidity [68]. Since squamous cell carcinoma of the cervix shows dose dependence with a greater response to higher doses of radiation, this can be expected to lead to increases in local control and survival.

11.3 Conclusion

Understanding the radiobiological principles of brachytherapy allows a more informed choice of dose rate, fractionation, and prescription with improved prediction of expected toxicity and control. Now that radiobiological treatment planning has been encompassed in 3D treatment planning it is perhaps time to focus on the integration of translational research to allow tissue-modifying factors to be used, which can enhance the radiobiological responses to improve brachytherapy response in specific patients.

References

1. Stitt JA, Fowler JF, Thomadsen BR, et al. High dose rate intracavitary brachytherapy for carcinoma of the cervix: the Madison system: I. Clinical and radiobiological consideration. Int J Radiat Oncol Biol Phys. 1992;24:335–48.
2. Brenner DJ, Huang Y, Hall EJ. Fractionated high dose rate versus low dose rate regimens for intracavitary brachytherapy of the cervix:equivalent regimens for combined brachytherapy and external irradiation. Int J Radiat Oncol Biol Phys. 1991;21:1415–23.
3. Eifel PJ. High-dose-rate brachytherapy for carcinoma of the cervix: high tech or high risk? Int J Radiat Oncol Biol Phys. 1992;24:383–6.
4. ICRU 38. Dose and volume specifications for reporting intracavitary therapy in gynecology. Bethesda: International Commission on Radiation Units and Measurements; 1985. pp. 1–23.
5. Dale RG, Fowler JF. Radiation repair mechanisms. In: Dale RG, Jones B, editors. Radiobiological modelling in radiation oncology. London: British Institute of Radiology; 2007.
6. Fu KK, Ling CC, Nath R, et al. Radiobiology of brachytherapy. In: Interstitial brachytherapy: Physical, Biological and Clinical Considerations (Interstitial Collaborative Working Group). Eds Anderson LL and the Interstitial Collaborative Working Group. New York: Raven Press Ltd; 1990.
7. Dale RG, Jones B. The clinical radiobiology of brachytherapy. Br J Radiol. 1998;71:465–83.
8. Mason KA, Thames HD, Ochran TG, et al. Comparison of continuous and pulsed low dose rate brachytherapy: biological equivalence in vivo. Int J Radiat Oncol Biol Phys. 1994;28:667–71.
9. Armour EP, White JR, Armin A, et al. Pulsed low dose rate brachytherapy in a rat model: dependence of late rectal injury on radiation pulse size. Int J Radiat Oncol Biol Phys. 1997;38:825–34.
10. Visser AG, van den Aardweg GJ, Levendag PC. Pulsed dose rate and fractionated high dose rate brachytherapy: choice of brachytherapy schedules to replace low dose rate treatments. Int J Radiat Oncol Biol Phys. 1996;34:497–505.
11. Fowler JF, van Limbergen EFM. Biological effect of pulsed dose rate brachytherapy with stepping sources if short half-times of repair are present in tissues. Int J Radiat Oncol Biol Phys. 1997;37:877–83.

12. Dale RG. The application of the linear quadratic dose-effect equation to fractionated and protracted radiotherapy. Br J Radiol. 1985;58:515–28.
13. Joiner MC, van der Kogel AJ. The linear quadratic approach to fractionation and calculation of isoeffect relationships. In: Steel GG, editor. Basic clinical radiobiology. 3rd ed. London: Hodder Arnold; 1997. p. 106–22.
14. Bentzen SM, Joiner MC. The linear quadratic approach in clinical practice. In: Joiner MC, van der Kogel A, editors. Basic clinical radiobiology. 4th ed. London: Hodder Arnold; 2009. p. 120–34.
15. Pop LA, van den Broek JF, Visser AG, et al. Constraints in the use of repair half times and mathematical modelling for the clinical application of HDR and PDR treatment schedules as an alternative for LDR brachytherapy. Radiother Oncol. 1996;38:153–62.
16. Bentzen SM, Saunders MI, Dische S. Repair halftimes estimated from observations of treatment-related morbidity after CHART or conventional radiotherapy in head and neck cancer. Radiother Oncol. 1999;53:219–26.
17. Steel G. Basic Clinical Radiobiology, vol. 1. 3rd ed. London: Arnold; 2002.
18. Potter R, Haie-Meder C, Van Limbergen E, et al. Recommendations from gynaecological (GYN) GEC ESTRO working group (II): concepts and terms in 3D image-based treatment planning in cervix cancer brachytherapy-3D dose volume parameters and aspects of 3D image-based anatomy, radiation physics, radiobiology. Radiother Oncol. 2006;78:67–77.
19. Noda SE, Ohno T, Kato S, et al. Late rectal complications evaluated by computed tomography-based dose calculations in patients with cervical carcinoma undergoing high-dose-rate brachytherapy. Int J Radiat Oncol Biol Phys. 2007;69:118–24.
20. Clark BG, Souhami L, Roman TN, et al. The prediction of late rectal complications in patients treated with high dose rate brachytherapy for carcinoma of the cervix. Int J Radiat Oncol Biol Phys. 1997;38:989–93.
21. Yoshimura R, Hayashi K, Ayukawa F, et al. Radiotherapy doses at special reference points correlate with the outcome of cervical cancer therapy. Brachytherapy. 2008;7:260–6.
22. Guerrero M, Li XA. Extending the linear–quadratic model for large fraction doses pertinent to stereotactic radiotherapy. Phys Med Biol. 2004;49:4825–35.
23. Fowler JF. Is repair of DNA strand break damage from ionizing radiation second-order rather than first-order? A simpler explanation of apparently multiexponential repair. Radiat Res. 1999;152:124–36.
24. Millar WT, Canney PA. Derivation and application of equations describing the effects of fractionated protracted irradiation, based on multiple and incomplete repair processes. Part 1L: Derivation of equations. Int J Radiobiol. 1993;64:275–91.
25. Orton C. High dose rate brachytherapy may be radiobiologically superior to low dose rate due to slow repair of late responding normal tissue cells. Int J Radiat Oncol Biol Phys. 2001;49: 183–9.
26. Denham JW, Hamilton CS, Simpson SA, O'Brien MY, Ostwald PM, Kron T, et al. Acute reaction parameters for human oropharyngeal mucosa. Radiother Oncol. 1995;35:129–37.
27. Roberts SA, Hendry JH, Swindell R, et al. Compensation for changes in dose-rate in radical low-dose-rate brachytherapy: a radiobiological analysis of a randomised clinical trial. Radiother Oncol. 2004;70:63–74.
28. Bentzen SM, Ruifrok AC, Thames HD. Repair capacity and kinetics for human mucosa and epithelial tumors in the head and neck: clinical data on the effect of changing the time interval between multiple fractions per day in radiotherapy. Radiother Oncol. 1996;38:89–101.
29. Bentzen SM. Design of clinical trials in radiation oncology: saving lives not grays. In: JB DR, editor. Radiobiological modelling in radiation oncology. London: British Institute of Radiology; 2007. p. 196–211.
30. Jones B, Dale RG. The potential for mathematical modelling in the assessment of the radiation dose equivalent of cytotoxic chemotherapy given concomitantly with radiotherapy. Br J Radiol. 2005;78:939–44.

31. Jones B, Dale RG, Gaya AM. Linear quadratic modelling of increased late normal-tissue effects in special clinical situations. Int J Radiat Oncol Biol Phys. 2006;64:948–53.
32. Meredith WJ. Radium dosage: the Manchester system. Baltimore: Williams & Wilkins; 1949.
33. Hoskin PJ, Rembowska A. Dosimetry rules for brachytherapy using high dose rate remote afterloading implants. Clin Onc. 1998;10:226–30.
34. Mai J, Erickson B, Rownd J, et al. Comparison of four different dose specification methods for high dose rate intracavitary radiation for treatment of cervical cancer. Int J Radiat Oncol Biol Phys. 2001;51:1131–41.
35. Lee SW, Suh CO, Chung EJ, et al. Dose optimization of fractionated external radiation and high dose rate intracavitary brachytherapy for FIGO stage IB uterine cervical carcinoma. Int J Radiat Oncol Biol Phys. 2002;52:1338–44.
36. Foroudi F, Bull CA, Gebski V. Radiation therapy for cervix carcinoma: benefits of individualized dosimetry. Clin Onc. 2002;14:43–9.
37. Pierquin B, Dutreix A, Paine CH, et al. The Paris system in interstitial radiation therapy. Acta Radiol Oncol Radiat Phys Biol. 1978;17:33–48.
38. Teshima T, Inoue T, Ikeda H, et al. High dose rate and low dose rate intracavitary therapy for carcinoma of the uterine cervix. Final results of Osaka University Hospital. Cancer. 1993;72:2409–14.
39. Patel FD, Sharma SC, Negi PS, et al. Low dose rate vs. high dose rate brachytherapy in the treatment of carcinoma of the uterine cervix: a clinical trial. Int J Radiat Oncol Biol Phys. 1993;28:335–41.
40. Lertsanguansinchai P, Lertbutsayanukul C, Shotelersuk K, et al. Phase III randomized trial comparing LDR and HDR brachytherapy in treatment of cervical carcinoma. Int J Radiat Oncol Biol Phys. 2004;59:1424–31.
41. Hareyama M, Sakata K, Oouchi A, et al. High dose rate versus low dose rate intracavitary therapy for carcinoma of the uterine cervix. Cancer. 2002;94:117–24.
42. Stewart AJ, Viswanathan AN. Current controversies in high-dose-rate versus low-dose-rate brachytherapy for cervical cancer. Cancer. 2006;107:908–15.
43. Shrivastava S, Dinshaw K, Mahanshetty U, et al. Comparing low-dose-rate and high-dose-rate intracavitary brachytherapy in carcinoma cervix: results from a randomized controlled study. Int J Radiat Oncol Biol Phys. 2006;66:S42.
44. Viani GA, Manta GB, Stefano EJ, et al. Brachytherapy for cervix cancer: low-dose rate or high-dose rate brachytherapy-a meta-analysis of clinical trials. J Exp Clin Cancer Res. 2009;28:47.
45. Stewart AJ, Jones B. Radiobiological concepts for brachytherapy. In: Devlin P, editor. Brachytherapy: applications and techniques. 1st ed. Baltimore: Lippincott, Williams & Wilkins; 2006.
46. Ling CC, Spiro IJ, Mitchell J, et al. The variation of OER with dose rate. Int J Radiat Oncol Biol Phys. 1985;11:1367–73.
47. Dale RG. The use of small fraction numbers in high dose-rate gynaecological afterloading: some radiobiological considerations. Br J Radiol. 1990;63:290–4.
48. Dale RG, Coles IP, Deehan C, et al. Calculation of integrated biological response in brachytherapy. Int J Radiat Oncol Biol Phys. 1997;38:633–42.
49. Haie-Meder C, Kramar A, Lambin P, et al. Analysis of complications in a prospective randomized trial comparing two brachytherapy low dose rates in cervical carcinoma. Int J Radiat Oncol Biol Phys. 1994;29:953–60.
50. Lambin P, Gerbaulet A, Kramar A, et al. Phase III trial comparing two low dose rates in brachytherapy of cervix carcinoma: report at 2 years. Int J Radiat Oncol Biol Phys. 1993;25: 405–12.
51. Au SP, Grigsby PW. The irradiation tolerance dose of the proximal vagina. Radiother Oncol. 2003;67:77–85.

52. Kirisits C, Lang S, Dimopolous J, et al. The Vienna applicator for combined intracavitary and interstitial brachytherapy of cervical cancer: design, application, treatment planning, and dosimetric results. Int J Radiat Oncol Biol Phys. 2006;65:624–30.
53. van den Berg AP, van Geel CAJF, van Hooije CMC, et al. Tumor hypoxia – a confounding or exploitable factor in interstitial brachytherapy? Effects of tissue trauma in an experimental rat tumor model. Int J Radiat Oncol Biol Phys. 2000;48:233–40.
54. Lindegaard JC, Tanderup K, Nielsen SK, et al. MRI-guided 3D optimization significantly improves DVH parameters of pulsed-dose-rate brachytherapy in locally advanced cervical cancer. Int J Radiat Oncol Biol Phys. 2008;71:756–64.
55. Wang KL, Yang YC, Chao KS, et al. Correlation of traditional point a with anatomic location of uterine artery and ureter in cancer of the uterine cervix. Int J Radiat Oncol Biol Phys. 2007;69:498–503.
56. Yaparpalvi R, Mutyala S, Gorla GR, et al. Point vs. volumetric bladder and rectal doses in combined intracavitary-interstitial high-dose-rate brachytherapy: correlation and comparison with published Vienna applicator data. Brachytherapy. 2008;7:336–42.
57. Kim HJ, Kim S, Ha SW, et al. Are doses to ICRU reference points valuable for predicting late rectal and bladder morbidity after definitive radiotherapy in uterine cervix cancer? Tumori. 2008;94:327–32.
58. Pelloski CE, Palmer M, Chronowski GM, et al. Comparison between CT-based volumetric calculations and ICRU reference-point estimates of radiation doses delivered to bladder and rectum during intracavitary radiotherapy for cervical cancer. Int J Radiat Oncol Biol Phys. 2005;62:131–7.
59. Haie-Meder C, Potter R, Van Limbergen E, et al. Recommendations from the gynaecological (GYN) GEC ESTRO working group: concepts and terms in 3D image based 3D treatment planning in cervix cancer brachytherapy with emphasis on MRI assessment of GTV and CTV. Radiother Oncol. 2005;74:235–45.
60. Paley PJ, Goff BA, Minudri R, et al. The prognostic significance of radiation dose and residual tumor in the treatment of barrel-shaped endophytic cervical carcinoma. Gyn Onc. 2000; 76:373–9.
61. Eifel PJ, Thoms Jr WW, Smith TL, et al. The relationship between brachytherapy dose and outcome in patients with bulky endocervical tumors treated with radiation alone. Int J Radiat Oncol Biol Phys. 1994;28:113–8.
62. Sorbe B, Straumits A, Karlsson L. Intravaginal high-dose-rate brachytherapy for stage I endometrial cancer: a randomized study of two dose-per-fraction levels. Int J Radiat Oncol Biol Phys. 2005;62:1385–9.
63. Chatani M, Matayoshi Y, Masaki N, et al. A prospective randomized study concerning the point A dose in high dose rate intracavitary therapy for carcinoma of the uterine cervix. The final results. Strahlenther Onkol. 1994;170:636–42.
64. Okkan S, Atkovar G, Sahinler I, et al. Results and complications of high dose rate and low dose rate brachytherapy in carcinoma of the cervix: Cerrahpasa experience. Radiother Oncol. 2003;67:97–105.
65. Chen SW, Liang JA, Yang SN, et al. The adverse effect of treatment prolongation in cervical cancer by high dose rate intracavitary brachytherapy. Radiother Oncol. 2003;67:69–76.
66. Nag S, Erickson B, Thomadsen B, et al. The American Brachytherapy Society recommendations for high dose rate brachytherapy for carcinoma of the cervix. Int J Radiat Oncol Biol Phys. 2000;48:201–11.
67. Hama Y, Uematsu M, Nagata I, et al. Carcinoma of the uterine cervix: twice versus onceweekly high dose rate brachytherapy. Radiology. 2001;219:207–12.
68. Pötter R, Dimopoulos J, Georg P, et al. Clinical impact of MRI assisted dose volume adaptation and dose escalation in brachytherapy of locally advanced cervix cancer. Radiother Oncol. 2007;83:148–55.

Physics for Image-Guided Brachytherapy

12

Christian Kirisits, Kari Tanderup, Taran Paulsen Hellebust, and Robert Cormack

12.1 3D Image-Based Dose Specification

The integration of computed tomography (CT) and magnetic resonance (MR) imaging for brachytherapy treatment planning enables the use of dose and volume parameters that are more directly related to target structures and organs at risk (OARs). In the field of gynecological treatments, a detailed treatise has been introduced for cervix cancer brachytherapy. The gynecological GEC ESTRO recommendations part II [1] describe concept and terms for dose volume parameters. We emphasize that these recommendations include no explicit dose constraints or guidelines for treatment planning, as they are limited to dose recording and reporting. However, limited experience to date with the recommendations suggests that the dose parameters can also be helpful in prospective treatment. This chapter does not give the rationale and background of all parameters and is not a comprehensive summary of the GEC ESTRO guidelines. The chapter strives, however, to give an overview of the practical approach using these parameters for treatment planning.

C. Kirisits (✉)
Department of Radiotherapy,
Vienna General Hospital, Medical University of Vienna,
Währinger Gürtel 18-20, 1090 Vienna, Austria
e-mail: christian.kirisits@akhwien.at

K. Tanderup
Department of Oncology, Aarhus University Hospital,
Norrebrogade 44, 8000 Aarhus,
Denmark

T.P. Hellebust
Department of Medical Physics, Radiumhospitalet,
0310 Oslo, Norway

R. Cormack
Department of Radiation Oncology, Brigham & Women's Hospital,
75 Francis Street, Boston, MA 02115, USA

A.N. Viswanathan et al. (eds.), *Gynecologic Radiation Therapy*,
DOI: 10.1007/978-3-540-68958-4_12, © Springer-Verlag Berlin Heidelberg 2011

12.1.1 Dose to Target Structures (GTV, HR CTV, IR CTV)

The GYN GEC ESTRO recommendations define target structures and related dosimetric quantities. A number of target structures are defined: gross tumor volume (GTV), high-risk clinical tumor volume (HR CTV), and intermediate-risk clinical tumor volume (IR CTV). The primary dose volume parameters reported for target structures are D90, D100, and V100.

D90, defined as the dose received by at least 90% of the target volume, is currently the most used 3D cervix parameter for reporting and comparing dose values. The cumulative D90 for the whole treatment is defined as the sum of D90s from the individual fractions plus the dose from external beam treatment. The dose from external beam treatments is assumed to be homogeneous within the target structure, and only one fixed dose value is currently added. The dose might change if special inhomogeneous dose distributions are applied by IMRT techniques or boost fields. In most clinical approaches reported to date, the D90 is the prescribed dose for the whole treatment and a lower limit for the D90 values can be used as a dose constraint for prospective treatment planning [2–5].

D100 is much more sensitive to inaccuracies in contouring and dose calculation. However, it must be emphasized that this parameter represents the minimum target dose. Reaching a certain limit for the D90, but still having a low D100 due to single portions of the target that are not covered by an appropriate dose, might substantially decrease the probability for local control.

The V100 can be used to measure the coverage of the whole target volume. V100 reaches 100% only when all portions of the target are covered by the prescribed dose. While V100 cannot be used for comparison with other treatment schedules using a different prescribed dose, it can be useful in daily clinical practice for prospective treatment planning.

The use of more than one parameter is important for a comprehensive description of the dose distribution within the target volume. For example, the D90 can be much higher than the prescribed dose, but small parts of the target volume may be lower than the 100% dose. Increasing the dwell time would result in further dose escalation for the D90 while the coverage of all portions of the target is still not achieved. This coverage can be measured by reporting and optimizing on V100 or D100.

The term prescribed dose is less straightforward; it is the dose intended for the target volume. During treatment planning, dose optimization techniques attempt to cover the target volume to the prescribe dose. It remains unclear if the prescribed dose should be related to minimum covering dose such as the D100 (V100 = 100%), or the dose to a particular percentage of the target volume (e.g., the prescribed dose has to be reached with D90, V100 = 90%). Both approaches are used, and the individual approaches followed at different centers can be found in Section V.

Traditionally, the dose to Point A has been extensively used in gynecological brachytherapy. Point A is defined as a point 2 cm from the tandem, and 2 cm cranial to the upper surface of the vaginal applicator. Even if a point is not sufficient to specify the dose to a target volume it is recommended to report the dose to this point. It allows comparison between different treatment approaches, establishes a direct link to non-3D image-based approaches, and serves as a dose value for quality assurance. In addition, the normalization of the dose distribution to point A is an ideal starting point for any further treatment plan optimization. In cases of interstitial or combined intracavitary/interstitial applications, point A dose may become useless, as dwell positions close to this point result in dose values of several hundred Gy or undefined situations.

The total reference air kerma (TRAK), a value indicating the total dose delivered by a plan independent of the dose distribution, can be used for comparison and for quality assurance (QA) measures.

12.1.2 Dose to Organs at Risk

The dose to organs at risks is reported by the cumulative sum of the dose volume histogram (DVH) values. Due to the special dose distribution for brachytherapy, it is observed that dose values related to small absolute volumes are independent of contouring the wall structure or only the outer organ wall [6]. Therefore, the main parameters recommended by the GEC ESTRO and reported in recent publications are the D_{2cc} and $D_{0.1cc}$ values. The D_{xcc} is the minimum dose received by the most exposed × cm^3 volume of the analyzed organ. The dose can be directly measured from a cumulative DVH if the volume is given in absolute units (cm^3).

These DVH parameters were initially only recommended for bladder, rectum, and sigmoid colon. It seems feasible to use the same values for other intestine structures, as individual intestine loops, if they can be delineated accurately, similar to rectum or sigmoid. For the whole intestine structure and the whole bladder, other concepts are currently under investigation. Possible quantities are doses to relative volumes or volumes receiving some absolute dose (e.g., V50 Gy).

For the vagina, it is difficult to recommend representative parameters now. The vagina is within a very steep dose gradient because it is directly adjacent to the applicator. The dose gradient makes the vaginal DVH highly susceptible to variations in contouring. While there is a clear need for uniformity in vaginal contouring, there are no clear recommendations about the thickness of the vaginal wall that should be contoured. Any vaginal contour is like a cylinder around the sources. The most exposed volumes are often noncontiguously distributed over the entire circumference, in most cases on both lateral parts close to the vaginal sources. Asymmetric dose distributions, following a high exposure on one side, could result in the same DVH as calculated for symmetric distribution if the same amount of volume is exposed. Due to these uncertainties, DVH parameters are not feasible for prospective planning or for comparison between individual patients. They might be of clinical interest when comparing large patient cohorts or different applicators [7]. Currently, in many centers, dose constraints are applied for dose points related to the surface of the applicator as, e.g., the vaginal surface and/or at 5-mm depth.

It must be emphasized that there are many more critical organs that are not explicitly contoured, including the normal tissue outside the uterus, nerves, vessels, ureter, and urethra. Such structures are often indirectly taken into account by using loading patterns and dose distributions linked to traditional standards. The same is true for high-dose regions within the volume to be treated. D50, V200, and V300 may limit the amount of volume irradiated with very high-dose values. However, review of the spatial dose distribution is essential (Sect. 12.4).

12.2 Applicator Reconstruction

12.2.1 Introduction to Applicator Reconstruction

To calculate the dose to a specific point or to an anatomical structure, the location of the source dwell positions (source path) in relation to the point or structure must be determined. Because the source is not inside the applicator during the image acquisition, reference points in the applicator are used in this process. Often dummy sources or marker strands are placed inside the applicator. To indicate a potential dwell position, the location of these reference points or the geometry of the marker strands has to be extracted from the images in the treatment planning system (TPS). This process is referred to as applicator reconstruction.

12.2.2 Library Reconstruction

Inaccuracy in the reconstruction process could potentially lead to uncertainties in definition of source positions. These uncertainties could alter the calculated dose distribution both to target volumes and organs at risk, as well as dose to specific points (Point A, ICRU reference points). Preclinical commissioning of the applicator and TPS is crucial [8,9]. During this process, the location of dwell positions is found in relation to one another or in relation to reference points in the applicator, e.g., the distance from the tip of the tandem applicator to the first dwell position. The geometry of the applicator, or more correctly the source path, can be stored as library files and later used clinically. The procedure for importing these library files is critical. It is important to realize that even a correctly reconstructed applicator positioned incorrectly in the 3D study will lead to an incorrect estimate of the dose distribution in the patient. At least three well-defined points must be identified in the applicator to merge the library file with the clinical 3D study (Fig. 12.1). This reconstruction method is usually referred to as the library reconstruction method (LIB).

Note that the LIB approach may not be applicable to applicators with variable geometry such as flexible needles. If ovoids with variable separation are us ed, the LIB method has to be applied for each of the applicators separately. Furthermore, there may be situations in which patient anatomy will distort the applicator, resulting in a disparity between the applicator and its reconstruction in the TPS. Procedures should be established to verify applicator reconstruction. In situations where the LIB reconstruction method is insufficient, a direct digitization approach should be performed.

12.2.3 Digitization

The applicator may also be reconstructed by digitizing the track of the source directly in the acquired images. Using this method it is important to identify the first dwell position correctly.

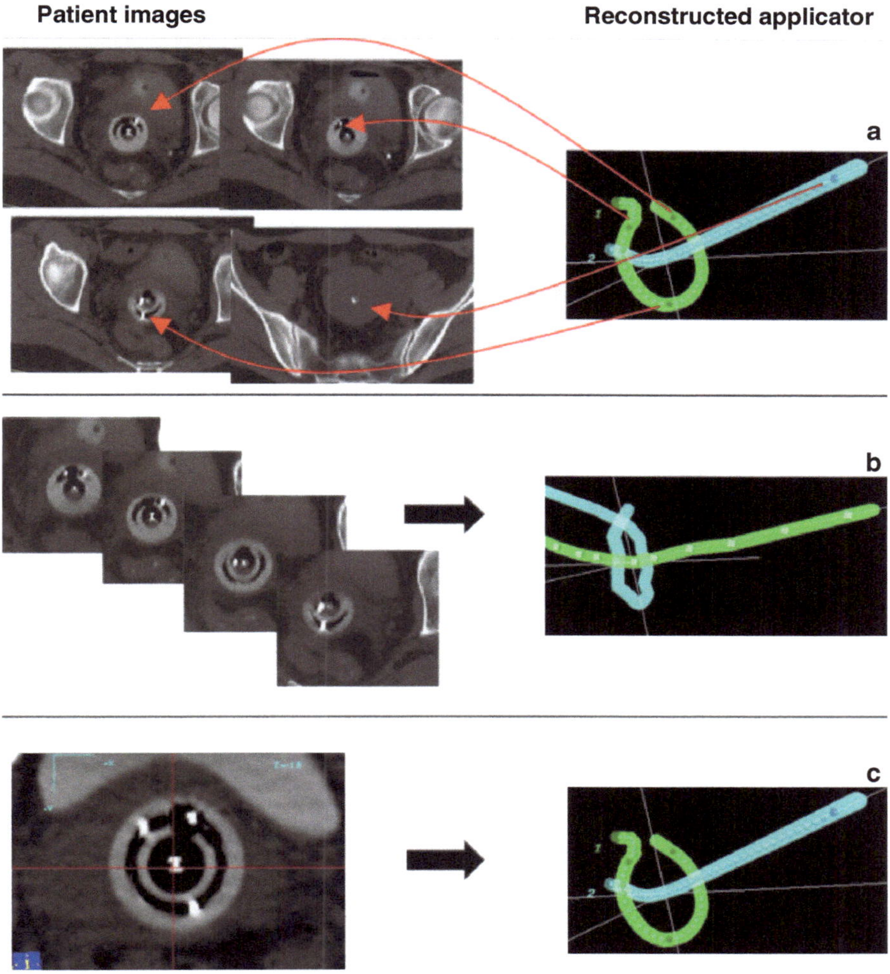

Fig. 12.1 Illustration of different reconstruction methods using (**a**) library reconstruction method (LIB), (**b**) direct reconstruction (DR), and (**c**) multiplanar reconstruction (MPR) images. The jagged shape of the reconstructed applicator in (**b**) is a result of digitalization in each image and does not reflect the true source path. As a consequence, the dwell position will be not be located correctly in relation to each other with potential inaccuracies in the dose distribution

If this position is located between two images, a correction can be applied. When transverse (or para-transverse) images are used, a lateral view is a valuable tool to determine the magnitude of this correction. Even if the first dwell position is correctly identified, it is also important to digitize the track of the source correctly. By digitizing a curved applicator in several images there is an inherent risk of reconstructing too long or too short a track. When many points are used, a jagged-shaped applicator is often the result (Fig. 12.1), which would result in incorrect dwell locations as well as incorrect determination of the length of the source path.

Modern brachytherapy TPSs can produce resampled oblique views that are not constrained to the principal axes of the image set. Such multiplanar reconstruction (MPR) images, derived from the originally acquired images, can be produced in any plane based upon the originally acquired images. The quality of these MPR images depends on the distance between the original images and usually they are a very useful tool in the reconstruction process. If the relevant part of an applicator, e.g., a ring applicator, could be visualized in a single MPR image, the problems with the direct reconstruction (DR) described above are eliminated (Fig. 12.1). Since the quality of the MPR images is sometimes a limitation, the reconstruction of straight, rigid applicators should preferably be performed by using the DR method. To avoid a tagged applicator, only two points should be used in this situation.

12.2.4 Applicator Reconstruction Using CT Images

It is easy to visualize the track of the source in CT images as illustrated in Fig. 12.1. Often the lumen of the applicator is well visualized and this means that a marker string is not always necessary. The locations of the dwell positions inside the lumen have to be determined. Marker strings should be selected with care, as some X-ray catheters may produce artifacts in the CT images that may increase the uncertainties associated with the contouring and reconstruction process.

Hellebust and colleagues analyzed the impact of the applicator orientation on the calculated dose around a reconstructed ring applicator set using CT imaging [10]. They also included an analysis of the impact of the reconstruction method used. Their results showed that it was not possible to identify one applicator orientation that gave lower uncertainties with regard to the calculated dose around the applicator. Moreover, they found that the LIB reconstruction method gave significantly smaller standard deviations than the DR method looking at the data for all the applicator orientations. However, it is important to point out the standard deviation of the calculated dose for all orientations and all reconstruction methods was less than 4%. They concluded that using CT for applicator reconstruction would result in reconstruction uncertainties that are considerably smaller than other uncertainties in brachytherapy.

12.2.5 Applicator Reconstruction Using MR Images

Localizing the source path from MR images is challenging because conventional markers used for X-ray and CT cannot be used in magnetic resonance imaging (MRI). Special MR markers like catheters containing a fluid $CuSO_4$ solution [11], water [12], or glycerin [13] can be used in plastic applicators (Fig. 12.2), although the signal from these MR markers can be faint in T2-weighted images when using applicators with narrow entrance diameters. In titanium applicators, fluid contrast cannot be visualized inside the source guide tubes due to susceptibility artifacts. Slice thickness is an important parameter for reconstruction, since it has direct impact on the precision of reconstruction. It is recommended to perform reconstruction in image series obtained with a slice thickness less than or equal

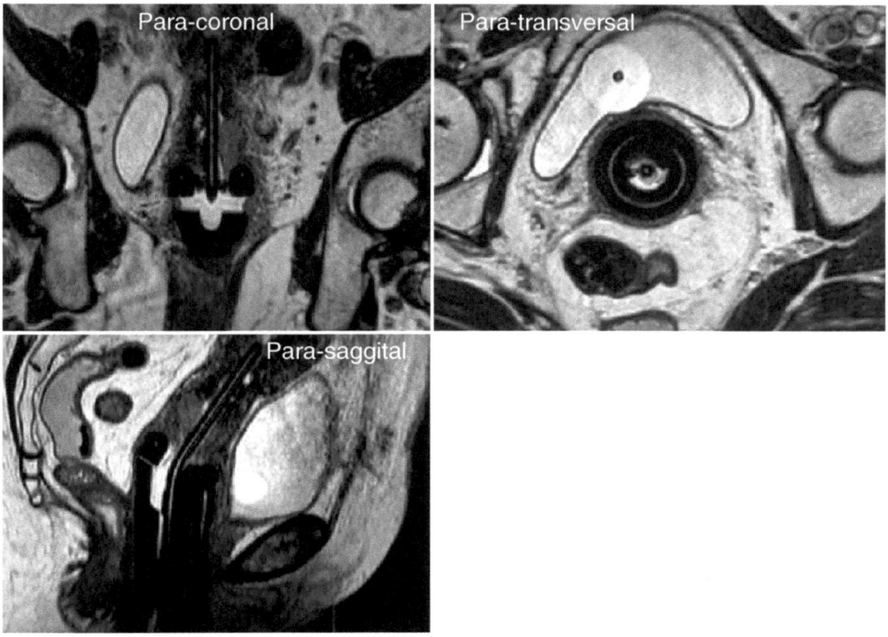

Fig. 12.2 Transversal and coronal (reconstructed) magnetic resonance (MR) images with a plastic tandem–ring applicator in situ. Thin catheters containing a $CuSO_4$ solution in water have been inserted into tandem and ring channels, and appear as bright contrast in the signal void of the applicator material

to 5 mm. Furthermore, para-transverse imaging visualizes the applicator better than with transverse imaging. 3D sequences with isotropic voxel sizes produce an excellent visualization of the applicator, and it is also possible to do contouring in certain T2-weighted 3D sequences [14]. Performing contouring and reconstruction in the same image series is an advantage when possible, because this eliminates uncertainties introduced by registering different image series. Moreover, it avoids uncertainties due to the artifact shifts that change with pulse sequence [15]. In many cases, an artifact is indicating the location of the applicator while the true applicator position is not directly visible. When using metallic applicators in particular, care should be taken to verify the geometric relationship between the true applicator position and the artifacts from the applicator.

Depending on the type of applicator, treatment planning system, and options for imaging, there are several possibilities for reconstruction procedures.

12.2.5.1
Single Image Set

Reconstruction can be done directly on T2-weighted images based on source channel markers. This is an option when the source channels (non-titanium) are visualized by inserting fluid contrast catheters [11–13]. In this case, library applicators or direct reconstruction are applied directly in the T2 images, although procedures should be developed to ensure the accurate localization of the applicator tip or other reference points. The signal from the marker catheters depends on the fluid lumen and on the field strength. When using applicators with narrow entrances (<1.5 mm) in low-field scanners (<1 T) it is difficult to establish a reasonable signal from MR markers, and one of the reconstruction approaches described below should be used.

12.2.5.2
Image Registration

Reconstruction can be performed by using registration of T2 images to images having superior applicator/source channels visualization. Such images include T1-weighted MR images, 3D MRI acquisitions, or CT images. The contouring is then performed in T2-weighted images, and reconstruction is done in the additional imaging sequences [2]. Uncertainties associated with the registration process must be considered when planning.

12.2.5.3
Applicator Reference Points

For rigid applicators, the reconstruction of the applicator can be performed in relation to the outer contour of the applicator or in relation to some reference points that are visible in T2 images. For the ring, the rotation is the limiting degree of freedom. Markers attached to the ring, holes used to guide needles (e.g., Vienna applicator illustrated in Fig. 12.3) [16], or liquid-filled marker tubes visible at the channel connected to the ring can be used to identify the accurate orientation. For both ovoids and rings the basis for this method is a template with the outer applicator geometry and the source path visible. The rotation of the ring could be adjusted manually according to a template printed on transparencies. However, more sophisticated methods have been recently integrated into the TPS, where a template, if predefined, can be translated and rotated until it fits to the outer shape, resulting in an automatic reconstruction of the source path.

12.3
Dwell Time Distributions

A loading pattern refers to the distribution of active dwell positions along the source path. Standard loading patterns were developed during years of clinical experience acquired without the aid of image guidance. These standard loading patterns most often were designed to mimic the dose distribution resulting from traditional radium tube loading. In order to maintain similar dose distribution, high dose rate (HDR) treatments developed

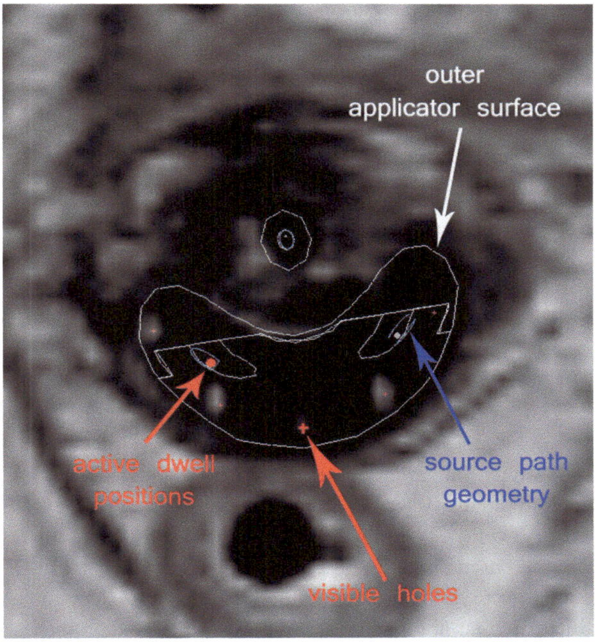

Fig. 12.3 Source path related to outer applicator surface in magnetic resonance imaging (MRI) images. The predefined outer applicator surface (*white*) containing the source path (*blue*) geometry is directly placed in the MRI dataset. Red dots indicate active dwell positions. Visible holes in the ring allow the practitioner to position the template precisely (*red crosses*)

dwell time distributions that were derived from historical activity distributions. The following characteristics of these distributions are highlighted here:

- The vaginal applicators are loaded symmetrically on each lateral side.
- The ratio between vaginal loading and uterine loading varies between different schools. Classical examples are Paris and Stockholm schools, where the ratio between vaginal loading and uterine loading is recommended to be around 1. With Fletcher loading, the ratio is within the range of 0.6–1.4. More recent American standard loading patterns use stronger constraints on vaginal dose, which means that the ratio between vaginal dose and uterine dose is lower – around 0.15–0.25 [17]. In some centers, no vaginal loading is used, and a single central tandem source is used.
- According to Fletcher loading (e.g., 15 mg, 10 mg, 10 mg, or 15 mg, 10 mg, 10 mg, or 15 mg, 10 mg) more positions are active at the tip of the tandem. Some loading patterns avoid any loading to the first cm of the tandem source path. Some loading patterns have dwell positions in the tandem down to the level of the vaginal sources, while others avoid any positions outside the cervix.

There are substantial differences of loading patterns for ovoids, where some approaches load until the tip of ovoids (close to the rectum), while others are shifted more anterior toward the bladder.

The width, height, and thickness of the pear-shaped isodose depend both on the applicator and on the standard loading pattern applied. A collection of standard loading patterns from seven different European and American institutions [18] showed that for the same tandem–ring applicator, the width of the point A isodose ranged from 4.8 to 6.0 cm at the level of the ring due to different loading patterns. An example of two different standard loading patterns is shown in Fig. 12.4. Both dose distributions are normalized in point A. The Vienna standard loading pattern has more dwell weight in the ring, resulting in a wider pear, compared with the Milwaukee standard loading. The ratio between vaginal loading and uterine loading is 1.0 and 0.16, respectively, and the width of the point A isodose is 6.2 and 4.3 cm, respectively.

According to French tradition and ICRU 38 (ICRU 38), it is recommended to evaluate the dimension of the 60 Gy isodose. The distance between the point A isodose and the 60 Gy isodose depends on the prescribed dose and fractionation of external beam radiotherapy and brachytherapy. Typically, the distance between the two pears is between 10–17 mm, when BT is combined with 45–50 Gy EBRT.

Due to the optimization process, which changes the loading pattern, these standard loading patterns become less important [19]. However, they are still a very good base to start any optimization process and a link to the standard dose distribution, which has been applied clinically for decades. New alternatives are anatomy-based loading patterns. The active dwell positions are not fixed to specific locations related to the applicator, but are defined based on margins around target structures and OARs. Sources are activated inside and close to the target, avoiding positions very close to OARs. For typical clinical situations such an approach often results in loadings comparable with standard loading patterns, i.e., no active dwell positions on the anterior (close to the bladder) and posterior part (close to the rectum) of the vaginal applicator, no active dwell positions at the tip of the tandem in case of a nearby sigmoid loop.

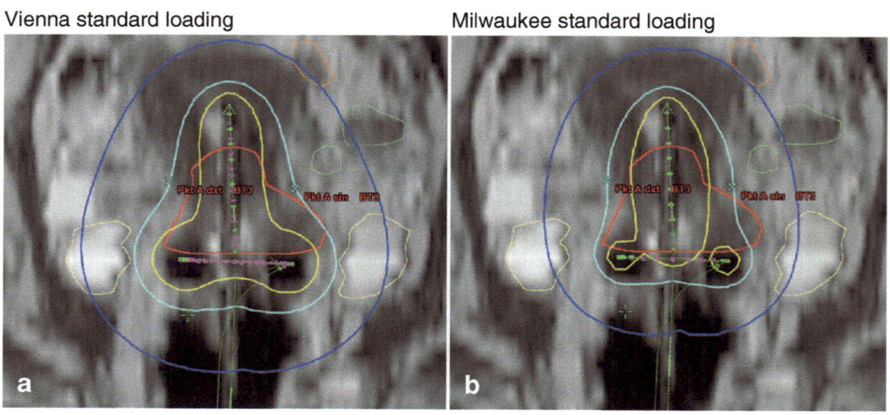

Fig. 12.4 Dose distribution corresponding to two different standard loading patterns: (**a**) Vienna and (**b**) Milwaukee. Isodose curves: 50%, 100%, and 200%. High-risk clinical tumor volume (HR CTV) is delineated in *red*

12.4 Optimization

In current clinical practice, the process of 3D treatment planning is similar as reported by different centers [2–5]. The optimization procedure starts by normalizing the dose to point A and with a defined loading pattern resulting in a pear-shaped isodose. The recommended DVH parameters are evaluated for target and organ structures. Based on defined dose constraints, the location of active dwell positions and dwell times are modified. In most centers this is performed manually, with or without graphical modification, while inverse optimization techniques have not been fully integrated into clinical practice.

12.4.1 Manual Optimization

Manual optimization involves changing the position of normalization points, the dwell position pattern, and each individual dwell time to achieve the clinically desired dose distribution. Bar graphs for changing relative dwell weights (with a normalization point) or absolute dwell times (without normalization) are ideal tools for quick optimization. In addition to DVH-based dose constraints, the manual stepwise dwell time modification can to guarantee a reproducible and safe treatment plan if:

- The optimization process starts with a standard dose distribution that is only changed when dose values are outside the tolerance limits.
- The use of a normalization point can be limited to certain distances from the applicator or a dwell time limit can be introduced. Both methods keep a limit for the total dose and high-dose volume.
- The differences in total volume encompassed by the prescribed dose (Vpd) and TRAK between actual plan and standard values are compared and related to the treated tumor volume and topography.

12.4.2 Graphical Optimization

Graphical optimization allows on-screen manipulation of isodose lines and is often an efficient tool to use during the optimization process. However, to use this software tool safely and to utilize its potential completely, it is important to be aware of the way this optimization modality works. The system automatically calculates dwell times or dwell weights when the user drags and drops the isodose lines. It is important to keep track of how the dwell times or the dwell weights change during the process. A display of the dwell times/dwell weights on the screen either numerically or graphically (if possible) is helpful. When using many applicators (e.g., intracavitary applicators combined with needles) it can be difficult to display all the dwell positions. Then extra care should be taken to follow the changes in the dwell positions that are not displayed. Prior to the optimization, high-dose levels isodoses should be displayed, such as the 300% and the 400% isodose lines.

During the graphical optimization process, the user can increase or decrease the number of sources that are affected by the modification performed. By using the "global" setting, manipulation of an isodose line will influence many source positions, while the "local" setting only will influence the dwell positions closest to the place of the modification. The local setting should be carefully used when an isodose curve is made larger. Even small alterations in the isodose lines can lead to severely blown-up dwell time in one single source position. However, the local setting can be useful when the purpose is to reduce the dose in one area with a minimal change in other regions.

It is important where to realize that-screen manipulation influences which source positions your operation will influence. For example, if you want to increase the contribution from one or two needles relative to the tandem applicator, your starting point should not be in between the needles and the tandem, but on the other side of the needles.

In principle, the graphical optimization can be performed in an absolute mode or in a relative mode. Using the absolute mode the normalization is changed, which means that the shape of the isodose is changed while the level of the isodoses will be kept constant. In the relative mode the normalization is kept constant, i.e., both the shape *and* the level of the isodose are changed. The way of dealing with this issue is different for a commercial treatment planning system. In some systems the mode has to be chosen before the graphical optimization starts, while in other systems the absolute mode is the default and the plan has to be renormalized if the original normalization needs to be kept. It is advisable to explore the graphical optimization tool regarding this issue before it is used clinically.

The ability to achieve all dose constraints is limited by the applicator geometry and patient anatomy. Dose optimization in intracavitary brachytherapy can reshape and expand the prescription isodose by up to around 5 mm depending on the surrounding OARs (Fig. 12.5). In general, the insertion of only intracavitary applicators is therefore not sufficient for clinical target volumes larger than 5 cm in width (level of point A) at the time of brachytherapy and for unfavorable topography of target and/or OARs. One possible solution is the insertion of additional needles, e.g., using the Vienna applicator for combined intracavitary/interstitial treatments [3,20]. The treatment concept starts with the standard dose distribution, dose optimization as far as possible, and then uses needles for small contributions compared with intracavitary loading. By using an optimization with a total sum of dwell times inside needles of about 10% to 20% compared with the total dwell times at all positions within tandem and ring results in substantial improvement of target coverage. The prescription isodose can be expanded by around 10–15 mm in the region of the needles, and it is possible to extend the width of treatable tumors to around 6–7 cm at level of point A and even more cranially [20]. The majority of the dose is still delivered from the intracavitary applicator, and therefore the dose distribution is similar to traditional plans, but with needles providing coverage to the peripheral regions of the target. Figure 12.6 illustrates a large tumor not covered by a standard pear-shaped isodose. Dose optimization using the intracavitary sources in the ring and tandem improves the dose distribution, but does not lead to sufficient coverage of the posterior extension of the tumor.

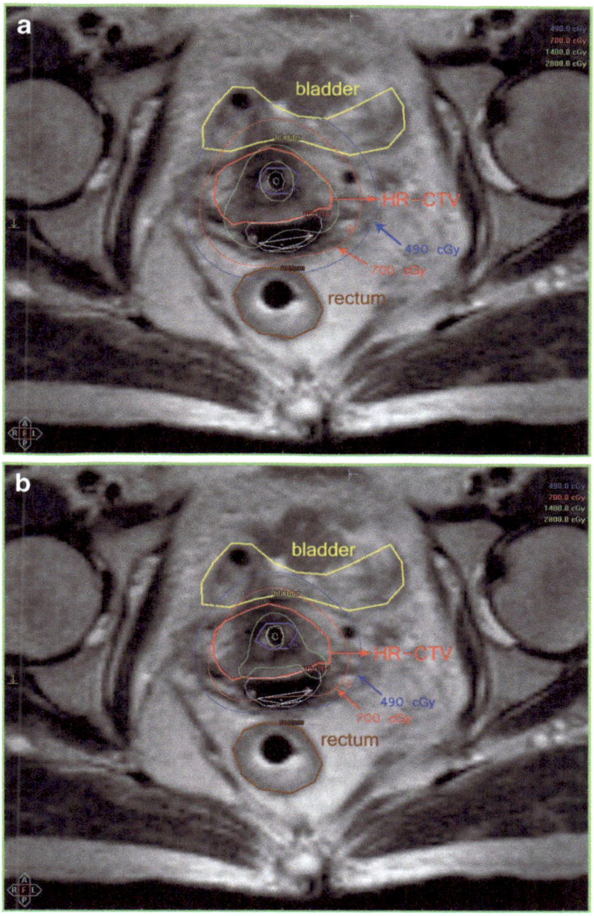

Fig. 12.5 Simple optimization for an intracavitary implant. The standard loading (**a**) resulted in high-dose values for the bladder and rectum. In the optimized plan (**b**) the prescribed isodose of 7 Gy is limited to the HR CTV to spare the organs at risk (OARs)

However, by loading additional interstitial needles it is possible to improve the dose distribution significantly and to cover the HR CTV.

For certain large target volumes the intracavitary concept has to be replaced completely by interstitial implants. Then the OAR DVH constraints are valid. Similar to intracavitary approaches the dose optimization process can be started with dose planning concepts such as the Paris system with definition and normalization to basal dose points.

12.4.3 Inverse Planning

The logical consequence to the developments in image-guided treatment planning for cervix cancer brachytherapy is to implement computer-based inverse planning to determine dwell times objectively. Such methods have been initially developed for prostate

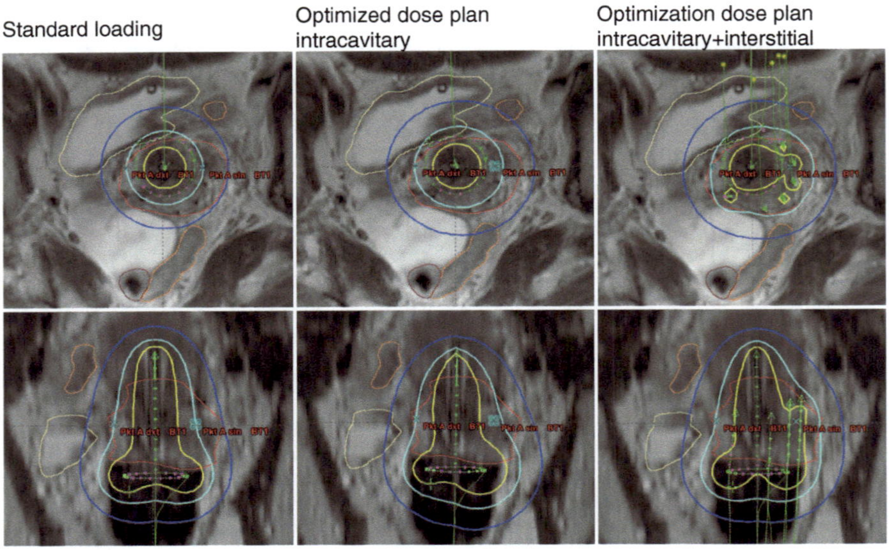

Fig. 12.6 Three different dose plans: (*Left*) intracavitary standard loading, (*middle*) optimized dose plan using intracavitary part (*tandem and ring*), and (*right*) optimized dose plan using both intracavitary and interstitial source positions. Isodose curves: 50%, 100%, and 200%. HR CTV is delineated in *red*

brachytherapy [21,22]. The objective is to improve the dosimetric results and decrease the time to prepare a treatment plan as well as to reduce subjectivity in the planning process. A small set of dosimetric parameters (D90, D100 for target, and D_{2cc} for OAR), is not sufficient to control the dosimetry for the whole involved region. Evidence-based dose constraints do not exist for different tissue types in the parametria, nerves, vessels, vagina, ureter, and urethra because 3D MRI-based treatment planning has only been applied for a limited time period. Multicenter trials have not been conducted. Currently, dosimetric and clinical results must be collected to obtain as much knowledge as possible, with the goal of developing constraints for future inverse planning tools.

Inverse planning concepts cannot always be limited to upper and lower dose constraints for different structures, because this may lead to dose plans that are very different from the standard dose distribution. This situation is pronounced for large tumors and combined intracavitary–interstitial implants because the DVH constraints on organs normally contoured will not restrict the algorithm from blowing up doses in needles and in the vaginal region. It is not feasible to contour many substructures (e.g., CTV inside uterus, CTV in parametrium, blood vessel or nerves, and the vaginal wall) in clinical routine. Therefore, limitations on the spatial distribution are essential. This can be handled by constraints on dwell time gradients, maximum dwell times, and/or by using different optimization rules for different parts of an implant (intracavitary versus interstitial applicators) while locking the dwell times and loading for the remaining already optimized dwell positions. Another option is to introduce help structures in the region of needles, tandem, and vaginal sources in order to control the dose delivered in the region close to the sources [13]. Help structures surrounding the target can also be introduced as avoidance volumes to increase the conformity of the dose distribution. The time spent contouring help structures should always be balanced with the time it would take to perform a manual optimization or a manual adaptation of an inversely optimized dose plan.

Inverse planning approaches look promising for small tumors in intracavitary treatments with regard to the speed of the dose planning procedure. However, for small tumors the dosimetric benefit of inverse dose planning is limited. In these cases, manual planning is already quite efficient because manipulation of source dwell times takes place in a limited number of source positions in only two channels. The impact of inverse planning is most likely greater in large tumors where a combined intracavitary–interstitial applicator is used. In these cases, the number of degrees of freedom for the dose planner is significantly increased, and the optimal solution may not be found by manual planning.

12.4.4 LDR/PB Optimization

As a last point, dose optimization may also involve that the total treatment time and dose per pulse/dose rate is varied when using pulsed brachytherapy (PB) or Low dose rate (LDR) treatment schedules. Decreasing the dose rate will reduce the EQD2 dose in target and OARs, but due to the difference in alpha–beta ratio, the reduction will be larger in OARs. This approach can be used to decrease dose to organs at risk in case of difficult topographies.

12.5 Uncertainties and Variations

Uncertainties and variations in delivered dose are correlated to all steps in the image-guided planning and delivery procedure: calculation uncertainties in the treatment planning system, contouring of target and OARs, reconstruction of applicator, and organ/applicator movement during irradiation or in between fractions.

12.5.1 DVH Calculation

Contours are entered into the system slice by slice and a 3D volume is reconstructed from the slice information. The approach for 3D volume reconstruction varies between dose planning systems. Kirisits and colleagues evaluated the impact of volume reconstruction on DVH parameters relevant for organs at risk in a phantom study [23]. They concluded that the volumetric variations between different TPSs are comparable to the interobserver variation related to contouring the phantom structures. Dosimetric variations amounted to standard deviations of 1–5% in phantom configurations, which were constructed to be relevant for OAR in gynecological brachytherapy. However, larger uncertainties appear when large dose gradients are present in the first or last slice of a contoured structure – a sigmoid loop passing along the slice orientation in a high-dose region.

The voxel size of the dose matrix influences the accuracy of the DVH calculation. The parameter voxel size or number of sampling points distributed within the volume to derive the DVH should be carefully adjusted to calculate reproducible and accurate dose and volume values. Depending on the algorithm of the TPS, this can be tested by repetitive calculation with different settings, and balancing the reproducibility versus calculation speed.

12.5.2 Contouring

Target contouring is of major importance for the reliability of the whole idea of image-guided brachytherapy. The concept of HR CTV and IR CTV has been developed and validated through small interobserver studies based on MRI [24]. MRI is recommended as the standard image modality for target contouring in image-guided brachytherapy. It has been shown that CT results in far more uncertainties for target contouring compared with MRI [25]. Hence, with CT there are significant differences in target dose assessment compared with MRI, both for the individual patient and for the mean dose in a patient population. Two MRI interobserver studies have been published [26,27], and both conclude that interobserver variations on target volumes assessed in MRI result in conformity indices of 0.7–0.8 for IR CTV and HR CTV. Petric and colleagues investigated the topographic variation, and evaluated a mean deviation of 1.6–2.3 mm between the contours of two different observers in eight different directions. The difference between DVH parameters was not presented, but keep in mind that the dose gradient is around 5–8% per mm in the region of the outer contour of the HR CTV.

The contouring of organs at risk can be done with reasonable accuracy on both CT and MRI. Saarnak and colleagues evaluated interobserver variation of delineation of rectum and bladder on CT images in ten patients [28]. They evaluated the interobserver variation of D_{2cc} to be 10% and 11% in the rectum and bladder, respectively. For single patients, there were variations seen even up to 27%, mostly in the region of the ovoids where the image quality was compromised. We emphasize that the image quality is important for limiting the contouring uncertainties in CT images. New CT-compatible applicators produce fewer artifacts and thereby more precise organ visualization. Viswanathan and colleagues compared OAR delineation in CT and MRI and concluded that there were no systematic differences in mean DVH values [25].

12.5.3 Reconstruction

Reconstruction uncertainties in BT are similar to set-up uncertainties in EBRT since both define uncertainties in the relation between the radiation source and the target and OARs. The impact of reconstruction uncertainties on delivered dose may be much greater than the impact of set-up uncertainties in EBRT because of the inherent dose inhomogeneities in BT, the size of reconstruction uncertainties, and the low number of BT fractions [29]. Systematic errors should be avoided as much as possible since they have greater impact on delivered dose than random errors. Typical systematic errors are errors in the applicator commissioning process (for instance, a wrong assessment of the thickness of the cap surrounding the vaginal sources) or systematic misinterpretations of MR images due to artifacts (for instance, in the assessment of the tip of a titanium needle). Random reconstruction errors are dependent on the visibility of the applicator in the images. With CT-based reconstruction, the visibility of the applicator is good and the variation in dose due to reconstruction is small. Hellebust and colleagues have shown that the variation between different reconstruction methods was below 4% (SD) in clinically relevant dose points [10]. With MRI-based reconstruction, it is essential to optimize the imaging sequence to improve the precision of applicator reconstruction. Para-transverse images result in a better visualization than pure transverse images. In general a small slice thickness is preferred, although long acquisition times should not be used to avoid patient movement during image uptake. By introducing appropriate applicator reconstruction methods and by eliminating systematic uncertainties, the uncertainties on DVH parameters (due to reconstruction) can be reduced to 5–10% in 90% of a patient population [29] (Fig. 12.7).

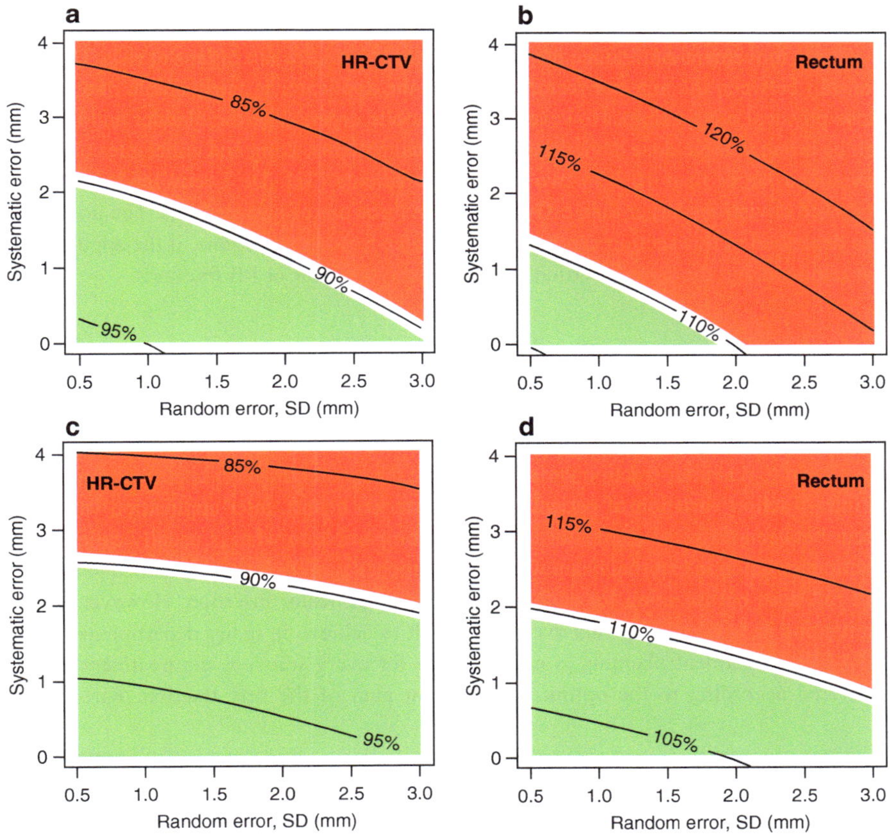

Fig. 12.7 Uncertainties of dose volume histogram (DVH) parameters may be reduced with reconstruction. Adapted from Tanderup et al. [29]

12.5.4 Applicator Stability and Organ Movement Within the Same Applicator Insertion

In daily clinical practice, there is always a risk of applicator or organ movement between imaging and irradiation. In a full 3D image-guided procedure, there will most often be at least 1–3 h between MR image uptake and start of irradiation. Furthermore, for PB irradiation time can be many hours. Finally, some treatment schedules involve delivery of several HDR fractions with one applicator insertion, i.e., delivery of one fraction on the day of applicator insertion and a second fraction the following day.

Stability of the applicator in relation to the target is essential to obtain the planned target dose. The type of applicator, the fixation, and the packing of the vagina (when this is performed) are crucial factors influencing the stability of the applicator. There have been reports of very stable applicator geometry during delivery of intracavitary brachytherapy treatment [30], but occasional applicator displacements have also been reported during PB, resulting in considerable changes in HR CTV D90 of 7 Gy in one patient out of nine [31]. When choosing the type of applicator and insertion technique, consider whether the applicator and the fixation are appropriate with regard to the institution work flow, i.e., patient transfer to CT/MR and duration of irradiation (HDR/PB).

Organ movement can induce deviations from planned dose in organs at risk. The relationship between the anterior rectum wall and the applicator is fairly stable due to their close physical relationship. However, highly mobile organs like the bladder and sigmoid can be prone to large dose deviations in individual patients. Lang and colleagues observed deviations larger than 10% in two out of ten patients [32]. De Leeuw and colleagues observed deviations larger than 5 Gy (EQD2) in three out of nine patients. The uncertainties described in this section can be related to inter-fraction variations, if the applicator is not removed, but the same insertion is used for several HDR or PB fractions.

12.5.5 Variations Between Fractions

In contrast to real inter-fraction variations, where the applicator stays in place (comparable to intra-fraction variation of patient setup in external beam), inter-application variations occur between different applicator insertions (comparable to what is usually called inter-fraction variation in external beam with a new patient setup). It is recommended to use MR and full dose optimization for each brachytherapy applicator insertion. However, due to limitations in MR capacity this may be difficult to achieve in many departments. When MRI-based treatment planning is not available for every fraction, the treatment can be delivered according to the optimized treatment plan of the first fraction. Kirisits and colleagues have discussed the consequences of using one MR plan for all brachytherapy fractions [33]. The delivered dose to the tumor/CTV will generally be higher than what was calculated from the first fraction due to tumor shrinkage; the mean D90 for the HR CTV was 6 Gy higher. For organs at risk the dose will also often be higher, since the dose optimization only takes into account the organ topography at the time of the first brachytherapy treatment. D_{2cc} in bladder, rectum, and sigmoid was higher by 3.5, 4.2, and 5.8, respectively. Hellebust and colleagues also investigated the inter-fraction (inter-application) variations of dose volume-related parameters for patients receiving fractionated HDR brachytherapy [34]. The variation in clinically relevant dose from fraction to fraction varied considerably from patient to patient for both the rectum and the bladder. For one patient, the relative standard deviation of D5% (~D_{2cc}) was 51.2% over 5 fractions. In average, the relative standard deviation was 15.0% and 17.5% for the rectum and bladder, respectively. In the absence of MR imaging for all fractions, the use of CT makes it possible to adapt the dose distribution to OAR. While OARs can be delineated accurately, the target contour can be obtained from the first MRI-based plan and transferred to subsequent CT plans. Such transfers can be based on dedicated registration procedures (e.g., related to the applicator) and can help to reduce the uncertainties in delineating the appropriate dimensions of the CTV on CT images (Fig. 12.8).

12.5.6 Dose Accumulation

Calculation of cumulative dose to organs at risk from succeeding BT fractions relies currently on a crude addition of D_{2cc} for subsequent BT fractions. For this assumption to be true, it is required that the part of the organ irradiated to a high dose in the first BT fraction will also be in the high-dose region for succeeding BT fractions. This approximation will lead to an overestimation of OAR dose when different parts of the organ are exposed to a high dose in different fractions, as for a moving sigmoid or a bladder with varying filling status. Therefore, assessment of total dose by addition of succeeding D_{2cc} will be a conservative estimate of the dose actually delivered to the organ. If the OAR is dose limiting, this might result in a decision to compromise target dose. On the other hand, one should be careful when it is obvious from the images that the same part of an organ is in the high-dose region in every fraction, e.g., a sigmoid loop fixed to the uterus.

In the future, deformable registration may become feasible for MR images from succeeding BT fractions. This method of registration can take into account organ deformation between fractions. By using deformable registration it is possible to track and accumulate dose, and this method has the potential to improve the assessment of dose in moving and deforming organs.

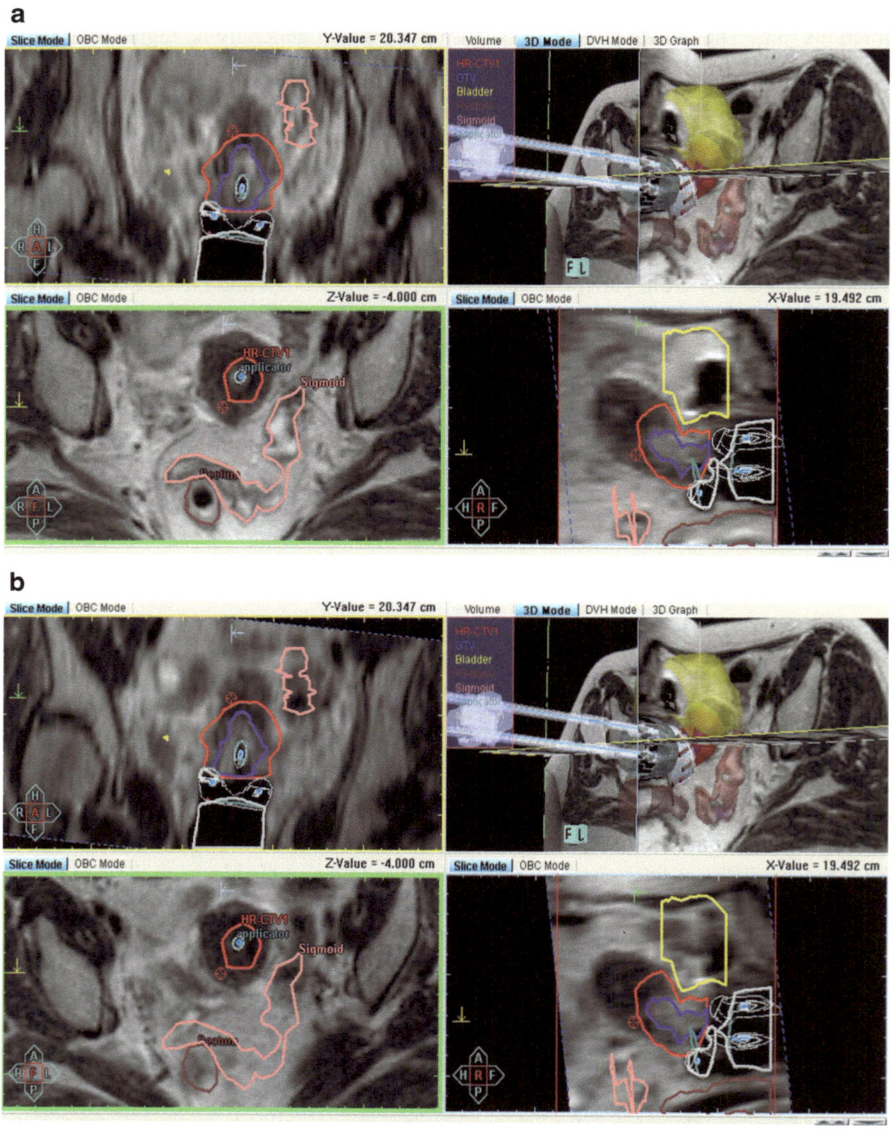

Fig. 12.8 All contours are based on the MRI anatomy at first implantation (**a**). The structures are transferred to the MRI of another fraction/implantation (**b**) by using the applicator geometry as the fixed coordinate system. While target volumes, bladder, and rectum show only slight deviations, the sigmoid has changed substantially

References

1. Pötter R, Haie-Meder C, Van Limbergen E, et al. Recommendations from gynaecological (GYN) GEC ESTRO working group (II): concepts and terms in 3D image-based treatment planning in cervix cancer brachytherapy-3D dose volume parameters and aspects of 3D image-based anatomy, radiation physics, radiobiology. Radiother Oncol. 2006;78:67–77.
2. Kirisits C, Pötter R, Lang S, Dimopoulos J, Wachter-Gerstner N, Georg D. Dose and volume parameters for MRI-based treatment planning in intracavitary brachytherapy for cervical cancer. Int J Radiat Oncol Biol Phys. 2005;62:901–11.
3. Lindegaard JC, Tanderup K, Nielsen SK, Haack S, Gelineck J. MRI-guided 3D optimization significantly improves DVH parameters of pulsed-dose-rate brachytherapy in locally advanced cervical cancer. Int J Radiat Oncol Biol Phys. 2008;71(3):756–64.
4. De Brabandere M, Mousa AG, Nulens A, Swinnen A, Van Limbergen E. Potential of dose optimisation in MRI-based PB brachytherapy of cervix carcinoma. Radiother Oncol. 2008;88:217–26.
5. Chargari C, Magné N, Dumas I, Messai T, Vicenzi L, Gillion N, et al. Physics Contributions and clinical outcome with 3D-MRI-based pulsed-dose-rate intracavitary brachytherapy in cervical cancer patients. Int J Radiat Oncol Biol Phys. 2009;74:133–9.
6. Wachter-Gerstner N, Wachter S, Reinstadler E, et al. Bladder and rectum dose defined from MRI based treatment planning for cervix cancer brachytherapy: comparison of dose-volume histograms for organ contours and organ wall, comparison with ICRU rectum and bladder reference point. Radiother Oncol. 2003;68:269–76.
7. Berger D, Dimopoulos J, Georg P, Georg D, Pötter R, Kirisits C. Uncertainties in assessment of the vaginal dose for intracavitary brachytherapy of cervical cancer using a tandem-ring applicator. Int J Radiat Oncol Biol Phys. 2007;67:1451–9.
8. Kubo HD, Glasgow GP, Pethel TD, Thomadsen BR, Williamson JF. High dose-rate brachytherapy treatment delivery: report of the AAPM Radiation Therapy Committee Task Group No. 59. Med Phys. 1998;25(4):375–403.
9. Nath R, Anderson LL, Meli JA, Olch AJ, Stitt JA, Williamson JF. Code of practice for brachytherapy physics: report of the AAPM Radiation Therapy Committee Task Group No. 56. American Association of Physicists in Medicine. Med Phys. 1997;24(10):1557–98.
10. Hellebust TP, Tanderup K, Bergstrand ES, Knutsen BH, Røislien J, Olsen DR. Reconstruction of a ring applicator using CT imaging: impact of reconstruction method and applicator orientation. Phys Med Biol. 2007;52:4893–904.
11. Haack S, Nielsen SK, Lindegaard JC, Gelineck J, Tanderup K. Applicator reconstruction in MRI 3D image-based dose planning of brachytherapy for cervical cancer. Radiother Oncol. 2009;91:187–93.
12. Perez-Calatayud J, Kuipers F, Ballester F, et al. Exclusive MRI-based tandem and colpostats reconstruction in gynaecological brachytherapy treatment planning. Radiother Oncol. 2009;91:181–6.
13. Chajon E, Dumas I, Touleimat M, et al. Inverse planning approach for 3-D MRI-based pulse-dose rate intracavitary brachytherapy in cervix cancer. Int J Radiat Oncol Biol Phys. 2007;68:955–61.
14. Petric P, Hudej R, Rogelj P, Logar HBZ. 3D T2-weighted fast recovery fast spin echo sequence MRI for target contouring in cervix cancer brachytherapy. Brachytherapy. 2008;7:109–10.
15. Gehl, HB, Frahm C, Passive visualization of needles in interventional magnetic resonance imaging, Debatin JF, Adam G Editors Springer Verlag 1997
16. Berger D, Dimopoulos J, Potter R, and Kirisits C, Direct reconstruction of the Vienna applicator on MRI images. Radiother Oncol, 2009. 93(2): p. 347–51.
17. Mai J, Erickson B, Rownd J, Gillin M. Comparison of four different dose specification methods for high-dose-rate intracavitary radiation for treatment of cervical cancer. Int J Radiat Oncol Biol Phys. 2001;51:1131–41.

18. Jürgenliemk-Schulz IM, Lang S, Tanderup K, de Leeuw A, Kirisits C, Lindegaard J, Petric P, Hudej R, Pötter R; Gyn GEC ESTRO network. Variation of treatment planning parameters (D90 HR CTV, D_{2cc} for OAR) for cervical cancer tandem ring brachytherapy in a multicentre setting: comparison of standard planning and 3D image guided optimisation based on a joint protocol for dose-volume constraints. Radiother Oncol, 2010;94:339–45.
19. Erickson B. The sculpted pear: an unfinished brachytherapy tale. Brachytherapy. 2003;2: 189–99.
20. Kirisits C, Lang S, Dimopoulos J, Berger D, Georg D, Pötter R. The Vienna applicator for combined intracavitary and interstitial brachytherapy of cervical cancer: design, application, treatment planning, and dosimetric results. Int J Radiat Oncol Biol Phys. 2006;65:624–30.
21. Lahanas M, Baltas D, Zamboglou N. A hybrid evolutionary algorithm for multi-objective anatomy-based dose optimization in high-dose-rate brachytherapy. Phys Med Biol. 2003; 48(3):399–415.
22. Pouliot J, Lessard É, and Hsu I-C. Advanced 3D planning. In: Brachytherapy physics. 2nd ed. M.P. Publishing; 2005. p. 393–413.
23. Kirisits C, Siebert FA, Baltas D, et al. Accuracy of volume and DVH parameters determined with different brachytherapy treatment planning systems. Radiother Oncol. 2007;84:290–7.
24. Lang S, Nulens A, Briot E, et al. Intercomparison of treatment concepts for MR image assisted brachytherapy of cervical carcinoma based on GYN GEC-ESTRO recommendations. Radiother Oncol. 2006;78:185–93.
25. Viswanathan AN, Dimopoulos J, Kirisits C, Berger D, Pötter R. Computed tomography versus magnetic resonance imaging-based contouring in cervical cancer brachytherapy: results of a prospective trial and preliminary guidelines for standardized contours. Int J Radiat Oncol Biol Phys. 2007;68:491–8.
26. Petric P, Dimopoulos J, Kirisits C, Berger D, Hudej R, Potter R. Inter- and intraobserver variation in HR CTV contouring: Intercomparison of transverse and paratransverse image orientation in 3D-MRI assisted cervix cancer brachytherapy. Radiother Oncol. 2008;89:164–71.
27. Dimopoulos JC, Vos VD, Berger D, Petric P, Dumas I, Kirisits C, et al. Inter-observer comparison of target delineation for MRI-assisted cervical cancer brachytherapy: application of the GYN GEC-ESTRO recommendations. Radiother Oncol. 2009;91:166–72.
28. Saarnak AE, Boersma M, van Bunningen BN, Wolterink R, Steggerda MJ. Inter-observer variation in delineation of bladder and rectum contours for brachytherapy of cervical cancer. Radiother Oncol. 2000;56:37–42.
29. Tanderup K, Hellebust TP, Lang S, Granfeldt J, Pötter R, Lindegaard JC, et al. Consequences of random and systematic reconstruction uncertainties in 3D image based brachytherapy in cervical cancer. Radiother Oncol. 2008;89:156–63.
30. Tanderup K, Christensen JJ, Granfeldt J, Lindegaard JC. Geometric stability of intracavitary pulsed dose rate brachytherapy monitored by in vivo rectal dosimetry. Radiother Oncol. 2006;79:87–93.
31. de Leeuw A, Lotz HT, Moerland MA, Teersteeg RHA, Jürgenliemk-Schultz IM. Displacements and resulting dose effects of tandem ovoid applicators during PB brachytherapy for cervical cancer. Brachytherapy. 2008;7(2):94–5.
32. Lang S, Georg P, Kirisits C, Dimopoulos J, Kuzucan A, Georg D, et al. Uncertainty analysis for 3D image based cervix cancer brachytherapy by repeated MRI examinations: DVH-variations between two HDR fractions within one applicator insertion. Radiother Oncol. 2006;81 Suppl 1:S79.
33. Kirisits C, Lang S, Dimopoulos J, Oechs K, Georg D, Pötter R. Uncertainties when using only one MRI-based treatment plan for subsequent high-dose-rate tandem and ring applications in brachytherapy of cervix cancer. Radiother Oncol. 2006;81:269–75.
34. Hellebust TP, Dale E, Skjonsberg A, Olsen DR. Inter fraction variations in rectum and bladder volumes and dose distributions during high dose rate brachytherapy treatment of the uterine cervix investigated by repetitive CT-examinations. Radiother Oncol. 2001;60:273–80.

Part IV

Institutional Experiences: Practical Approaches to Image-Guided Brachytherapy

Australia: Peter Maccullum Cancer Center, Melbourne

13

Kailash Narayan, Sylvia van Dyk, and David Bernshaw

13.1 Introduction

Transabdominal ultrasound (US) has been used to assist applicator placement at the Peter MacCallum Cancer Centre since 1985. Magnetic resonance imaging (MRI) was introduced in 2001 to assess tumor response to external beam treatment. The next logical step was to assess brachytherapy dosimetry on the MRI scan and develop an image-based planning and treatment protocol. Over time a strong correlation between the size and shape of the uterus and cervix, containing residual tumor, as seen on the US and MRI images, was observed. It became apparent that US could give an accurate depiction of the applicator within the cervix and uterus, and the cervix and uterus within the pelvis. Ultrasound was progressively incorporated into the protocol to avoid uterine perforation and to assist with the dosimetric coverage of the cervix, residual tumor, and uterus [1]. All patients receive external beam radiotherapy prior to intracavitary brachytherapy (ICBT). Patients without nodal metastasis and those with metastatic no des confined to the pelvis are treated with pelvic radiotherapy. The patients with upper common iliac or para-aortic nodes are treated with four-field Extended Field Radiotherapy (EFRT). Involved nodes received small AP-PA rectangular boosts of 6–10 Gy in 2 Gy fractions in between the intra-cavitary brachtherapy (BT), which was given always at the completion of External Beam Radiotherapy (EBRT). ICBT consisted of 30 Gy in five fractions or 28 Gy in four fractions, given twice weekly[2].

13.2 Applicators Available and Selection Parameters

The applicators available at Peter MacCallum Cancer Centre (PMCC) for MRI and US-based brachytherapy are Nucletron, standard CT – MR compatible tandem and ovoids (T&O) and

K. Narayan (✉), S. van Dyk, and D. Bernshaw
Division of Radiation Oncology, Australia, Peter MacCallum Cancer Centre, Melbourne, Locked Bag 1, A'Beckett Street, East Melbourne, VIC 8006, Australia
e-mail: mahaguru@petermac.org

A.N. Viswanathan et al. (eds.), *Gynecologic Radiation Therapy*,
DOI: 10.1007/978-3-540-68958-4_13, © Springer-Verlag Berlin Heidelberg 2011

the vaginal CT – MR compatible tandem and cylinders (T&C). Applicator selection is based on individual patient anatomy taking into account length of uterine canal, response to external beam treatment, capacity of vagina, and presence of gross vaginal disease at the time of brachytherapy. Where possible the T&O are used in preference to the T&C because the former consists of a straight intrauterine tube that is easier to identify on transabdominal ultrasound. The T&O set is limited to 4.0, 5.0, and 6.0 cm long intrauterine tubes. The T&C consists of 4.0, 6.0, and 8.0-cm long curved intrauterine tubes and vaginal rings forming vaginal cylinder.

13.3 Insertion Techniques

Applicator insertion is carried out under general or spinal anesthesia. The patient is placed in lithotomy position. A brief pelvic examination is carried out to determine the clinical status of disease. An 18–20 gauge Foley catheter is inserted and the bladder is filled with 300 cc of sterile saline. The uterus is sounded under transabdominal ultrasound, to ascertain the required length of the tandem and the cervical canal is dilated.

The selected tandem is inserted under ultrasound guidance confirming central placement in the uterine cavity. The ovoids and vaginal spatula are then positioned. Vaginal pack moistened with 1% chlorhexidine obstetric examination cream is firmly packed anteriorly, between the bladder and the ovoids, and posteriorly, between the ovoids and the spatula. At first insertion, following firm vaginal packing the system is pushed high in the pelvis and kept in place with the help of a large bilateral labio-gluteal suture tied to the coupling section of the system to avoid tandem displacement between the first treatment and planning MRI. Labial sutures are not used at subsequent treatments.

13.4 Imaging Protocol

The patient is rescanned with ultrasound in the treatment position with the legs resting on the table. The tandem is identified in the uterine canal and its position optimized to ensure central placement on the sagittal and axial views. The sagittal image is frozen for 2D planning. The tandem is identified based on its known geometry; it acts as an internal ruler. Measurements are taken from the tandem to the anterior and posterior surface of the uterus and cervix at fixed intervals along the tandem from external cervical os (flange) to end of uterine canal (tip of tandem).

Axial images (Fig. 13.1c) taken at the flange confirm the anterior–posterior dimensions of the cervix as seen in the sagittal plane (Fig. 13.1a) and also define the lateral dimensions. Axial images taken at the tip of the tandem (Fig. 13.1d) confirm the anterior–posterior and lateral dimensions of the uterine fundus. An axial image is also taken through the ovoids. This can be checked clinically. These images are saved to a disc and hardcopies are printed.

Patients undergoing their first insertion are transferred to the MR scanner following treatment for imaging. A full scan set using T1 and T2 sequences are taken. Uterine

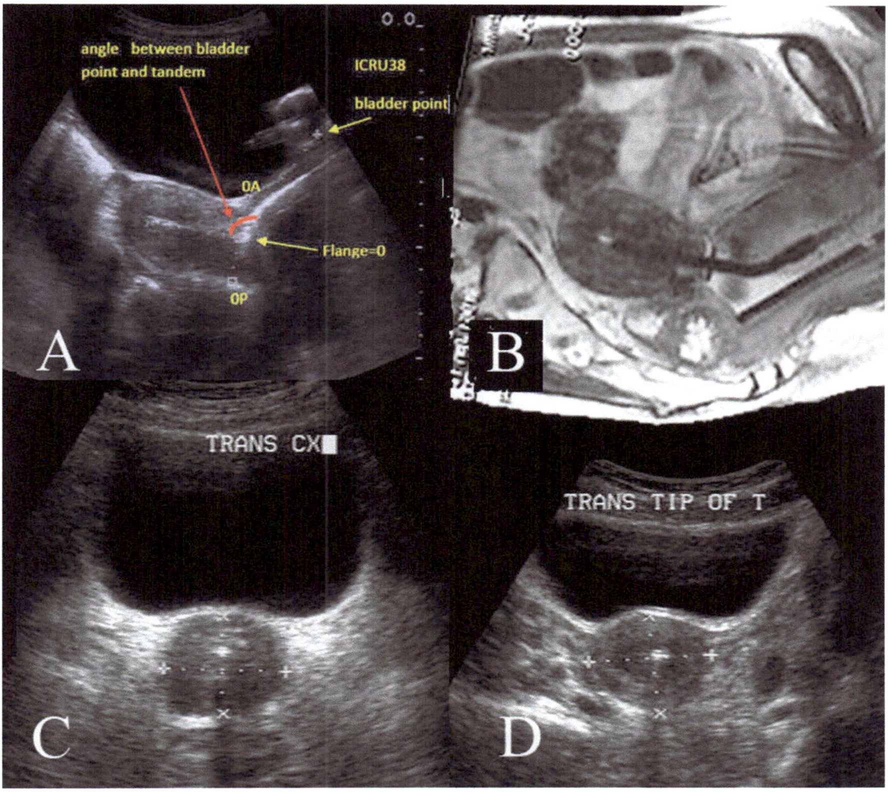

Fig. 13.1 (**a**) Trans-abdominal ultrasound sagittal view showing measurement points. (**b**) Planning magnetic resonance imaging (MRI) sagittal view showing position of tandem in the treatment position. (**c**) Trans-abdominal ultrasound axial view at flange (external os). (**d**) Trans-abdominal ultrasound axial view at tip of tandem (end of uterine canal)

dimensions are measured on the sagittal MR image (Fig. 13.1b) and compared to the ultrasound image (Fig. 13.1a). The isodose distribution based on ultrasound measurements is checked on the MR image. Modifications are made to the plan if necessary. The iso-coverage of this plan is checked on the ultrasound images on the subsequent insertions.

Ultrasound measurements of the uterus in the sagittal plane are taken at each insertion to check iso-coverage.

13.5 Caveats to Imaging

Claustrophobic patients may refuse to undergo scanning. MR imaging can be limited by patients who have ferromagnetic implants and pacemakers. Transabdominal ultrasound imaging can be limited by a large body habitus, but will always be attempted, particularly if MR imaging was not possible. A large abdominal pannus can be positioned away from the scan area to allow ultrasound scanning just above the pubic area.

13.6 Contouring Protocol

The target is initially mapped as an area on the 2D sagittal ultrasound image. The treatment volume is conceptualized in 3D by the brachytherapist and the radiation oncologist using clinical information and the measurements from the axial and sagittal ultrasound scans. Measurements are taken from the tandem to the anterior and posterior surface of the uterus and cervix at fixed intervals along the tandem from cervical os (flange) to end of uterine canal (tip of tandem). The usual measurements are distance from flange to ICRU 38 bladder point, diameter of the cervix at the plane of the flange (F), at the narrowest part of cervix/isthmus (X1), and along the length of tandem (X2, X3), and from the tip of the tandem to the external surface of uterine fundus (X4).

13.7 Treatment Planning

A library plan containing the tandem and ovoid combination used is retrieved on the planning computer using the Plato (Nucletron) radiotherapy planning system. The library plan is used only to obtain applicator geometry. Traditional dose points at Point A are used to start optimization. Source positions are activated along the tandem from first dwell to flange at 0.25–0.5-cm intervals depending on source strength. The ovoids typically contain three active dwell positions with dwell weights around 0.7. The tandem and ovoid dwell weights are manipulated to shape the 100% isodose to the known dimensions of the target as seen on ultrasound. The target consists of residual tumor contained within cervix, the uterus, and any clinically palpable disease in the vagina at the time of brachytherapy. Dose normalization is defined at the target and not at Point A. Points of interest are assessed. The ICRU 38 reference point for rectum is saved with each library plan for immediate assessment, as are vaginal mucosal points positioned on the surface of the ovoids. If these points are within tolerance, the sagittal isodose plot is printed and overlaid on the sagittal ultrasound image. Target coverage is assessed. The sagittal plane affords a good view of organs at risk along the length of the uterus such as rectum, bladder, small and large bowel. Once isodose coverage of the target is approved the first treatment takes place. The patient is then sent for planning MRI. A planning MRI is performed with the T&O still in treatment position.

For the second and subsequent treatments, the target and treatment volumes are assessed on the planning MRI imported in the treatment planning system. Adjustments are made if required to optimize the isodose pattern, coverage of the target volume, and limit dose to surrounding structures. Organs surrounding the cervix and uterus such as bladder, rectum, sigmoid, and small bowel loops are contoured on MRI. Organ boundaries are considered.

Ultrasound is performed at each subsequent insertion to reproduce and verify the tandem position in the uterus and in relation to catheter balloon in the bladder and to adapt the treatment plan according to tumor response if necessary.

13.8 Dose and Fractionation: GTV, CTV, OAR

Patients receive 40 Gy to the whole pelvis via four fields with external beam radiation therapy (EBRT) while positioned prone on a bellyboard. Total doses are calculated presuming the brachytherapy target and surrounding organs at risk receive 100% of the EBRT dose. Brachytherapy commences at the completion of EBRT. Brachytherapy consists of four fractions of 7 Gy to the 100% isodose line. Intent is to deliver a total of 80 Gy_{10}–96 Gy_3 to the clinical target volume (CTV). The target volume (CTV) as described above contains the gross tumour volume (GTV) or residual disease at brachytherapy and takes into account uterine invasion as determined on the pretreatment MRI. Original extent of disease other than corpus invasion is not taken into account in the brachytherapy volumes. Organs at risk are assessed through ICRU 38 bladder and rectal reference points, and vaginal mucosal points. Dose tolerances to these points are 75 Gy, 70 Gy, and 120 Gy respectively. Particular notice is taken of the isodose lines outside the target volume. These isodose lines describe dose to surrounding normal tissues. The target coverage is kept as conformal as possible to minimize the dose to these surrounding organs.

13.9 Documentation

External beam and brachytherapy physical doses are recorded on the brachytherapy prescription sheet. Total doses to the brachytherapy target volume, Point A, ICRU 38 bladder and rectal reference points, vaginal mucosal points, and any other points of interest are reported in EQD2 in the treatment folder. These dose descriptors are also stored electronically in a prospective database. Isodose distributions are printed onto hard copies of the sagittal and coronal MR images and the sagittal ultrasound image. The ultrasound image is filed in the patient's medical records. The MR images are stored on site.

13.10 Quality Assurance/Avoidance of Errors

Consent is obtained from all patients who are queried about their name, date of birth, and reason for treatment. A name band is attached to their wrist for the duration of the anesthetic and treatment procedures. Prior to starting the procedure the radiation oncologist and nurse cross-check the patient's identity and procedure. The patient's electronic medical history and image file are opened on screen in the operating room and brachytherapy planning room. All brachytherapy equipment is checked by two brachytherapists prior to being given to the nursing staff. Applicator insertion is confirmed both clinically and on transabdominal ultrasound. Applicator positioning and identification is confirmed by the brachytherapist and the radiation oncologist. Target area is measured by the brachytherapist performing the ultrasound scan and confirmed by the radiation oncologist. Library plan retrieval, source activity, dose per fraction, indexer length, step size, dwell positions, dwell weights, dose shaping, and point doses are checked by an independent brachytherapist. Plan approval is given by the radiation oncologist. Once the plan is sent to the treatment console the physical setup and plan are double checked by a brachytherapist and physicist. Treatment is monitored via audio and visual contact on a close circuit television by the anesthetist, radiation oncologist, brachytherapist, and physicist. At completion of each fraction of treatment the physicist enters the suite with a hand-held radiation monitor to ensure the source has retracted successfully from the patient. This is in addition to the independent radiation monitor housed in the suite and the built-in treatment machine safety mechanism. The plan is reviewed on both ultrasound images and 3D MR images if available and discussed at a weekly chart round attended by brachytherapists and radiation oncologists.

Reference

1. van Dyk S, Bernshaw D. Ultrasound-based conformal planning for gynaecological brachytherapy. J Med Imaging Radiat Oncol. 2008;52(1):77–84.

Austria: Medical University of Vienna, Vienna

14

Johannes C. Athanasios Dimopoulos, Christian Kirisits, and Richard Pötter

14.1 Introduction

At the Department of Radiotherapy, Medical University of Vienna 3D imaging for brachytherapy has been intensively investigated during the last decade. An open magnetic resonance image (MRI) scanner (0.2T Siemens Magnetom Open-Viva®) was installed in 1997/1998 at the division of brachytherapy in order to support image-guided brachytherapy, particularly for the treatment of gynecological cancers and prostate cancer. The MRI device was adapted to the needs of external beam radiotherapy (EBRT) and brachytherapy [1]. Specific image acquisition protocols were developed for prostate and gynecologic brachytherapy [1, 2]. At the beginning, the translation of the traditional experience based on X-ray assisted treatment planning into image-guided treatment planning was studied [3]. Finally, gynecological brachytherapy was performed MR image-guided [4, 5, 7, 10]. In cooperation with the GYN-GEC ESTRO group, concepts and terms for delineation of gross tumor volume (GTV) and clinical target volume (CTV) and organs at risk (OAR) [8], treatment plan optimization by adaptation of dwell times and locations [5, 7], integration of biological modeling [18], development of 3D image-based parameters to potentially evaluate dose volume relations for GTV and CTV as well as for OAR [9] and for dose escalation, as appropriate and feasible were developed [9, 10]. During these years, the departmental protocol for cervix cancer radiotherapy, and in particular for image-guided brachytherapy, was continuously developed [10]. Since 2001, a systematic approach, which enables prospective application of the different parameters for improvement of target coverage and dose escalation, is applied [10]. In 2007, based on the clinical experience collected during 1998–2003, the first mono-institutional study with clinical results on 145 patients treated

J.C.A. Dimopoulos (✉)
Director of Department of Radiation Therapy, Metropolitan Hospital
9 Ethn. Makariou & 1 El. Venizelou, 18547 Athens, Greece
e-mail: adimopoulos@metropolitan-hospital.gr

C. Kirisits and R. Pötter
Department of Radiotherapy, Vienna General Hospital,
Medical University of Vienna, Währinger Gürtel 18-20, 1090 Vienna, Austria
e-mail: christian.kirisits@akhwien.at

A.N. Viswanathan et al. (eds.), *Gynecologic Radiation Therapy*,
DOI: 10.1007/978-3-540-68958-4_14, © Springer-Verlag Berlin Heidelberg 2011

with MR image-guided brachytherapy was published [10]. Since 2008, dose-effect relationships for the target volumes and the OARs are available for this patient series [11–14].

14.2 Applicator Selection and Brachytherapy Application

The tandem/ring combination is traditionally used for intracavitary brachytherapy applications. The commercially available applicator (Nucletron, Veenendaal, The Netherlands) is used mainly with nominal ring diameters of 34, 30, and 26 mm, tandem lengths of 60 and 40 mm, and an angle of 60° (the version where the tandem is straighter than with 45°). In large tumors with insufficient response and/or unfavorable topography after external beam radiotherapy, combined intracavitary/interstitial techniques are systematically applied if adequate coverage of the target is not provided by a pure intracavitary method [15, 16]. In these patients, the intracavitary application technique is adapted according to the tumor extension at the time of brachytherapy and its relation to the intracavitary applicator. A modified in-house developed version with interstitial parametrial needles positioned inside guiding holes drilled into the ring (Vienna applicator) is used when: (1) unilateral tumor extension is exceeding 3.5 cm at the level of the ring, 2.5 cm at the level of point A, 2.2 cm at a distance 3–4 cm cranial to the ring surface, (2) tumor extension cannot be covered by the symmetrical dose distribution of the tandem alone without exceeding dose limits for OAR [15, 16]. In case of tumor extension up to the distal vagina, close to the pelvic sidewall or posterior along the anterior rectal wall other in-house made applicator types (e.g., combination of cylinder, tandem, perineal template for guidance of interstitial needles) are used.

The applicator insertion is performed under spinal or epidural anesthesia in the lithotomy position. The decision regarding the precise strategy of insertion is made based on the clinical assessment of tumor size, amount, and pattern of tumor regression during EBRT with or without chemotherapy and tumor topography. A urinary catheter is inserted and fixed against the bladder neck. The physician performs gynecologic examination to assess tumor topography (dimensions) with regard to the location of the cervical os (symmetric/asymmetric tumor spread). Depending on the length of the uterine cavity as measured by a semiflexible hysterometer and the topography of vagina and cervix as clinically evaluated, the appropriate size, length, and curvature of the uterovaginal applicator is chosen, if the tandem/ring applicator is used.

For interstitial implantations with the Vienna applicator, the number of needles and their position in the ring, are determined based on the clockwise representation of the parametrium by the ring taking into consideration the extension and the side of parametrial invasion (e.g., left, clockwise at 1–4, 3–6, and 1–6). The planned depth of needle placement in the parametria is determined by the cranial extent of the HR CTV and is usually 3–4 cm above the upper ring surface [15, 16]. After implantation of the tandem–ring applicator or the Vienna applicator and the needles, the vagina is packed with gauze to push away the rectum and bladder and to fix the applicator. This gauze is filled with diluted gadolinium (Pro-Hance, dilution 1:10). Rectum and bladder probes are inserted for in vivo dosimetry (PTW AM6 diodes, PTW Freiburg, Germany).

If more complex interstitial application techniques are used, the number of needles and their position in, e.g., the perineal template, are determined based on the representation of the parametrium by the template, taking into consideration the extension and the side of parametrial invasion. Under these challenging clinical conditions a complete "MRI-guided" approach, with the application at the dedicated MRI unit is performed [17]. In some patients, the number of needles placed in the parametria is changed after the first application to tailor the dose distribution to the critical organs [15, 16].

The MRI verification of the implant position takes place directly after the applicator placement, or in case of complex interstitial techniques, step by step during the implantation procedure ("image guided"). If the applicator positioning is inadequate, or if the uterus is perforated, the implantation procedure is adapted. The positioning is corrected with the assistance of the imaging information about topography of target, needles, and organs at risk. Due to the lithotomy position of the gynecologic patient during implantation and the limited space of the MRI gantry, a MRI-assisted real-time implantation with direct visualization of the needles at the time of application is hardly possible at present. During tandem/ring applications and in case of challenging anatomic situations the flexible hysterometer is inserted with the assistance of trans-abdominal ultrasound. Ultrasound-guided applications are at present only helpful for paravaginal insertions due to technical and imaging limitations of ultrasound at present (probe dimensions, field of view, and soft tissue contrast).

Appropriate measures to prevent venous thrombosis and infection are taken for the duration of the implant. After irradiation, the gauze and the tandem are removed in the operation theatre. In case of interstitial implants, this procedure is followed by removal of the ring together with all the needles, or the template with the needles, or the cylinder with the needles by a resolute pull. The patients are discharged 24 h later after clinical examination to exclude bleeding.

14.3 Imaging Protocol

MR imaging is obtained before EBRT and at each brachytherapy application. MRI is performed using a pelvic surface coil. Fast spin–echo technique, with a repetition time of 4.500 ms and an echo time of 96 ms for T2-weighted images and with a repetition time of 680 ms and an echo time of 15 ms for T1-weighted images, is used. The displayed field of view (DFOV) is 38 × 38 cm, and data collection is performed with a matrix of 256 × 256 [1, 2]. MRI at diagnosis includes T2 FSE–weighted sequences in axial, sagittal, coronal, paraaxial, and paracoronal planes; T1 SE–weighted sequences in axial orientation; and axial and sagittal dynamic contrast-enhanced T1 SE sequences after bolus injection of 0.1 mmol/kg gadoteridol (Prohance, Bracco s.p.a, Milan, Italy), followed by 20 ml of normal saline solution. Section thickness is 5 mm, with an intersection gap of 1 mm. At time of brachytherapy, images are acquired after placing the applicators, with T2-weighted (FSE) sequences in axial, sagittal, and coronal orientation, as well as paraaxial and paracoronal slices orientated orthogonal and parallel to the applicator axis [2, 17]. Slice thickness is 5 mm without an intersection gap. Axial images are obtained from the level above the uterine fundus to the inferior border of the symphysis pubis below any vaginal tumor extension; sagittal images are obtained between internal obturator muscles. Coronal, paracoronal, and paraaxial images include the tumor, entire cervix, corpus uteri, parametria, and vagina.

14.4 Caveats to Imaging

In case of involvement of the distal vagina, the entire organ is scanned. Applicator, vaginal packing, bladder balloon, and rectal probe are displayed with low signal intensity on T2-weighted images [2]. To achieve reproducible filling conditions for the urinary bladder, the empty bladder is filled with 50 cm^3 saline solution prior to MRI and brachytherapy dose delivery using a syringe connected to the catheter. The catheter remains open during the entire imaging and planning process, which results in reproducible bladder filling of 50–100 cm^3. Marking gel in the vagina is used for the pretreatment scans to produce contrast between the vaginal lumen and the organ walls. The gauze used for vaginal packing is filled with diluted gadolinium (Pro-Hance, dilution 1:10) and the balloon of the urinary catheter is filled with 7 ml of diluted gadolinium (ProHance, dilution 1:1) [2, 7]. Therefore, both appear with low signal intensity on T2-weighted images.

14.5 Contouring Protocol

Contouring is performed on T2-weighted axial slices directly on the treatment planning system. The outer organ contours are delineated [6]. For the rectum, the delineation includes the entire organ from the anorectal junction up to the rectosigmoid flexure. For the sigmoid colon, contouring is performed from the rectosigmoid flexure up to the level of the uterine fundus. If small bowel is in the proximity (<2 cm) of the uterus, this is also contoured. The outer contour of the urinary bladder, also including the bladder base and neck, is delineated.

The GTV, HR CTV, and IR CTV are contoured according to our in-house protocol and the GYN GEC-ESTRO group recommendations [8].

14.6 Treatment Planning

Treatment planning has been performed in the past with PLATO planning system and now with OncentraGYN (both Nucletron, Venendaal, The Netherlands). Reconstruction of tandem/ring applicators in MR images has always been based on library plan techniques [3]. The registration of the applicator geometry to the MRI dataset was initially performed by radiographs, later on by manual application of templates directly on the MRI image, and nowadays using software solutions to directly place the applicator with automatically registered source path into the 3D dataset [19]. This became possible after all our ring applicators were adapted with holes, which are visible like markers in MRI and help to determine the exact orientation of the ring.

The optimization procedure starts with a standard loading containing four dwell positions on each lateral side of the ring, and several positions in the tandem with increasing dwell position density in the direction of the tandem tip. This loading is adapted based on the applicator position and anatomy, by shifting, adding, or deleting dwell positions. This process results mainly in changing positions in the ring, due to the ring orientation in relation to the rectum, and less positions at the tandem tip due to nearby sigmoid loops. This concept is currently replaced by a full anatomy-based loading pattern, which is based on margins between organs, target structures, and the possible active source positions.

The final dose distribution is shaped by dwell time optimization using manual bar graph optimization. In case of interstitial applicators, the additional available dwell positions are activated and fine-tuned after the intracavitary part is optimized. Using new inverse planning solutions (HIPO) this concept is reproduced with dedicated tools of inverse optimization, dwell time gradient restriction, and locking of already optimized parts of the implant.

14.7 Dose and Fractionation: GTV, CTV, OAR

In addition to 45 Gy of external beam without midline shielding, four brachytherapy fractions with two insertions are applied. The reference dose is 7 Gy per fraction. The prescribed dose is 80–90 Gy (EQD2) for the HR CTV. This dose is achieved by trying to cover the whole HR CTV with the reference dose, resulting in a V100 of 100%. However, due to the constraints for organs at risk this dose is hardly achieved for all cases. The D90 should be in any case higher than the prescribed dose.

The D_{2cc} for bladder is limited to 90 Gy, but can be allowed up to 100 Gy. The rectum D_{2cc} is nowadays limited to 70 Gy to maximum 75 Gy. For the sigmoid the same constraints are applied as for rectum; however, the dose distribution is studied in detail in relation to the moving sigmoid. If there is clear evidence that the most exposed part of the sigmoid is not the same for a subsequent fraction, the dose limit is adjusted accordingly.

There are a number of additional intrinsic dose constraints based on the conservative optimization process. The vaginal dose is limited by dwell time gradient restriction, not allowing overexposure due to single dwell positions with high dwell time. The reference isodose resulting from the intracavitary part alone is never exceeding a distance of 25 mm from the tandem at level of point A, thus limiting the high dose regions inside the implant. The loading of dwell positions in needles is not closer than 1 cm to the ring source level, reducing additional dose to the vagina. The total dwell time in all needle positions is usually between 10 and 20% of the total dwell time of all positions in the tandem–ring applicator. This is limiting high dose regions from additional needles, located mainly in the parametrial tissue with additional healthy structures not contoured explicitly.

14.8 Documentation

Values for all dose and volume parameters are inserted into a spreadsheet, which is also calculating the total EQD2 dose.

14.9 Quality Assurance/Avoidance of Errors

Acceptance tests and constancy tests are performed regularly for all involved treatment planning systems, afterloader devices, and applicators. Most tasks of the treatment planning approach are double-checked by a second person or performed in close cooperation with the treatment team. A dedicated spreadsheet documents the dose and volume parameters prospectively for each individual fraction; thereby, deviations from predefined constraints can be identified quickly. Evaluation of the resulting treatment plan by the radiooncologist and physicist is essential. In addition to dose volume histogram parameters, the isodose distribution, the dwell time characteristics, the loading pattern, the reconstruction accuracy, and contouring have to be discussed and approved. A simple check of DVH numbers is not sufficient for approval. This approach depends very much on a well-trained and experienced team. At the treatment console, technicians are checking essential parts of the plan, including total reference air kerma, loading pattern, and treatment times before irradiation begins.

References

1. Fransson A, Andreo P, Pötter R. Aspects of MR image distortion in radiotherapy treatment planning. Strahlenther Onkol. 2001;177:59–73.
2. Dimopoulos JCA, Schard G, Berger D, et al. Systematic evaluation of MRI findings in different stages of treatment of cervical cancer: potential of MRI on delineation of target, Pathoanatomic structures, and organs at risk. Int J Radiat Oncol Biol Phys. 2006;64:1380–8.
3. Fellner C, Pötter R, Knocke TH, Wambersie A. Comparison of radiography- and computed tomography-based treatment planning in cervix cancer in brachytherapy with specific attention to some quality assurance aspects. Radiother Oncol. 2001;58:53–62.
4. Gerbaulet A, Pötter R, Haie-Meder C. Cervix cancer. In: Gerbaulet A, Pötter R, Mazeron JJ, Meertens H, Van Limbergen E, editors. The GEC ESTRO handbook of brachytherapy. Brussels: ESTRO; 2002. p. 301–63.
5. Wachter-Gerstner N, Wachter S, Reinstadler E, et al. The impact of sectional imaging on dose escalation in endocavitary HDR-brachytherapy of cervical cancer: results of a prospective comparative trial. Radiother Oncol. 2003;68:51–9.
6. Wachter-Gerstner N, Wachter S, Reinstadler E, et al. Bladder and rectum dose defined from MRI based treatment planning for cervix cancer brachytherapy: comparison of dose-volume histograms for organ contours and organ wall, comparison with ICRU rectum and bladder reference point. Radiother Oncol. 2003;68:269–76.

7. Kirisits C, Pötter R, Lang S, Dimopoulos J, Wachter-Gerstner N, Georg D. Dose and volume parameters for MRI based treatment planning in intracavitary brachytherapy of cervix cancer. Int J Radiat Oncol Biol Phys. 2005;62:901–11.
8. Haie-Meder C, Pötter R, Van Limbergen E, et al. Recommendations from Gynaecological (GYN) GEC-ESTRO Working Group (I): concepts and terms in 3D image based 3D treatment planning in cervix cancer brachytherapy with emphasis on MRI assessment of GTV and CTV. Radiother Oncol. 2005;74:235–45.
9. Pötter R, Haie-Meder C, Van Limbergen E, et al. Recommendations from gynaecological (GYN) GEC ESTRO working group (II): concepts and terms in 3D image-based treatment planning in cervix cancer brachytherapy-3D dose volume parameters and aspects of 3D image-based anatomy, radiation physics, radiobiology. Radiother Oncol. 2006;78:67–77.
10. Pötter R, Dimopoulos J, Georg P, et al. Clinical impact of MRI assisted dose volume adaptation and dose escalation in brachytherapy of locally advanced cervix cancer. Radiother Oncol. 2007;83:148–55.
11. Dimopoulos J, Lang S, Kirisits C, et al. Dose-volume histogram parameters and local tumor control in MR image guided cervical cancer brachytherapy. Int J Radiat Oncol Biol Phys. 2009;75:56–63.
12. Dimopoulos J, Lang S, Kirisits C, et al. Dose-effect relationship for local control of cervical cancer by magnetic resonance image guided brachytherapy. Radiother Oncol. 2009;93:311–5.
13. Georg P, Kirisits C, Goldner G, et al. Correlation of dose-volume parameters, endoscopic and clinical rectal side effects in cervix cancer patients treated with definitive radiotherapy including MRI-based brachytherapy. Radiother Oncol. 2009;91:173–80.
14. Georg P, Dimopoulos J, Kirisits C, et al. Dose volume parameters in cervical cancer patients treated with MRI based brachytherapy and their predictive value for late adverse side effects in rectum, sigmoid and bladder. Radiother Oncol. 2006;81(S1):S38–9.
15. Dimopoulos JC, Kirisits C, Petric P, et al. The Vienna applicator for combined intracavitary and interstitial brachytherapy of cervical cancer: clinical feasibility and preliminary results. Int J Radiat Oncol Biol Phys. 2006;66:83–90.
16. Kirisits C, Lang S, Dimopoulos J, et al. The Vienna applicator for combined intracavitary and interstitial brachytherapy of cervical cancer: design, application, treatment planning and dosimetric results. Int J Radiat Oncol Biol Phys. 2006;65:624–30.
17. Pötter R. Modern imaging in brachytherapy. In: Gerbaulet A, Pötter R, Mazeron JJ, Meertens H, Van Limbergen E, editors. The GEC ESTRO handbook of brachytherapy. Brussels: European Society of Therapeutic Radiology and Oncology; 2002. p. 123–51.
18. Lang S, Kirisits C, Dimopoulos J, Georg D, Pötter R. Treatment planning for MRI assisted brachytherapy of gynecologic malignancies based on total dose constraints. Int J Radiat Oncol Biol Phys. 2007;69:619–27.
19. Berger D, Dimopoulos J, Pötter R, Kirisits C. Direct reconstruction of the Vienna applicator on MR images. Radiother Oncol. 2009;93:347–51.

Belgium: University Hospital, Leuven 15

Marisol De Brabandere and Erik Van Limbergen

15.1 Introduction

At Leuven University (UZL) we started magnetic resonance imaging (MRI)-guided intracavitary BT in 2002. After a learning period where we prescribed the dose according to our standard 2D X-ray-based protocol, and changed source positions and dwell times to correct for overdoses on organs at risk [1], we went to full 3D dose prescription and dose escalation of the high risk CTV (HR CTV) according to the GEC-ESTRO protocol [2, 3].

15.2 Applicators Available and Selection Parameters

At UZL, the Nucletron MR/CT compatible standard applicator is used. This Fletcher-type applicator consists of plastic-carbon endo-uterine and endovaginal ovoid tubes. The curvature of the uterine applicator is 30°, and different lengths of 40, 50, and 60 mm are available. Ovoids have a standard anteroposterior thickness of 20 mm, and can be 30, 25, or 20 mm in width. The medial sides of the ovoids have a slit to immobilize the endo-uterine tube centrally in between the ovoids.

15.3 Insertion Techniques

Applications are performed under general anesthesia. After clinical examination, the uteri ostium is dilated. In case of retroversion of the uterus, a destroyed cervical canal, or in any

M. De Brabandere and E. Van Limbergen (✉)
Department of Radiation Oncology, University Hospital Gasthuisberg,
Herestraat 49, 3000 Leuven, Belgium
e-mail: marisol.debrabandere@uzleuven.be; erik.vanlimbergen@uzleuven.be

A.N. Viswanathan et al. (eds.), *Gynecologic Radiation Therapy*,
DOI: 10.1007/978-3-540-68958-4_15,

case of difficult access, the endo-uterine tube is placed under ultrasonographic guidance to avoid perforations. For the choice of the ovoids, always the largest possible ovoids are used to expand the irradiated volume as far as possible to the lateral sides. In case of insufficient coverage of anterior, posterior tumoral extensions in the vaginal walls, or lateral tumor extension, interstitial plastic tubes are inserted in the vaginal wall, and/or the parametria.

For lower vaginal or paravaginal extensions, tubes are positioned under manual control. In case of high parametrial extensions, tubes are inserted under laparoscopic control, to manipulate the position of the uterus and to control the depth of the needle insertions in the parametria.

15.4 Imaging Protocol

For delineation of the organs of interest, MR images are acquired on a 1.5T Siemens Sonata scanner. Patients are scanned in supine position. Axial, paraxial, parasagittal, and para-coronal fast spin echo (FSE) T2-weighted images are acquired with the applicator in place using following parameters: TE = 120 ms, TR = 6,000 ms, slice thickness 4 mm without interslice gap.

Applicator reconstruction is performed using two orthogonal digital X-ray images at gantry 0° and 90°. Radiopaque dummy markers allow identification and reconstruction of the source positions.

15.5 Caveats to Imaging

In Leuven, we have tried to visualize the source channels on transversal MR-T2 images by inserting plastic tubes (outer diameter 1.0 mm) filled with water. It was possible to identify the source channels on the MR images by an increased signal in those slices where the tubes were perpendicular to the slice plane (parallel to the scanning direction). However, in those slices where the tubes curve away the signal was too low, even with increased scanning times. Using tubes with a larger diameter (and hence a larger volume of water) was not possible due to the limited dimension of the applicator channel. Hence, in the crucial areas where channel identification is most difficult (at the level of the ovoids) the plastic tubes did not provide useful information to visualize the source channels. For that reason, direct applicator reconstruction on T2-weighted MR images was found not to be reliable.

15.6 Contouring Protocol

Contouring is carried out according to the GYN GEC-ESTRO recommendations. GTV, HR CTV including cervix and paracervical grey zones, and intermediate risk CTV (IR CTV) extending at least 50 mm anteroposteriorly and 10 mm laterally and craniocaudally beyond the HR CTV are delineated.

The outer wall of the whole bladder, the whole rectum, and the sigmoid and the small bowel adjacent to the uterus are delineated.

15.7 Treatment Planning

Treatment planning is performed in Plato BPSv14.3 and Plato EVALv3.1 (Nucletron, Veenendaal, The Netherlands) using a combination of X-ray and MRI data. After reconstruction of the three source channels on the X-ray images, a symmetrical standard loading pattern with equal dwell times in the intra-uterine and ovoid dwell positions is applied. In the ovoids the first 2 cm starting from the tip is loaded. The intra-uterine tandem is loaded starting at 1 cm from the first source position unto the intersection with the catheters. As a starting point, a preliminary dose of 35 Gy is normalized to point A.

The X-ray images are registered to the axial MR images using four manually defined matching points: the tip of the three catheters and an additional point at the top of the bladder balloon. The dose distribution as created in the X-ray-based plan is then evaluated in relation to patient anatomy in the Plato-EVAL module.

Patients are treated in one pulsed dose rate (PDR) fraction. The aim is to prescribe a total D90 of 85 $Gy_{\alpha\beta10}$ to the HR CTV and to fully cover the IR CTV with 60 $Gy_{\alpha\beta10}$, respecting the tolerance doses in the organs at risk. The tolerance limits applied are $D_{2cc} <$ 90 $Gy_{\alpha\beta3}$ on the bladder, $D_{2cc} < 75$ $Gy_{\alpha\beta3}$ on the rectum, and $D_{2cc} < 75$ $Gy_{\alpha\beta3}$ on the sigmoid colon and small intestines. Priority is given to the organs at risk. In general, these dose criteria are not fulfilled with the standard loading pattern. Depending on the tumor extent and location, the source positions and dwell times are manually optimized in the BPS planning module. If necessary, the dose at point A is renormalized. After each adjustment, the resulting dose grid is projected onto the MR images again for a visual inspection of the isodoses and calculation of the dose-volume parameters. This stepwise optimization procedure is repeated until the dose constraints are fulfilled as close as possible.

15.8 Dose and Fractionation: GTV, CTV, OAR

In a recent optimization study performed in Leuven, the dose in GTV, CTV, and the organs at risk was analyzed in detail for 16 patients [1]. A selection of the studied parameters is given in Table 15.1. During optimization, the D90 in the HR CTV is increased as high as possible, while respecting the D_{2cc} tolerance values in the organs at risk. In practice, the doses in the rectum are usually much lower than the applied restriction, while bladder and sigmoid colon (or small intestines) often form a major limitation to a dose increase in the target. Due to the strict priority given to the organs at risk, the criterion D90 ≥ 85 $Gy_{\alpha\beta10}$ in

Table 15.1 Dose values (mean ± 1SD) for the organs at risk and the target volumes as obtained with magnetic resonance imaging (MRI)-based dose optimization. V(60 $Gy_{\alpha\beta10}$) represents the volume receiving 60 $Gy_{\alpha\beta10}$

	Bladder	Rectum	Sigmoid colon
D_{2cc} [$Gy_{\alpha\beta3}$]	82 ± 6	62 ± 4	68 ± 7
	GTV	HR CTV	IR CTV
D100 [$Gy_{\alpha\beta10}$]	89 ± 19	64 ± 6	58 ± 3
D90 [$Gy_{\alpha\beta10}$]	103 ± 24	79 ± 7	69 ± 4
V(60 $Gy_{\alpha\beta10}$) [%]	–	–	99 ± 2

the HR CTV is not always achieved. The dose requirements of the IR CTV are however easier to fulfill than those of the HR CTV. Our results showed that in patients where D90 > 80 $Gy_{\alpha\beta10}$ for the HR CTV, coverage of the IR CTV with the 60 $Gy_{\alpha\beta10}$ isodose was automatically guaranteed. The dose objective for the HR CTV is generally more difficult to accomplish than the dose objective for the IR CTV. Therefore, we decided that dose optimization in the target should be mainly guided by the dose recorded in the HR CTV.

The number of pulses is decided during the optimization process and usually it varies between 65 and 85 pulses. By increasing the number of pulses (lower dose rate) the radiobiologically normalized dose in the targets and organs at risk is decreased. Due to the lower α/β ratio, the dose reduction is more pronounced in the organs at risk than in the target volumes, hence enabling an additional "radiobiological" optimization. Increasing the number of pulses cannot be done unlimited however, as dose gain and patient comfort always need to be balanced. Moreover, the applied radiobiological model carries some uncertainties, e.g., in the values of α/β and $T_{1/2}$. Large deviations from the "reference" dose rate (i.e., 50 cGy/h) are therefore applied and interpreted with caution.

15.9 Documentation

All patients and treatment parameters are recorded according to the GEC-ESTRO protocol [2, 3].

15.10 Quality Assurance/Avoidance of Errors

General quality assurance checks are executed as a part of the commissioning program and for any major upgrade of the brachytherapy system. The clinical performance of the treatment planning system and afterloader was tested by postal external audits in the frame of EQUAL-ESTRO (Estro Quality Assurance Network) [4]. More in particular, the geometric accuracy of applicator reconstruction, including image acquisition, image data transfer,

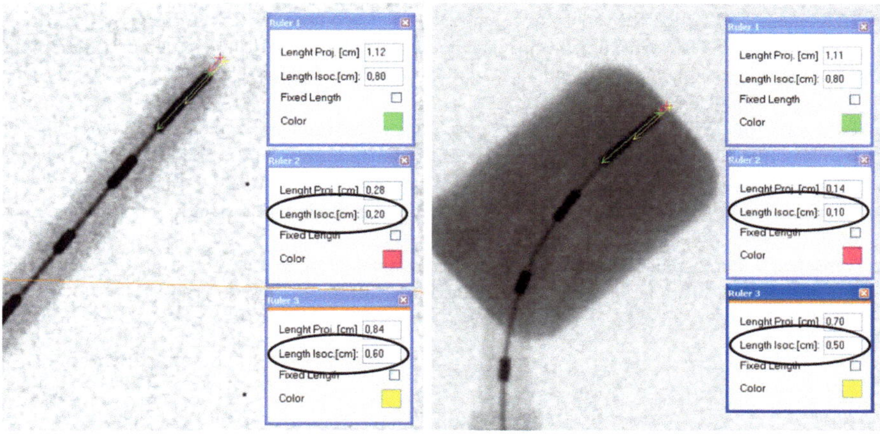

Fig. 15.1 X-ray images of the Nucletron Standard CT/MR tandem–ovoid applicator containing radiopaque markers (dummy sources). Sleeve thickness and distance from tip to first source position were measured digitally in the treatment planning system

and source position definition, was tested with the Baltas phantom for X-ray-based and 3D image-based reconstruction. Dosimetric checks were performed with a remote thermoluminescence detector (TLD) monitoring phantom designed to identify discrepancies in dosimetry data and dose calculation algorithms.

Besides general quality control checks, additional technique specific tests are necessary to exclude systematic and occasional errors in the treatment process. A potential source of systematic errors is applicator reconstruction. Accurate reconstruction is only possible when the applicator dimensions are known and correctly applied. Although nominal values are specified by the vendor, the most important applicator dimensions (e.g., sleeve thickness, distance from first source position to outer applicator tip) were verified independently in Leuven using X-ray images. An example is shown in Fig. 15.1.

The dose distribution is optimized by the physicist in close cooperation with the radiotherapist. The DVH values are entered in an electronic sheet in order to have an overview of the radiobiologically normalized doses in targets and organs at risk.

To intercept occasional errors a second physicist who was not involved in the original planning reviews the patient plan, both on print and on screen, with specific attention for the source data (type and strength), applicator reconstruction, source positioning and dwell times, dose prescription, and total reference air kerma (TRAK).

References

1. De Brabandere M, Mousa AM, Nulens A, Swinnen A, Van Limbergen E. Potential of dose optimisation in MRI based PDR brachytherapy of cervix carcinoma. Radiother Oncol. 2008;88(2):217–26.

2. Haie-Meder C, Pötter R, Van Limbergen E, et al. Recommendations from Gynaecological (GYN) GEC-ESTRO Working Group. (1) Concepts and terms in 3D image based 3D treatment planning in cervix cancer brachytherapy with emphasis on MRI assessment of GTV and CTV. Radiother Oncol. 2005;74(3):235–45.
3. Pötter R, Haie-Meder C, Van Limbergen E, et al. Recommendations from gynaecological (GYN) GEC-ESTRO Working group (II): Concepts and terms in 3D image-based treatment planning in cervix cancer brachytherapy - 3D dose volume parameters and aspects of 3D image-based anatomy, radiation physics, radiobiology. Radiotherapy and Oncology, Vol 78: 67–77, 2006.
4. Venselaar J, Perez-Calatayud J. Chapter 10: A practical guide to quality control of brachytherapy equipment. In: Venselaar J, Perez-Calatayud J, editors. Estro Booklet 8. 1st ed. Brussels: ESTRO; 2004. p. 233–40.

Denmark: Aarhus University Hospital, Aarhus

16

Kari Tanderup and Jacob C. Lindegaard

16.1 Introduction

Magnetic resonance imaging (MRI)-guided brachytherapy for locally advanced cervical cancer was introduced at Aarhus University Hospital in December 2005. Until then two-dimensional (2D) X-ray based planning had been performed with prescription of dose to point A. With X-ray based planning, doses to ICRU rectal and bladder points were calculated, and in a minority of cases, the applicator position or the loading of the applicator was modified. During a short learning period of 2 months, we retrospectively contoured on the magnetic resonance (MR) images and recorded dose from standard plans, before we moved to full prospective MRI-guided dose planning and optimization for every brachytherapy fraction [1].

16.2 Applicator Selection and Brachytherapy Application

Based on the agreement of a multidisciplinary conference, cases with locally advanced cervical cancer staged as IB2-IVA receive definitive radio-chemotherapy. Cases with limited metastatic para-aortic nodes (stage IVB) are also treated with curative intent on an individual basis. Staging involves biopsy and gynecologic examination in general anesthesia performed together with our gynecological oncology colleagues. Cystoscopy and rectoscopy are performed in cases of suspected stage IVA disease. The clinical findings are documented by use of the Embrace cartoons (www.embracestudy.dk). Further diagnostic investigations involve whole-body 18FDG-PET-CT and MRI of the pelvis.

Clinical assessment of the tumor volume and topography is repeated at each brachytherapy (BT) fraction, and a clinical drawing is made using the standardized EMBRACE

K. Tanderup (✉) and J.C. Lindegaard
Aarhus University, Norrebrogade 44, 8000 Aarhus C, Denmark
e-mail: karitand@rm.dk; Jacolind@rm.dk

A.N. Viswanathan et al. (eds.), *Gynecologic Radiation Therapy*,
DOI: 10.1007/978-3-540-68958-4_16, © Springer-Verlag Berlin Heidelberg 2011

cartoons. The application technique is planned on the basis of clinical examination in general anesthesia and a pretreatment MRI planning scan 1 week prior to the first BT application. The planning scan is performed with an intracavitary applicator (tandem–ring) in situ.

The applicator is inserted under US guidance with the patient under general anesthesia. In case of limited disease and/or good response to external beam radiation therapy (EBRT), an MRI-compatible intracavitary plastic tandem–ring applicator (GammaMed, Varian) is used. For patients with vaginal tumor extension at the time of BT a custom-made multichannel vaginal cylinder is attached to the tandem/ring applicator to allow for irradiation in the vagina. When the pretreatment MRI planning scan indicates that parametrial extension would lead to insufficient coverage by an intracavitary application, a combined intracavitary–interstitial (IC/IS) applicator is used with blunt-ended titanium needles (Acrostack, Wintherthur, Switzerland) inserted into the parametria either through steering holes in the ring or as free needles. The number of needles and the insertion depth is planned prior to insertion based on a provisional treatment plan with virtual needles on the pretreatment planning MRI. A Foley catheter with 7-mL of X-ray diluted contrast is placed in the bladder, and the vagina is packed with gauze soaked in diluted gadolinium (Magnevist 469 mg/mL, 7.5 mL in 100 mL NaCl). A 20-cm drainage tube is inserted 15 cm into the rectum to allow for the introduction of rectal diodes for in vivo dosimetry during pulsed dose rate (PDR) BT. Orthogonal X-rays are taken to check the implant geometry before the patient wakes from anesthesia and leaves the operating room.

16.3 Imaging Protocol

Magnetic resonance imaging is performed on the awake patient using a 1.5 Tesla scanner (Siemens Magnetom Symphony) about 45–60 min following the implant procedure. Plastic tubes filled with a copper sulphate solution ($CuSO_4$) are inserted in the applicator channels to serve as “dummy wires” [2]. All MRI sequences are oriented according to the axis of the applicator. The MRI protocol includes a T1-weighted (Turbo Spin Echo) paratransverse scan with a 3-mm slice thickness and no gap. T2-weighted (Turbo Spin Echo) sequences in all three planes: para-transversal, parasagittal, and para-coronal are produced with a slice thickness of 4 mm and a 1-mm gap.

16.4 Contouring Protocol

Contouring is performed on the T2-weighted para-transversal sequence supported by the clinical drawings and the MRI studies from diagnosis and at BT. The HR CTV, IR CTV, as well as the outer wall of the bladder, rectum, sigmoid, and bowel are contoured. Delineation of the HR CTV is aided by “copy-paste” of the HR CTV contour drawn in the T2-weighted para-coronal and parasagittal planes. The Point A and ICRU bladder and rectal points are positioned directly in the three-dimensional (3D) study.

16.5 Treatment Planning

Applicator reconstruction is performed in BrachyVision (Varian Medical Systems) on the para-transversal T2-weighted sequence. The T1-weighted images are fused with T2 to aid in the reconstruction. Due to smaller slice thickness, the T1-weighted sequence is superior to T2 with regard to visualization of CuSO4 dummy wires, needles, and the black void corresponding to the plastic applicator. However, to minimize the impact of fusion uncertainties, contouring and reconstruction is performed in the same image sequence (T2-weighted images) and T1 is only used for visualization. Tandem–ring library applicators with predefined geometry are introduced with guidance from CuSO4 dummy wires and by measuring the distance from the ring surface to the ring channel and from the tip of the tandem to the first stopping position in the tandem. Needles are introduced by direct reconstruction. However, an additional computed tomography (CT) scan is needed when free needles are employed.

Each BT fraction is planned individually and is always initiated using a standard library plan. The Aarhus standard plan contains three lateral stopping positions spaced by 5 mm in each side of the ring, and stopping positions each 5 mm in the tandem from the tip to the level of the ring with equal dwell times in all stopping positions. Optimization is first performed by manually adding or removing stopping positions and adjusting the dwell times. Fine tuning of the dose plan is done with a combination of graphical and manual dose optimization. The intention is to reach D90 of at least 85 Gy to the HR CTV, but keeping D_{2cc} of bladder and rectum/sigmoid at below 90 and 70–75 Gy, respectively. In this process, we pay attention to the high-dose volumes (i.e., 200% and 400% isodose lines). Also, we avoid to extend the prescription isodose curve to >25 mm from the center of the tandem at the level of Point A for intracavitary treatment. For patients receiving combined intracavitary/interstitial treatment, we aim for a loading of the parametrial needles less than 10–20% of the dwell times used in the tandem/ring so that the main part of the dose is delivered from the intracavitary applicator. After inspecting the isodoses at all image levels, we obtain the cumulative Dose Volume Histogram (DVH) parameters from BrachyVision. The resulting dose is recalculated into EQD2 in a spreadsheet. The EQD2 of EBRT and BT is then added to evaluate the optimized plan with regard to the DVH constraints. In case of four-field box, EBRT it is assumed that the organs at risk (OARs) receive the full EBRT prescribed dose. For IMRT a more detailed assessment of OAR dose is done, particularly to evaluate whether the parts of the OAR, which receive large BT dose, is also in a high-dose region during IMRT. Furthermore, a worst-case scenario is used, where it is assumed that it is the same 2 cm^3 of the OARs, which receive the maximal BT dose at each BT fraction.

We routinely record the DVH parameters of non-optimized standard dose plans. In this way, we keep track of the changes we are introducing by doing 3D dose optimization and are able to quantify and monitor the DVH changes over time for our patient cohort (Fig. 16.1). Using this analysis, we have shown that MRI-guided 3D optimization significantly improves the DVH parameters of PDR BT [3].

We have further observed that this improvement is not related to a significant overall BT dose escalation for the whole patient group, since the mean TRAK across the entire patient population is slightly decreased by 8% in optimized plans as compared to standard

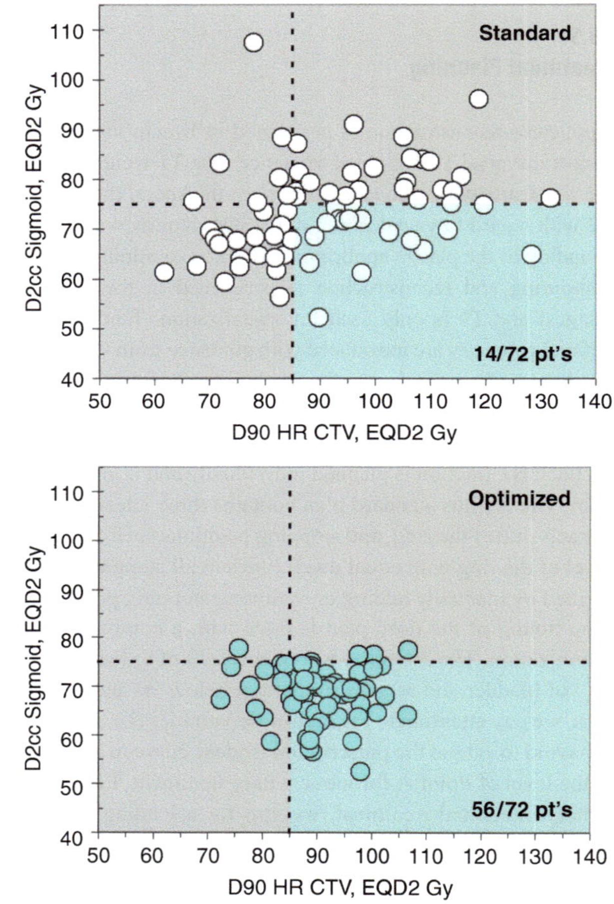

Fig. 16.1 Dose-volume histogram evaluation of standard (*top*) versus optimized (*bottom*) BT observed in 57 patients with locally advanced cervical cancer treated at the Aarhus University Hospital with EBRT and PDR BT. The figure shows D_{2cc} for sigmoid plotted against D90 of the HR CTV. DVH constraints for sigmoid (<75 Gy) indicated by the *horizontal dotted line*. *Vertical dotted line* indicates the desired D90 to HR CTV (i.e., >85 Gy). Symbols within the box fulfilled DVH constraints with respect to both sigmoid and tumor. When similar evaluation was performed for bladder and rectum it was found that all DVH constraints were met in 14/72 patients for standard versus 56/72 patients with optimized plans ($p < 0.001$)

plans. Optimization leads to an individualization of the source positions and loading and makes it possible to shape the dose individually to small and large tumors. Thus, the general trend is that dose optimization often decreases the point A dose in small tumors where the OAR are situated very close to the applicator. For larger tumors with the OAR at further distance, it is most often possible to increase target coverage without violating the DVH constraints, in particular with the use of interstitial needles.

16.6 Dose and Fractionation: GTV, CTV, OAR

The diagnostic PET-CT signal is fused with the CT simulation to aid the contouring of primary and nodal Gross Tumour Volume at diagnosis (GTV-TD and GTV-N). The contouring of GTV is further refined by the findings obtained by the clinical examination and MRI. Relevant Nodal Clinical Target Volume (CTV-N) is contoured and finally the Elective

Clinical Target Volume CTV-E is established, which always completely respect GTV-TD and CTV-N. A 10–15 mm anterior–posterior margin at the level of GTV-TD is added to encompass internal movement of the uterus. No margin is used for internal movement of the elective or pathological nodes. For Elective Planning Target Volume (PTV-E) an additional 5-mm margin is added to CTV. Daily cone-beam CT (CBCT) is used for image guidance of all EBRT fractions.

The prescribed standard dose of EBRT to PTV-E is 45 Gy in 25 fractions delivered by use of a conformal box technique (MLC equipped Varian Linacs, 6–10 MV). The Nodal Planning Target Volume (PTV–N), when present, is treated with 60 Gy in 30 fractions and in this situation, the prescribed dose to PTV-E is raised to 50 Gy in 30 fractions. IMRT with a simultaneous integrated boost (SIB) is used to obtain differential dose levels for the PTV-E and PTV–N. Concomitant chemotherapy (weekly cisplatin, 40 mg/m^2) for a maximum of six courses is given to all patients with sufficient kidney and bone marrow function.

PDR BT is initiated during the last 1–2 weeks of EBRT, with two fractions given with a 1-week interval, aiming for a total treatment including both EBRT and BT of no more than 50 days. Weekly blood tests are performed and blood transfusion is used to keep the hemoglobin above 7 mmol/L during the 6–7 week treatment period. EBRT or concomitant cisplatin is not given on BT treatment days. The prescribed dose for each BT fraction is 15–17.5 Gy to the HR CTV delivered in 15–20 pulses with 1 pulse per hour. The overall aim is to reach a D90 of at least 85 Gy EQD2 in the HR CTV. EQD2 is calculated using the mono-exponential repair half time model with $\alpha/\beta = 10$ for tumor, $\alpha/\beta = 3$ for OARs, and a repair half time of 1.5 h. DVH constraints for OARs are 90 Gy EQD2 for bladder and 70–75 Gy EQD2 for rectum and sigmoid. There are rarely any problems to keep bladder and rectum dose below 90 Gy and 70 Gy EQD2, respectively. In our institute, sigmoid is the OAR that most often challenges the DVH constraint, and 75 Gy or even a bit higher is justified if the target would otherwise be considerably under-dosed.

16.7 Documentation

Dose and volume parameters are recorded in a spreadsheet. Calculation of total EBRT + BT EQD2 dose is done automatically in the spreadsheet. For GTV, HR CTV, and IR CTV the following parameters are recorded: volume, D90, D100, and V100 (for HR CTV). For OARs (bladder, rectum, sigmoid, and bowel when required): volume, D0.1 cc, D2 cc and dose to ICRU points (for bladder and rectum). Additionally, point A dose and TRAK are reported.

16.8 Quality Assurance/Avoidance of Errors

Applicator commissioning related to MR image guidance involves some extra steps since the source channel is not directly visible on the images as in CT. MR and CT imaging of the applicator in a phantom is performed to characterize the geometry of the source channel relative to the appearance of the applicator on MRI. These scans are used to create library applicators.

In vivo dosimetry is used as an overall check of delivery of dose. A fivefold PTW rectal diode dosimeter is placed in the drainage tube in the rectum before coupling of the applicators to the afterloader. For each pulse, the dosimeter will show a distinctive dose pattern based on the position of the diodes in relation to the source positions. In addition, the accumulated dose throughout the PDR treatment is recorded. During BT treatment, planning the maximal dose to the diodes is estimated in the dose planning system. After the first pulse, the measured rectal dose is compared to the estimated dose and a decision by the medical doctor in charge is taken as to continue treatment. For each succeeding pulse, the implant is visually inspected and the stability of the measured doses is monitored by the nursing staff. Treatment is interrupted for renewed review if there are single pulse deviations of more than 30% or deviation in accumulated dose of more than 15%. In this case, the dose pattern of the diodes in the specific pulse is helpful in order to evaluate the nature and severity of the accumulated dose deviation. Currently a new and more patient friendly micro dosimeter system based on luminescence dosimetry is being investigated.

References

1. Lindegaard JC, Tanderup K, Nielsen SK, Haack S, Gelineck J. MRI-guided 3D optimization significantly improves DVH parameters of pulsed-dose-rate brachytherapy in locally advanced cervical cancer. Int J Radiat Oncol Biol Phys. 2008;71:756–64.
2. Haack S, Nielsen SK, Lindegaard JC, Gelineck J, Tanderup K. Applicator reconstruction in MRI 3D image-based dose planning of brachytherapy for cervical cancer. Radiother Oncol 2009;91:187–93.
3. Tanderup K, Nielsen SK, Nyvang GB, Pedersen EM, Røhl L, Aagard T, Fokdal L, Lindegaard JC. From point A to the sculpted pear: MR image guidance significantly improves tumour dose and sparing of organs at risk in brachytherapy of cervical cancer, Radiother Oncol, 2010; 94(2):173–180.

France: Institut Gustave-Roussy, Paris 17

Christine Haie-Meder and Isabelle Dumas

17.1 Introduction

In our institution, there has been a long tradition of brachytherapy, especially in gynecological tumours. From the beginning, there was an attempt to adapt the brachytherapy dose to the volume and the shape of the tumour and to take the anatomy of the vagina into account. The first step to achieve this goal was the use of the vaginal mould, performed for each patient. It was initially used with low dose-rate brachytherapy. When MRI images became available, we had the opportunity to use these MRI data with the mould in, as this applicator was perfectly MRI-compatible. The first step was to collect all the MRI images and to retrospectively look at the tumour coverage, without modifying our dosimetric policy. In any case, the potential dosimetric modification would have been limited as low dose-rate brachytherapy was performed using cesium sources. Almost 120 patients had MRI images without dosimetric modifications. In 2004, after the introduction of pulse dose-rate brachytherapy in our department, it became possible to adapt brachytherapy doses to MRI findings, using the European Gynecological Brachytherapy Group/European Society for Therapeutic Radiology and Oncology (GEC-ESTRO) recommendations.

17.2 Applicators: Mould Technique

At the Institut Gustave-Roussy, there has been a long tradition of personalized applicator adapted to each patient, based on the fabrication of moulded applicator realized from a vaginal impression [1, 4]. This mould technique was used in the former time for low dose-rate brachytherapy and is used nowadays for pulse dose-rate brachytherapy. The first step is the

C. Haie-Meder (✉) and I. Dumas
Brachytherapy Service, Institut Gustave Roussy,
Rue Camille Desmoulins, 94800 Villejuif, France
e-mail: Christine.haiemeder@igr.fr

A.N. Viswanathan et al. (eds.), *Gynecologic Radiation Therapy*,
DOI: 10.1007/978-3-540-68958-4_17, © Springer-Verlag Berlin Heidelberg 2011

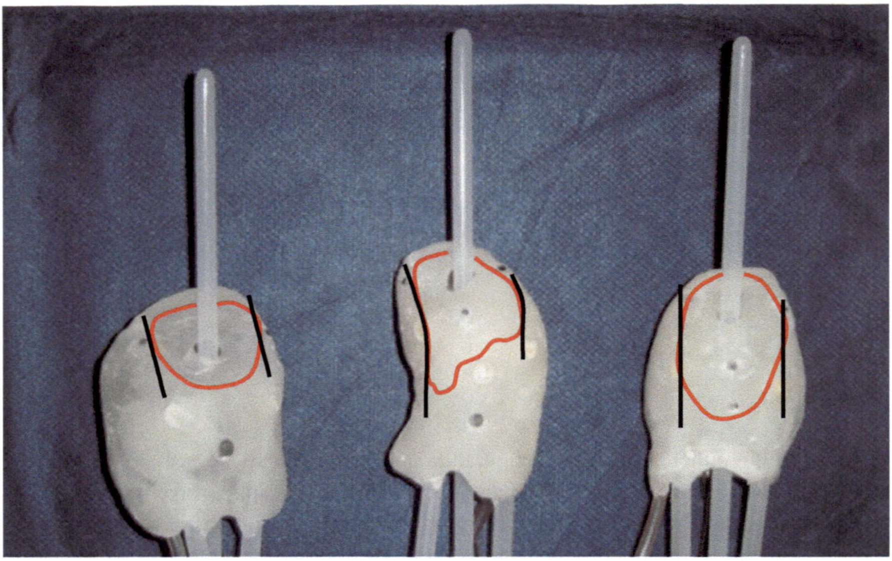

Fig. 17.1 The mould technique: these 3 examples show tandem with different vaginal moulds that were created at the time of diagnosis. Vaginal catheter placements and lengths are determined based on tumour extension and size

vaginal impression, with injection of a liquid paste into the vagina after the placement of two strips of gauze into each lateral vaginal fornix. After solidification, the impression is extracted from the vagina. This procedure does not require any anaesthesia, apart from performed in children. The tumour topography, the size of exo cervical tumour, the extension within the vagina are perfectly identified on the vaginal impression. The second step consists of acrylic moulded applicator fabrication, performed by technicians. The vaginal impression is plunged into liquid plaster. When dry, the plaster is cut into two pieces, the vaginal impression removed, and after reconstitution of the plaster, a synthetic autopolymerized resin is poured in a thin layer. When this resin (Palapress) is dry, the two plaster pieces are removed and the applicator is ready. The position of the two vaginal catheters, decided by the radiation oncologist, is drawn according to the tumour limits. Vaginal catheters are basically located on each side of the cervical limits. Their length depends on the tumour size and the vaginal extension (Fig. 17.1). These catheters are fixed into the applicator. One hole is made at the level of the cervical os for the uterine tube insertion and different holes are made in the applicator, allowing daily vaginal irrigation and vaginal mucosal herniation that prevents mould displacement [9].

17.3 Insertion Techniques

The mould insertion is performed under spinal anaesthesia or under general anaesthesia. The first step of the application consists of a careful gynecological examination materialized by a cartoon, which will be used at the time of target delineation. After insertion of a bladder catheter with the balloon filled with 7cc of radiopaque solution, a smooth hysterometer is inserted through the cervical os to measure the length of the uterine cavity precisely and to document its curvature. The position of the hysterometer is systematically checked with trans-abdominal ultrasound in order to avoid perforation. The dilatation is progressively performed up to the size required for the intrauterine catheter, which is inserted through the cervical os into the uterine cavity. The mould is then introduced into the vagina. No packing is necessary, as the mould by itself expands the vaginal walls. With this mould applicator, the patient systematically moves out of the bed at least twice a day, without any risk of mould displacement, avoiding bed rest complications.

17.4 Imaging Protocol/Caveats to Imaging

3-D MRI-based pulse dose-rate brachytherapy is systematically performed, allowing dose adaptation to the targets with optimization, taking dose to organs at risk into account. After the implantation, the patient is transferred to the MRI-scanner. Homemade MRI-compatible dummy sources (filled with glycerin) are inserted into the catheters to visualize the intrauterine and vaginal positions of the sources. Patients are scanned without any bladder filling to reproduce the treatment conditions. Fast spin-echo T2-weighted images (TE 120s, TR 4100s) are acquired on a General Electric Signa Excite 1.5T MRI machine. Axial and sagittal images are acquired with 3-mm slice thickness, no interslice gap, and a matrix size of 256 × 224. Immediately after MRI imaging, orthogonal X-rays are systematically performed to check imaging reconstruction of the applicator on MRI. Appropriate geometry of the implant is evaluated and reference points (right and left points A, pelvic wall points, ICRU bladder and rectal points, and one point 1.5 cm cranial to the ICRU bladder point) are identified on X-ray films. The next step is the three-dimensional (3D) reconstruction. Axial images are imported into the Plato brachytherapy planning system (BPS) treatment planning system, (Nucletron, The Netherlands) and a 3D set is reconstructed. All reference points are digitized and transferred from the X-ray images into the treatment planning system. To identify the dwell positions, the dummy source images are digitized in each axial MRI slice. The size length to be activated is secondarily defined according to the target volume (intermediate-risk CTV) delineated on MRI images, as in our experience the length of radioactive sources is not predetermined and directly depends on the tumour extension.

17.5 Contouring Protocol

The gross tumour volume (GTV), high-risk (HR-CTV) and intermediate-risk clinical target volumes (IR-CTV), and OAR are delineated (GEC-ESTRO) [7, 8]. This delineation process integrates the clinical findings and the MRI images at the time of diagnosis. The entire bladder and sigmoid are contoured. The rectum is contoured 3 cm from the anal margin to the sigmoid flexure.

17.6 Treatment Planning/Dose and Fractionation: GTV, CTV, OAR

In our standard protocol, a total dose of at least 15 Gy is prescribed to the IR-CTV for additional brachytherapy, after 45 Gy of external beam radiation therapy to the pelvis with weekly cisplatin (40 mg/m^2). In limited disease, stage IB1 cervix cancer, preoperative brachytherapy is used, with a prescription of 60 Gy to the IR-CTV. The first treatment plan is generated using point A as a reference point, without any optimization and the resulting dose distribution is evaluated in terms of target volume coverage and doses to the most exposed 2 cm^3 received by the OAR. The limits for doses to OAR are 75 Gy EQ2Gy total dose to the rectum and 85 Gy EQD2Gy total dose to the bladder [2]. After generating the first treatment plan, manual optimization is performed to obtain the best dose distribution covering the target. In all cases, we try to maintain differences between neighbouring dwell times no greater than a factor of 2, especially in vaginal sources. This approach is based on clinical experience and results following low-dose rate brachytherapy [5, 6]. After each modification, isodose distribution is evaluated and a detailed analysis of the dose-volume parameters (DVH) for CTVs and OAR is systematically performed. Finally, the dose-rate is corrected if the limit of 0.50 Gy per h to the OAR is exceeded, by decreasing the dose-rate in the isodose prescription and increasing the number of pulses [3]

17.7 Quality Assurance/Avoidance of Errors

Patients are regularly followed during brachytherapy, on a twice-daily basis. Clinical assessment is performed and systematic X-rays are performed on day 2 to check the absence of mould position modification. In order to avoid errors in the 3D reconstruction, as stated before, all reference points are digitized and transferred from the X-ray images into the treatment planning system. A systematic study of accordance between transferred points and their situation in the 3D image reconstruction is performed to avoid errors in reconstruction. The delineation results are systematically reviewed and validated by a senior radiation oncologist prior to the start of the dosimetric procedure. Dosimetry is validated by both physicist and physician. The pulse size and pulse number are double-checked.

References

1. Albano M, Dumas I, Haie-Meder C. Curiethérapie à l'Institut Gustave Roussy: applicateur moulé vaginal personnalisé: modification et amélioration techniques. Cancer Radiothér. 2008;12:822–6.
2. Briot E, de Crevoisier R, Petrow P, et al. Dose-volume histogram analysis for tumor and critical organs in intracavitary brachytherapy of cervical cancer with the use of MRI. Radiother Oncol. 2001;60 Suppl 1:S3.

3. Chargari C, Magné N, Dumas I, et al. Physics contributions and clinical outcome with 3D MRI based pulsed dose-rate intracavitary brachytherapy in cervical caner patients. Int J Radiat Oncol Biol Phys. 2009;74:133–9.
4. Gerbaulet A, Bridier A, Haie-Meder C, et al. Curiethérapie des cancers du col utérin. Méthode de l'Institut Gustave-Roussy. Bull Cancer Radiother. 1992;79:107–17.
5. Gerbaulet A, Kunkler I, Kerr GR, et al. Combined radiotherapy and surgery: Local control and complications in early carcinoma of the uterine cervix. The Villejuif experience, 1975–84. Radiother Oncol. 1992;23:66–73.
6. Gerbaulet A, Michel G, Haie-Meder C, et al. The role of low dose rate brachytherapy in the treatment of cervix carcinoma. Experience of the Gustave-Roussy Institute on 1245 patients. Eur J Gynaecol Oncol. 1995;16:461–75.
7. Haie-Meder C, Pötter R, Van Limbergen E, et al. Recommendations from Gynaecological (GYN) GEC-ESTRO Working Group: concepts and terms in 3D image based 3D treatment planning in cervix cancer brachytherapy with emphasis on MRI assessment of GTV and CTV. Radiother Oncol. 2005;74:235–45.
8. Pötter R, Haie-Meder C, Van Limbergen E, et al. Recommendations from gynaecological (GYN) GEC ESTRO working group (II): concepts and terms in 3D image-based treatment planning in cervix cancer brachytherapy-3D dose volume parameters and aspects of 3D image-based anatomy, radiation physics, radiobiology. Radiother Oncol. 2006;78:67–77.
9. San Filippo N, de Crevoisier R, Kafrouni H, et al. Three dimensional assessment of applicator movement in brachytherapy for cervical carcinoma. Radiother Oncol. 2001;60:S23.

Great Britain: Mount Vernon Cancer Center, Middlesex

18

Peter Hoskin, Gerry Lowe, and Rachel Wills

18.1 Introduction

High dose rate brachytherapy was initiated at Mount Vernon Hospital in 1992 prior to which low dose rate manual afterloading Cesium treatment had been in use for gynaecological treatments. The high dose rate system was a Gammamed 12i machine and an intrauterine tube and Manchester ovoid applicators were used using orthogonal films for dosimetry and ICRU reference points. The standard dose at that time was 14 Gy in two fractions to Point A after 50 Gy external beam.

In 2003, image-guided three-dimensional (3D) planning was introduced and the applicator was changed from a tube and ovoids to a tube and ring. Initially computed tomography (CT) was used moving to magnetic resonance (MR) imaging in February 2004. With the advent of three-dimensional planning the dosimetry has also evolved from a standard atlas based on Point A doses (defined using the Abacus system supplied with the Gammamed unit) to individualised applicator reconstruction and 3D dosimetry using Brachyvision (Varian Medical Systems, Crawley UK). In 2006, an open bore MR was installed in the brachytherapy suite and MR image-guided brachytherapy has become our standard of care using the tube and ring applicator and interstitial parametrial implants. With the advent of image-guided brachytherapy, the doses used have increased initially to 18 Gy in 3 fractions and currently 21 Gy in 3 fractions, which is to be further escalated to 24 Gy in 4 fractions with the external beam dose remaining standard at 50 Gy in 25 fractions.

P. Hoskin (✉), G. Lowe, and R. Wills
The Mount Vernon Hospital NHS Trust Mount Vernon Centre for Cancer Treatment, Mount Vernon Hospital, Rickmansworth Road, Northwood, Middlesex, HA6 2RN, UK
e-mail: peterhoskin@nhs.net

A.N. Viswanathan et al. (eds.), *Gynecologic Radiation Therapy*,
DOI: 10.1007/978-3-540-68958-4_18, © Springer-Verlag Berlin Heidelberg 2011

18.2 Applicator Selection

The initial experience was with the MR-compatible Varian system composed of plastic utilising the intrauterine sleeve as a conduit for the central source tube (Varian Medical Systems, Crawley, UK). These system have now been replaced by titanium intrauterine applicators and ring (Varian), which are used for all insertions. Recognizing the limitations of the ring, although more flexible than the two ovoids of the Manchester system, we have in the past 3 years been using interstitial implantation in addition to the tube and ring applicators to provide added dose into the parametrium as required for bulky stage 2B and 3B tumours. For this, flexible plastic interstitial needles are used (Varian).

18.3 Insertion

Since the inception of HDR brachytherapy at Mount Vernon in 1992, Smit sleeves have been used to enable multifraction HDR treatments to be delivered with only one general anaesthetic to place the sleeve. This practice has been continued as we have moved to the tube and ring applicator with interstitial boost.

First insertions are undertaken in the operating room with general anaesthetia unless there is a significant medical contraindication when a spinal anaesthetic will be used. Patients are placed in the lithotomy position, the cervix identified and the cervical canal and intrauterine cavity dilated. Trans-abdominal ultrasound may be used to confirm the presence of the tube within the cavity in cases where this is uncertain or difficult. The canal is dilated to Hegar size 7, the appropriate length of the sleeve is chosen from the available range (2, 4 or 6 cm) and this is then inserted in the cervical canal and stitched in position using an absorbable suture to the cervix or lateral vaginal fornix as practicable.

If interstitial applicators are to be used then these are placed at this point. Freehand implant is performed introducing the applicator through the lateral vaginal wall at the junction of the upper and middle third and running the applicator submucosally into the fornix and from there to the parametrium. Two or three applicators may be used depending upon the extent of tumour to be implanted and bilateral interstitial implants are undertaken if clinically indicated.

Following this procedure, the intrauterine tube is placed within the sleeve and the ring positioned at the vaginal fornices. Prior to implantation, aqueous gel is inserted into the spacer cap, which is then fitted onto the ring, and also into the cervical sleeve. This action improves localisation of the titanium applicators on MR imaging. The Varian applicators are rigid, and the tube and the ring are located together and fixed. Rectal displacement is achieved using either the rectal spatula provided with the applicator or, in patients where there is no room for this, gauze packing. The interstitial applicators, the tube and the ring are fixed in position using padded dressings and a perineal bandage.

18.4 Imaging

Following recovery from general anaesthetia, patients return to the radiotherapy department where they undergo an MR scan. The brachytherapy unit includes an open bore 0.35 T scanner (Siemens Magnetom C!, Siemens Medical Systems, Camberley, UK) on which T2 images in the para-transverse (3 mm slices with no inter-slice gap) and sagittal planes are obtained. By acquiring these images in two concatenations, patient motion artefacts are more easily visible and taken into account. The images are examined by the brachytherapy physicist. If satisfactory, no further scans are taken; if there is uncertainty with regard to location of any of the applicators then a CT scan is taken to augment the MR scan. Currently, a CT scan will also be taken if interstitial applicators are present. CT is reconstructed with 3-mm slice spacing, and registered to the MR using the applicators themselves as fiducial markers.

We have validated our MR scanner to provide a volume of 14 cm × 14 cm × 14 cm inside which geometric image distortion is less than or equal to 2 mm, for the coils and sequences used. Care is taken to ensure that the applicator set is within this volume, which is defined relative to the room lasers and magnet, and centred within the coil. This, and the other validation measurements and applicator dimensions used in this process, should be undertaken by each centre for the individual scanner, sequences, coils, and applicator sets to be used.

18.5 Contouring

Contouring proceeds with the identification of the HR CTV [1] and organs at risk (OARs): bladder, bowel, sigmoid colon, and rectum. The PTV is taken as the HR CTV. Following planning and dosimetry (see below) and immediately before treatment delivery the MR is repeated to detect any gross changes in position or size of the OARs. Subsequently, for all but the final fraction, the images are registered to the planning MR, recontoured, and the dosimetry revised to take account of changes.

18.6 Treatment Planning

Localization of the applicators on the MR is performed with reference to the spacer cap. The cranio-caudal position of the ring is best determined using sagittally acquired images. The positions of both caudal and cranial faces of the spacer cap are determined, with prior knowledge of its size (Fig. 18.1). The cranio-caudal level of the ring can then be established with prior knowledge of its position in the cap and, because the tandem is fixed relative to the ring, the tandem too can be localized in the cranio-caudal direction. The use of an applicator library on the treatment planning computer enables geometrical information about the applicators to be pre-stored. The aqueous gel inserted into the cervical sleeve can be used as a check of the previously ascertained tandem position (Fig. 18.2).The artefact pattern visualised on the MR from the tandem has been characterised. Figure 18.3 shows the para-transaxial position of the tandem as determined by phantom measurements relative to the artefacts seen on MR from the scanner.

The ring reconstruction is aligned rotationally in the para-transaxial plane, using the aqueous gel inserted into the spacer cap, which marks the outside of the distal end of the ring (Fig. 18.4). This can be checked with reference to the tube as it enters the ring, and also with reference to the mounting bracket attaching the ring to the tandem; both of these provide good rotational landmarks for the ring. Finally, any flexing of the tandem is accounted for by moving the distal end of the tandem reconstruction to overlie the visualised position.

Once the applicators are reconstructed in the treatment planning system, a standard plan is set up (or recalled from a library). This acts as a starting point for the dosimetry

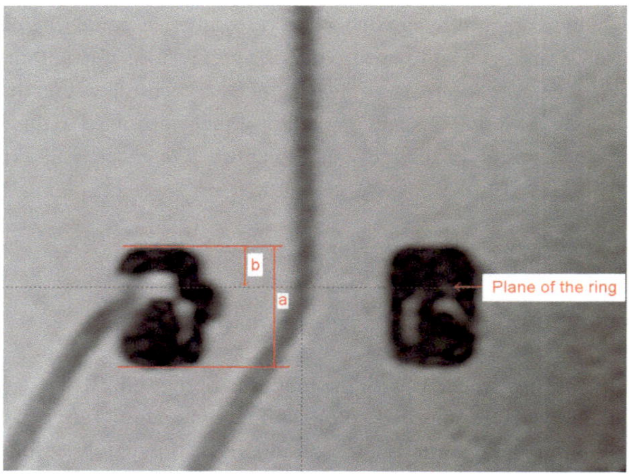

Fig. 18.1 Localisation of the spacer cap in a phantom on a sagittally acquired image. Although signal from the patient makes clinical images harder to interpret, the principle remains unchanged. Distances measured at Mount Vernon: black spacer cap, a = 15 mm, b = 4.8 mm; white spacer cap, a = 17.5 mm, b = 7.3 mm

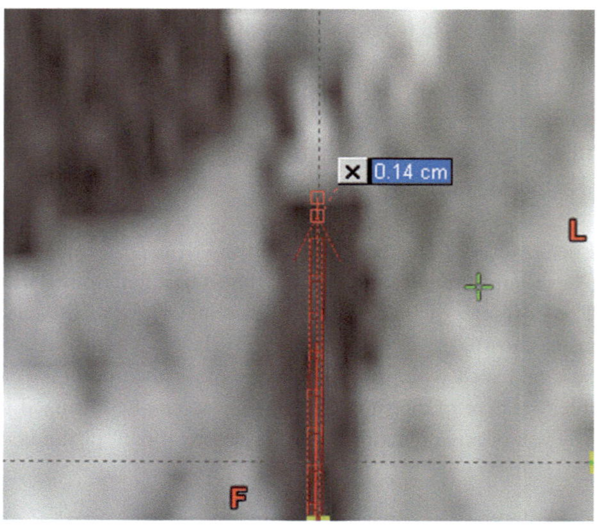

Fig. 18.2 Verification of the distal end of the tandem. The distance from the top of the red reconstruction overlay to the visualised gel inserted into the cervical sleeve is 0.14 cm (as measured at Mount Vernon)

Fig. 18.3 Para-transaxial alignment of the tandem applicator. The *red* cross wires mark the position at which to place the reconstruction

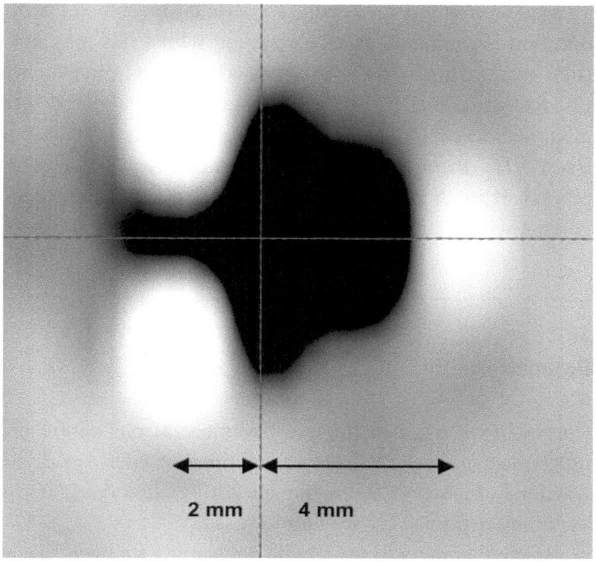

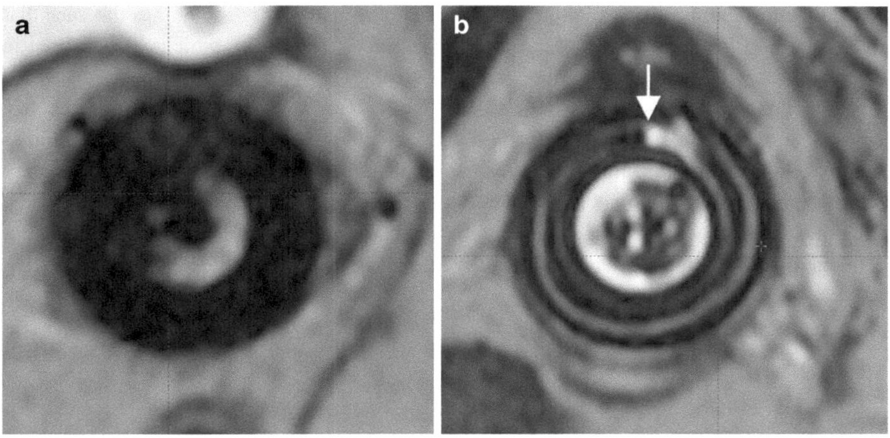

Fig. 18.4 Imaging the end of the ring applicator, (**a**) with no gel, and (**b**) aided by aqueous gel inserted into the spacer cap. The *white arrow* in (**b**) marks the position of the end of the ring

calculation; it has dwell positions along the length of the tandem from its distal end to the level of the ring, and also in the ring at the lateral extents (roughly where ovoid dwell positions would lie). A dwell spacing of 3 mm is used. From this point, the plan is optimised to maximise the coverage of the PTV whilst keeping the critical structures within tolerance. It is imperative to review carefully the results of the optimiser, and often necessary to adjust the final plan by hand. If the PTV is irregular in shape, it may be necessary to deviate markedly from the standard loadings. Interstitial needles, if used, are loaded sparingly to increase coverage where required.

In assessing critical structure DVHs it is assumed that the same portion of the organ in question is irradiated at each fraction; whilst this may not be true for a mobile structure (like the small bowel) it is a safe assumption on which to work. Following the GEC-ESTRO guidelines [2], PTV coverage is evaluated at D100 and D90; V100 and V150 are also considered. Critical structure dose constraints are defined at D_{2cc} points on the respective DVHs (the GEC-ESTRO guidelines suggest also consideration of the D_{1cc} and $D_{0.1cc}$ points). Point A and ICRU reference points (bladder, rectum) are also reported for comparison with historical data, but are not used to assist in plan optimisation.

18.7 Dosimetry

Current dose regimes for this treatment at our centre are 21 Gy as a minimum dose prescribed to the PTV in three fractions of HDR brachytherapy, following 50 Gy in 25 fractions of external beam. This gives just less than 80 Gy equivalent in 2 Gy fractions, assuming α/β is 10 Gy for tumour tissue.

Brachytherapy will usually be delivered with each fraction on a different day, although sometimes, for logistical reasons, two fractions are delivered on the same day with a minimum of 6 h between fractions. This can arise, for example, if interstitial needles are used, and there is a desire to minimize the time that the needles are in place. It is sometimes the case that interstitial needles cannot be kept in place for all three fractions, in which case dosimetric compromises will be required for the fractions delivered with just the intracavitary sources.

For second and subsequent fractions, the applicators may be left in situ, particularly where interstitial implantation has been undertaken and this is an important contribution to the final dose distribution. In other cases the applicators will be removed; the patient may return home and continue subsequent fractions as an outpatient. Second and subsequent fractions undergo MR imaging in the para-transaxial and sagittal planes and, if necessary, CT imaging. The images are analysed in the same way as done for the first fraction.

18.8 Quality Assurance

Before treatment, an independent check of the dosimetry is performed using a spreadsheet to calculate the dose expected at a reference point, given the source dwell positions and times as input.

Rigorous commissioning, and ongoing quality assurance is necessary, at least for the following:

- Magnetic resonance imaging (MRI) scanner (including geometrical properties, specifically assessing the image distortion of the individual scanner, and image artefact patterns).

- Treatment planning system (usual checks of dosimetry for an HDR planning system, and also checks of imported image geometry and orientation are required).
- Treatment unit (interlocks, transit time, source strength, and positional checks as usual for an HDR treatment unit).
- Applicator system. Here a specific issue is the backlash of the source cable in the ring applicator, which can distort the position of the source in the ring, and this must be checked by autoradiography on each individual ring and possibly each source. Since reproducibility of the source position within the ring must also be checked, multiple autoradiographs should be taken of each individual ring (Fig. 18.5a).
- It must be checked that the library applicator in the planning system places the source dwell positions close to the actual positions measured from an autoradiograph. In particular, a small error in the ring radius can lead to a large error in dwell position placement around the ring's circumference. One way to do this check is to superimpose a life-size printout from the planning system with an autoradiograph of the ring (Fig. 18.5b).
- Geometry of the applicator reconstruction (dimensions of the applicator as will be used during applicator reconstruction should be checked for each individual applicator).

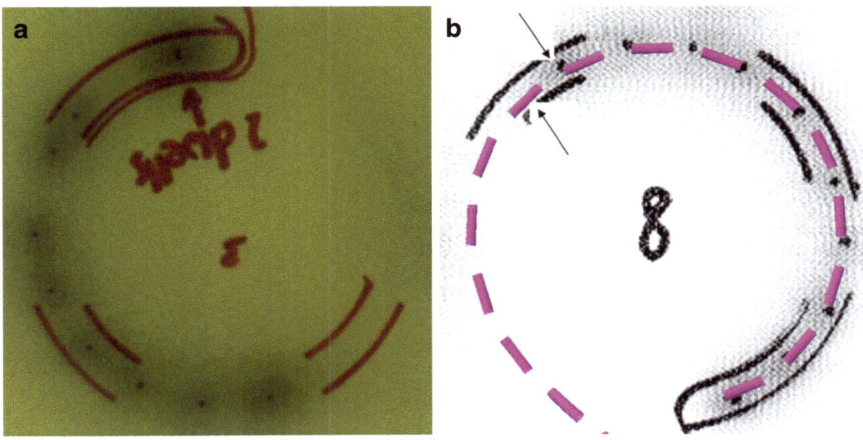

Fig. 18.5 Specific problems that can arise in QA of the ring applicators. (**a**) Dwell positions irregularly spaced because of backlash of the source cable in the ring; (**b**) incorrect dwell spacing round the circumference of the ring. *Black dots* represent observed dwell positions from autoradiograph; *pink rectangles* represent dwell positions placed by the planning system. The highlighted pair should correspond[1]

[1]Courtesy of David Polley, Mount Vernon Hospital

References

1. Recommendations from Gynaecological (GYN) GEC-ESTRO Working Group (I): concepts and terms in 3D image based 3D treatment planning in cervix cancer brachytherapy with emphasis on MRI assessment of GTV and CTV, *Radiotherapy and Oncology* 74 (2005) p235–245.
2. Recommendations from Gynaecological (GYN) GEC-ESTRO Working Group (II): Concepts and terms in 3D image based treatment planning in cervix cancer brachytherapy – 3D dose volume parameters and aspects of 3D image-based anatomy, radiation physics, *Radiotherapy and Oncology* 78 (2006) p67–77

India: Tata Memorial Hospital, Mumbai

19

Umesh Mahantshetty, Jamema Swamidas, and S.K. Shrivastava

19.1 Introduction

Cervical cancers constitute 15–51% of all female cancers, and rates of age-standardized incidence range from 17.2 to 55 per 100,000 women in different regions of India [1]. More than 80% of cases are diagnosed at an advanced stage [1]. At Tata Memorial Hospital, every year 1,200–1,300 new cervical cancer cases are registered, and 500–600 patients are treated with radical intent. The remaining are referred to facilities closer to their home or for palliative care [2]. Magnetic resonance (MR) image-based brachytherapy for cervical cancer was introduced in May 2006 at Tata Memorial Hospital.

19.2 Applicators Available and Selection Parameters

Cervical cancer patients undergoing radical treatment with radiation therapy +/− concomitant cisplatin chemotherapy are offered MR-based brachytherapy. After joint evaluation with GYN oncologists and FIGO staging, these patients undergo an MR of the pelvic region to substantiate the loco-regional disease documentation. During intracavitary brachytherapy, application selection is done depending on the examination under anesthesia (EUA), pretreatment and current disease extent on imaging, and its relation to the applicator configuration. If the coverage with intracavitary configuration is inadequate,

U. Mahantshetty (✉), J. Swamidas, and S.K. Shrivastava
Department of Radiation Oncology and Medical Physics,
Tata Memorial Hospital, Mumbai, India
Dr. E Borges Marg, Parel, Mumbai, 400 012, India
e-mail: drumeshm@gmail.com

A.N. Viswanathan et al. (eds.), *Gynecologic Radiation Therapy*,
DOI: 10.1007/978-3-540-68958-4_19, © Springer-Verlag Berlin Heidelberg 2011

then combined intracavitary and interstitial brachytherapy using Martinez Universal Perineal Interstitial template [MUPIT] with stainless needles followed by CT-based planning is performed.

We have standard CT/MR applicators (Nucletron, Veenendaal, the Netherlands) with intrauterine tubes (40 mm, 50 mm, and 60 mm with fixed angulations of 45°), ovoids of 20 mm, 25 mm, and 30 mm, and a rectal retractor of 30-mm and 40-mm width. We also have the CT/MR tandem and ring set – Stockholm type with 26-mm ring diameter and 45° with wide bore channels so that 6F catheters filled with water can be used as dummies for catheter reconstruction on MR images.

19.3 Insertion Techniques

Intracavitary brachytherapy procedure is performed under general anesthesia. After dilatation of the cervical os, the uterine tandem and ovoid/ring set with/without rectal separator is inserted followed by vaginal packing. The radio-opaque gauze used for vaginal packing is soaked with betadine solution and gadolinium (10:1 dilution) to aid the visualization of vaginal mucosal disease, if present. The urinary bladder is kept empty until the treatment is completed. In the combined intracavitary and interstitial approach, one insertion under spinal with epidural analgesia is preferred with multiple treatments spread over 2–3 days. At times we have placed 6F plastic catheters adjacent to the ovoid/ring surface to improve the lateral coverage of medial parametrial disease.

19.4 Imaging Protocol

Patients undergoing MR-based brachytherapy are transferred to the MR suite and a magnetic resonance imaging (MRI) (1.5 T, Signa, GE Systems) is performed using a body coil. Fast spin echo (FSE) T1 axial and FSE T2 axial (true), sagittal, and coronal (in the plane of central tandem) sequences are obtained with 3–4-mm thick slices and 0–1-mm slice gap. T1 axial images assist in catheter identification and reconstruction. The FSE T2 series helps to identify and delineate the residual disease at the cervix and parametrium, and reconstruct the water-filled dummies.

19.5 [Caveats] of Imaging

The inability to obtain MRI scans with the conventional, stainless-steel afterloading applicators used for implantation has discouraged the implementation of MRI for gynecologic brachytherapy treatment planning to a large extent. Also, with the applicator in situ there are some uncertainties in target volume delineation, especially in partial/poor responders with intra procedure local bleeding obscuring the true tumoral region. The transition zone termed as “grey zone” (between the disease and the normal parametrial tissue) identification is subjective and dependent on imaging parameters and the window settings.

19.6 Contouring Protocol

Contouring is usually done on Oncentra (V 3.1.2.9 Nucletron, Veenendaal, the Netherlands). Clinical examination, EUA, and MRI findings are used for accurate target volume delineation. For practical purposes and reporting, we usually define the high-risk clinical target volume (HR CTV) and sometimes the gross tumor volume (GTV). GTV is defined as residual disease visible or palpable on EUA and hyperintense region on FSE T2 MR images. HR CTV is the combination of GTV and grey zones (intermediate intensity lesion on FSE T2 axial) in the parametrial region, which corresponds to pretreatment parametrial disease. The rectum, bladder, and sigmoid loop are contoured as organs at risk (OARs).The outer walls of the organs are contoured based on the GYN GEC ESTRO recommendations on each slice at least 2–3 cm below the HR CTV to 2–3 cm above the uterus. (Fig. 19.1a)

19.7 Treatment Planning

Axial images along with a structure set are transferred from Oncentra contouring workstation (V 3.1.2.9) to Brachytherapy Plato Sunrise treatment planning system (V 14.3.5).

19.7.1 Reconstruction

Multiplanar reconstruction (MPR) is used to reconstruct the catheters where sagittal and coronal images are reconstructed as a three-dimensional volume from the original (raw) axial images. To circumvent the problem of catheter reconstruction, we tried using catheters filled with water, coconut oil, vitamin E oil, etc., as dummies. The major limitation was the narrow lumen of the applicators, resulting in very thin dummies for reconstruction. Finally, we requested wide bore applicators, which allowed 6F plastic catheters filled with water as dummies and provided an excellent visualization of catheters (Fig. 19.1b). The first dwell position is calculated as 7 mm from the tip of the catheter, which was extrapolated from conventional orthogonal radiographs of the applicator with the dummy markers.

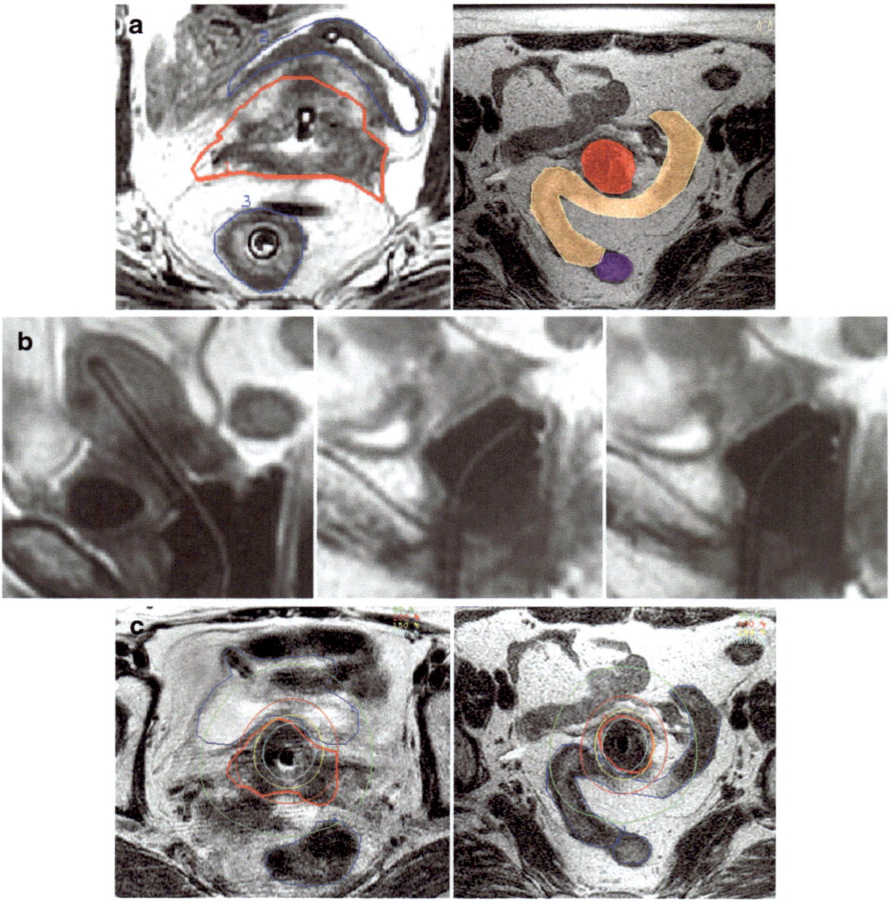

Fig. 19.1 Figure showing our MR-based brachytherapy principles. (**a**) Contouring of high-risk clinical target volume (HR CTV), rectum, bladder, sigmoid, and proximity of sigmoid to HR CTV. (**b**) Sagittal sections at the level of central tandem, right, and left ovoid showing the dummies (6F plastic catheters filled with water) as seen on FSE T2 series for catheter reconstruction. (**c**) Axial sections showing point A prescription with poor HR CTV coverage and high sigmoid doses

19.7.2 Definition of Point A

For the ovoid applicator, the presence of a flange makes it easy to position the origin of the coordinate system. However, for the ring applicator, the surface of the cap (5 mm anterior to the ring source channel) is considered the origin of the coordinate system. Point A is defined as 2-cm superior and 2-cm lateral to the origin.

19.7.3 Source Loading

The Fletcher loading pattern is generally used in our institution. However, changing the dwell positions up to a maximum of 2.5–5.0 mm is accepted to improve the target coverage and reduce the dose to the OARs. Table 19.1

19.7.4 Normalization and Optimization

Dose is normalized at point A (both right and left). Evaluation of cumulative dose–volume histogram (DVH) parameters using the GEC ESTRO recommendations is carried out. Manual optimization in terms of changing the dwell time/dwell weight and the dwell positions is carried out such that the dose to the OARs is minimal without compromising the HR CTV coverage. The acceptability criteria for OARs are as follows: D_{2cc} of bladder, rectum/sigmoid are 80% and 60% of point A dose, respectively. In some situations when the acceptability criteria for the OARs are not met, the clinician makes the decision considering the stage of the disease, extent of disease on EUA, and remaining fractions of brachytherapy (Fig. 19.1c) . After this initial experience we have now contemplated HR CTV–based optimization and prescription with adequate doses to D90.

Table 19.1 Standard Loading Pattern used at Tata Memorial Hospital, Mumbai, India

Applicator	Length of the uterine tandem in mm	Diameter of the ovoid /ring in mm	Active dwell positions (2.5 mm step size)
Nucletron Standard CT/ MR Compatible	40		1,3,5,7,10,13
	50		1,3,5,7,10,13,16
	60		1,3,5,7,10,13,16,20
		20	4,5,6
		25	4,5,6
		30	4,5,6,7
Nucletron Ring CT/MR Compatible	40		1,3,5,7,10,13
	50		1,3,5,7,10,13,16
	60		1,3,5,7,10,13,16,20
		26	4,6,8,10,21,23,25,27
		30	5,7,9,11,24,26,28,30
		34	7,9,11,13,28,30,32,34

19.8 Dose and Fractionation

For stage I and II patients a total dose of 40 Gy in 20 fractions over 4 weeks is delivered. A 4-cm wide divergent 5 HVL alloy step wedge (midline block) is used after initial 20 Gy in 10 fractions over 2 weeks to shield the central structures. For stage III a total of 50 Gy in 25 fractions over 5 weeks is delivered with 40 Gy in 20 fractions without midline block and the remaining 10 Gy in 5 fractions over 1 week with the midline block. Patients with early stage (I and II) receive 5 × 7 Gy to point A once weekly from the third week onward, while patients with stage III receive 3 × 7 Gy to point A once weekly starting from the fourth to fifth week of external radiation.[3] The treatment is delivered using the high-dose rate remote afterloading 192 Iridium micro-Selectron machine, with a dose rate of 50–100 cGy per minute.

Summation of EBRT and BT doses is calculated using a biologically equivalent dose in 2 Gy per fraction (EQD2) with the linear-quadratic model with $\alpha/\beta = 10$ Gy for tumor effects and $\alpha/\beta = 3$ Gy for late normal tissue damage. The repair half time is assumed to be 1.5 h.

DVH parameters for HR CTV and the doses delivered to 90% and 100% of the HR CTV D90, D100 are calculated and documented. For OARs the doses to 0.1 and 2 cc for rectum, bladder, and sigmoid bowel volumes are calculated and correlated with ICRU rectal and bladder doses, whenever possible and noted. Since this was our initial experience, optimization to reduce doses to rectal and bladder volumes was attempted and sigmoid doses were documented accordingly. Table 19.2 shows the summary of various DVH parameters calculated. In our experience, our HR CTVs are higher, total doses to D90 are lower, rectal doses are within tolerance limits while doses to bladder and sigmoid are higher. With more judicious use of combined intracavitary and interstitial brachytherapy, we are trying to deliver higher doses to HR CTV. The dose constraints we try to achieve for OARs are as follows: 65–70 Gy EQD2 for 2-cc rectum, 90–100 Gy EQD2 for 2-cc bladder, and for 2-cc sigmoid we are attempting to keep it <80 Gy EQD2 in prospective cohort patients, though there are no clear data on the dose–volume effect on the bladder and sigmoid. Table 19.2

19.9 Documentation

A spreadsheet containing the patient's name, hospital identification number, disease status, dose to the external beam radiation, dose to the brachytherapy fractions with GEC ESTRO dose–volume parameters such as D90, D100, V100 of HR CTV and D_{2cc}, D_{1cc}, $D_{0.1cc}$ of rectum bladder and sigmoid in terms of EQD2 are documented. Both hard-copy and electronic format are available. System backup of the treatment planning system in the internal hard disk is carried out periodically.

Table 19.2. Point A, ICRU point doses and DVH parameters in our series of 24 patients and 32 ICA-HDR applications

	Point A based with optimization to reduce rectal and bladder doses	Point A based with optimization for all OAR's including sigmoid
HRCTV		
D100	53.9 (41.0–73.1)	65±5
D90	70.3 (56.5–101.3)	75.1±6.2
Avg. Pt A dose	73.4 (62.5–78.8)	68.3±8
Bladder		
ICRU Bmax	80.4 (52–208)	76.8±15
$D_{0.1cc}$	136.0 (75.7–332)	129±21
D_{2cc}	91.4 (65.5–182.0)	89±7
Rectum		
ICRU Rmax	63.5 (48–84)	65±4
$D_{0.1cc}$	67.2 (52.8–97.5)	69±6
D_{2cc}	57.9 (44–74)	63±4
Sigmoid		
$D_{0.1cc}$	101.9 (62–266)	93±9
D_{2cc}	74.4 (50–140)	70.3±21

19.10 Quality Assurance

Quality assurance (QA) and avoidance of errors: QA could be patient-related, planning, and treatment-specific. The QA specific to the patient includes appropriate selection, MRI and accurate target delineation, findings during brachytherapy procedure, appropriate selection of applicator type, and reduction of uncertainties during treatment sessions.

It is imperative to ensure that the images belong to the correct patient name and hospital identification number. The brachytherapy fraction number and the date are entered correctly to avoid discrepancy. Target volume delineation has many uncertainties. MRI has the limitation of distinguishing the residual disease from post-treatment normal residual tissues because of inflammation, fibrosis, and edema. The definition, accurate identification, and demarcation of gray zones are arbitrary and highly dependent on imaging quality, parameters settings, etc. Finally, the HR CTV delineation is subjective; the radiation oncologist needs experience to interpret MR images. For OAR, contouring the outer walls of the rectum and sigmoid is not difficult; however, accurate identification of the rectosigmoid junction still needs standardization and consensus. Finally, maintaining a constant and small bladder volume and accurate contouring remains a challenge and needs to be individualized at each center.

In treatment planning, the following parameters are checked to ensure that the error in the reconstruction is minimized. The acceptability criteria for the reconstruction are ±2 mm. The following points help us to achieve this:

- Exact catheter numbering during reconstruction is essential.
- Ensure that the reconstruction of the tandem and the ovoid is from the tip of the applicator.
- A negative offset of 7 mm is to be applied for the tandem, ovoid, and ring.
- For tandem/ovoid applicator, the length of the tandem is measured from the tip of the applicator to the flange. Alternatively, the length between the first dwell positions to the flange level should be the length of the tandem minus 0.7 cm, for example, for 6-cm tandem it should be 5.3 cm. For the ring applicator, the distance between the first dwell position and the source channel in the ring should be equal to the length of the tandem minus 2 mm.

For dosimetric evaluation,

- Ensure that the origin of the coordinate system is fixed properly and determine the location of point A.
- Ensure that the source loadings are done according to standard protocol, and then optimized.
- Check for the DVH parameters and the documentation of the same.

An independent check of the entire planning process by another physicist is done before data transfer to the treatment console.

Successful treatment delivery requires

- Selection of appropriate patient
- Countercheck of the plan name and date of planning transferred from Treatment Planning System [TPS]
- Countercheck of the treatment time with that of TPS before treatment
- Extra cable check-run through the intracavitary tubes and/or interstitial tubes

19.11 Treatment Outcome and Toxicities

As mentioned earlier, we have reported on initial 24 patients treated with MR Based Brachytherapy and the dosimetric parameters as mentioned in the table 9.2. In these 24 patients, with a median follow-up of 10 months (Mean 12 months; Range 4–29 months), 21 are loco-regionally controlled. One patient failed locally after 6 months and is on palliative chemotherapy. Another patient developed histologically proven para-aortic nodal relapse and received palliative chemotherapy, however was locally controlled. The third patient failed in distant visceral organs (liver and lung) and left supraclavicular nodes. None of the patients on follow up have had late rectal, bowel and bladder grade III sequelae so far.

References

1. Nandakumar A. National Cancer Registry programme, Indian Council of Medical Research, consolidated report of the population based cancer registries. New Delhi, India; 1990–96. p. 60.
2. Dinshaw KA, Rao DN, Ganesh B. Tata Memorial Hospital cancer registry annual report. Mumbai, India; 1999. p. 52.
3. Tongaonkar HB, Shrivastava SK, Parikh PM, Dinshaw KA. Evidence based management guidelines, gynecological cancers. Vol. III. Tata Memorial Centre. Mumbai, India. ISBN: 81-7525-583-8; 2004: p. 7–9.

The Netherlands: University Medical Center, Utrecht

20

Ina M. Jürgenliemk-Schulz and Astrid A.C. deLeeuw

20.1 Introduction

In Utrecht, brachytherapy for cervical cancer is delivered using tandem and ovoid applicators. Point-based treatment planning has traditionally been performed according to the International Commission on Radiation Units (ICRU) 38 guidelines. Until December 2005, treatment plans were generated using standard loading patterns with adaptation if the dose to the ICRU bladder and/or rectum point exceeded our institutional constraints. The dilemma of this strategy is that the organ at risk (OAR)-related dose reduction decreases the tumor dose and may diminish tumor control. Since 2006, dosimetric improvement has been achieved using magnetic resonance imaging (MRI)-guided treatment planning according to the GEC ESTRO recommendations. Individual dose modulation produces an optimized dose-volume relationship between tumor and OAR. In 2007, we developed a new applicator, the "Utrecht Interstitial Fletcher Applicator" (Nucletron, Veenendaal, the Netherlands), for patients with large tumor remnants at the time of brachytherapy in order to increase the target dose and to spare the OAR.

20.2 Applicator Selection

For cervical cancer we routinely use the commercially available Fletcher CT/MR Applicator Sets from Nucletron (Veenendaal, the Netherlands), which contain a tandem part with an adjustable length (10–80 mm) and two different angles (15° and 30°). The ovoid pairs differ in diameter to allow ovoid tube separation from 15 to 30 mm. If necessary, asymmetrical ovoid placement is possible. Based on this applicator type a modification was

I.M. Jürgenliemk-Schulz (✉) and A.A.C. deLeeuw
Radiation Oncology, Utrecht University Medical Center, Heidelberglaan 100, 3584 CX, Utrecht, The Netherlands
e-mail: I.M.Schulz@umcutrecht.nl; a.a.c.deleeuw@umcutrecht.nl

A.N. Viswanathan et al. (eds.), *Gynecologic Radiation Therapy*,
DOI: 10.1007/978-3-540-68958-4_20,

developed together with Nucletron, which allows the use of additional needles for a combined intracavitary/interstitial approach. This modification consists of MRI compatible blunt plastic needles (Proguide Needles, 2 mm in diameter, 6F), which are equipped with a guiding system that is anchored in drilled holes in the ovoids. The ovoids are used as a template for needle placement. Each ovoid is modified with five guide holes, which allow for needle insertion with an angle of 15° to the orthogonal plane through both the ovoids. Three of the guide holes are located in the lateral part of the ovoids with a distance of 7 mm from each other and two holes are located in the ventral and dorsal part (Fig. 20.1). The holes allow placement of needles into the parametria or asymmetric tumor remnants at time of brachytherapy and allow for an adapted dose distribution, if necessary. In order to produce an applicator signal on the MR images the entrances of the source channels in

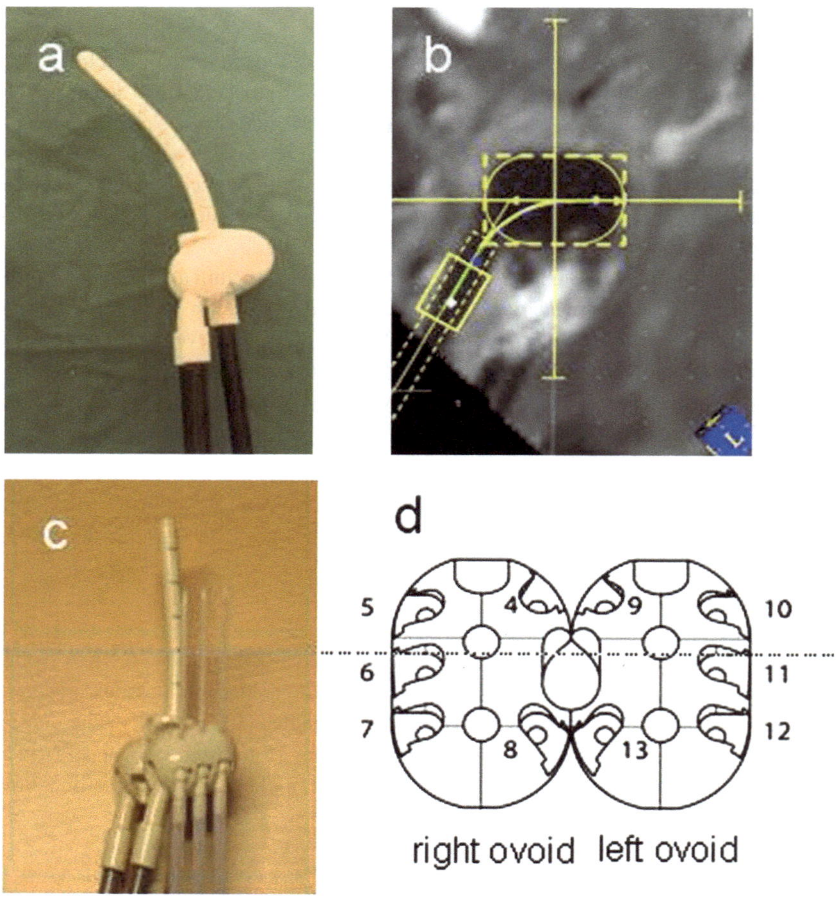

Fig. 20.1 Tandem ovoid applicators, (**a**) intracavitary type, (**b**) ovoid template projected on the black signal void on bSSFP MRI, (**c**) intracavitary/interstitial applicator modification, (**d**) position of guide holes in the ovoids

tandems and ovoids were enlarged to an inner diameter of 2.4 mm to allow placement of fluid-filled plastic MR dummy catheters. For special cases of cervical cancer with distant vaginal invasion or vaginal tumors we have a Vaginal CT/MR Applicator available.

20.3 BT Application

Brachytherapy is delivered either in two pulsed dose rate (PDR) or in four high dose rate (HDR) fractions. Adequate individual analgesia during application and during PDR or HDR treatment is realized by using a combined spinal and epidural approach. A foley catheter with 7-mL diluted X-ray contrast is inserted into the bladder before each insertion. Dilatation of the cervical canal and placement of the applicator parts is performed under ultrasound guidance. Vaginal packing consists of gauze soaked with gadolinium (7 mL, Magnevist 469 mg/mL) diluted in a combined NaCl/paraffin solution (100 mL).

20.4 Imaging

After each application orthogonal X-ray images are taken on the treatment couch. MR images at time of diagnosis and BT are made using a 1.5-T MRI scanner (Gyroscan NT Intera, Philips Medical Systems, Best, the Netherlands). Images are acquired according to a protocol that consists of axial, sagittal, and coronal T2-weighted Turbo Spin Echo (TSE) scans with a slice thickness of 4.5 mm that are generated using a Synbody coil [1]. A balanced Steady State Free Precession (bSSFP) scan consisting of 100 slices with thickness of 1.5 mm is added for applicator reconstruction purposes. All 4 scans have the same origin and are obtained in 1 session that takes about 20 min. MRI is performed within 2 h after the application. The complete MRI data set is imported into our homemade contouring tool (VolumeTool [2]) and the bSSFP data set into the treatment planning system (PLATO, Nucletron, Veenendaal, the Netherlands).

20.5 Caveats to Imaging

Special attention is needed to define vaginal involvement at time of BT. In order to differentiate between tumor and packing on the MR images, the gauze is soaked with diluted gadolinium as described above. During PDR treatments the bladder is nearly empty due to an open urinary catheter. During MRI, however, the bladder filling status can change due to the fact that the urinary sac has to be placed on the imaging couch and gets into equilibrium with the bladder filling. As differences in bladder filling can have impact on DVH parameters we try to empty the bladder before the start of MRI as good as possible. For HDR treatments we choose for a fixed bladder filling of 50 cc for imaging procedures and treatments.

20.6 Contouring

The assessment of tumor volume and topography is performed clinically and by repeated MRI at time of diagnosis and before each BT. Contouring of tumor targets and OAR is performed on T2-weighted TSE MR axial images in VolumeTool, which allows the registration of different imaging data sets and a direct 3D correction of individual points taking into account the sagittal and coronal information. Clinically defined tumor extension as documented on cartoons at time of diagnosis and at each brachy insertion are also taken into account. Target and OAR contours are generated according to the GEC ESTRO recommendations. In addition to the OAR mentioned in the GEC ESTRO recommendations, we also delineate the outer contour of the remaining bowel in the vicinity of the uterus.

20.7 Treatment Planning

Based on the X-ray images a standard plan is produced with standard loading patterns and dwell times, and dose prescription to point A. A technologist performs the applicator reconstruction. Each individual part of the applicator is reconstructed by combining its black signal void on bSSFP MR images with the knowledge of the geometrical dimensions using an applicator template (Fig. 20.1). Based on the delineations of the targets and the OAR the standard plans are evaluated in terms of DVH parameters. If the standard plans do not fulfill the demands of dose to high risk clinical target volume (HR CTV) or OAR, we take them as starting point for MRI-based optimization to produce the definitive treatment plans (optimized plans). Optimization is performed either manually by changing dwell positions and dwell times, by geographical scaling and/or by dragging and dropping of isodose lines, or a combination of these techniques. The effect on dwell times is controlled visually and continuously and excessive dwell time differences are avoided. The high dose volumes are controlled visually and the 400% isodose is preferably kept within or in close relation to applicator and HR CTV. The dose to the unaffected vagina is controlled by trying to keep the prescribed dose within 3–8 mm of the mucosa. In an individual fraction the dose to 2 cc of an OAR is allowed to exceed the constraint by 10%, but we keep the sum of all fractions within the total dose constraint. For the first PDR or HDR treatment the intracavitary applicator parts (tandem and ovoids) are used. Depending on the DVH analysis of the first treatment plan we use either the intracavitary or the combined intracavitary/interstitial approach for following BT insertions. Needles are placed if target coverage is insufficient or if OAR needs to be better spared. The choice for additional needles depends on the DVH parameters of the first application. Needles are placed if the dose to 90% of the HR CTV does not meet the prescribed dose. The choice of the number of needles and the needle positions is based on the spatial dose distribution. We prefer to keep the amount of dose coming from interstitial needles low (not more than 10% per needle). The Utrecht experience in MRI-guided treatment planning and optimization is described in a recent paper by Jürgenliemk-Schulz et al. [3]).

20.8 Dose and Fractionation

PDR treatment consists of two fractions given in two consecutive weeks. One fraction consists of 32 pulses of 60 cGy and is administered in a 24-h schedule at 1 pulse per hour. HDR treatment is delivered in four weekly fractions. The dose per fraction is 19.2 Gy in case of PDR treatments and 7 Gy for HDR treatments. The goal of combined external beam radiotherapy (EBRT) and BT is to achieve a total dose ≥84 $Gy_{\alpha\beta10}$ in 90% of the HR CTV (D90) with an EBRT dose of 45 Gy in 1.8-Gy fractions (EQD2 = 44.3 $Gy_{\alpha\beta10}$). The D_{2cc} of the bladder should not exceed a total of 90 $Gy_{\alpha\beta3}$ and the D_{2cc} of rectum, sigmoid, and bowel 75 $Gy_{\alpha\beta3}$, respectively. A worst-case scenario is assumed in these calculations suggesting that the 2 cc of the OAR receiving the maximal BT dose had received the full-prescribed EBRT dose.

20.9 Documentation

Documentation is routinely performed individually for EBRT and each BT fraction and also in total physical dose and total EQD2. We register the D90 and D100 of gross tumor volume (GTV), HR CTV, intermediate risk clinical tumor volume (IR CTV), the D50 of the HR CTV, the D_{2cc} and $D_{0.1cc}$ of the OAR as well as the dose to points A at the left and right side and the ICRU rectum and bladder point dose. Furthermore, we document the percentage of the GTV and HR CTV that receives 100% of the prescribed dose (V100), the volumes that per application receive one or two times the prescribed dose (VPD and V2PD), and the Total Reference Air Kerma (TRAK). In order to document the spatial gain of combined intracavitary/interstitial treatment over intracavitary treatment alone we perform an analysis of the dose distribution based on distance maps (Fig. 20.2).

20.10 Quality Assurance

Treatment planning and treatment itself are performed according to the protocols that are part of our institutional quality assurance program. The treatment planning system fulfills the demands as described in the recommendations of the Tax Group 43 for dose calculations.

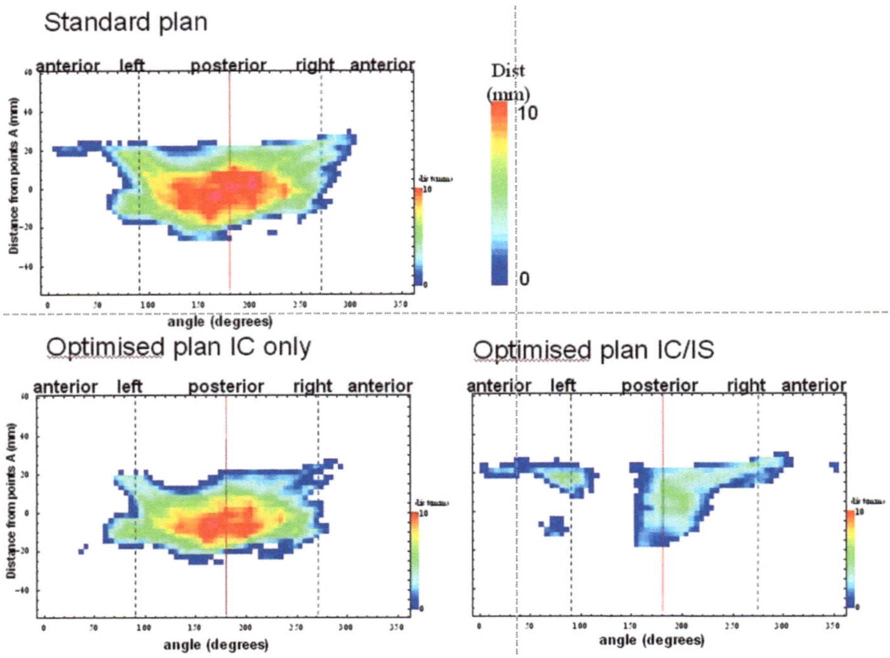

Fig. 20.2 Distance maps derived for the standard and two optimized plans of a typical application, intracavitary (IC) and combined intracavitary/interstitial approach (IC/IS). Distance maps give 2D representations of volumes and/or 3D dose distributions. For each point along the tandem of the applicator the distance to a particular volume is presented using a color code. This results in a plot with the X-axis ranging from 0° to 360° around the tandem, and the Y-axis ranging from the tip to the distal segment of the tandem. The color code is a measure of the distance between the HR CTV and the outer contour of the prescription isodose line in a plane perpendicular to the tandem. In this particular case, the lack of dose in the latero-posterior part was diminished by using four interstitial needles (implantation to a depth of 30 mm from the ovoid surface in the dorsally located guide holes)

MRI protocols have been developed together with a radiologist with special interest in gynecology and are adapted if new technology allows improvement. Trained technologists from the radiology and radiotherapy departments together perform the MRI. The applicator reconstruction is performed by technologists and is controlled by a physicist. In order to define the source track in the applicator parts and especially the first source position, X-ray images were taken from all applicator sets with dummy loads in the tandems and ovoids, as well as autoradiographs with the stepping source. A radiation oncologist trained in gynecologic oncology delineates the targets and the OAR and a second radiation oncologist controls the derived contours. A brachytherapy technologist and physicist together perform the dose-volume analyses and a radiation oncologist accords the definitive treatment plan. The relation between the TRAK and the volume that receives the prescribed dose is monitored for each treatment plan by comparing with the data of former applications.

References

1. Van de Bunt L, van der Heide UA, Ketelaars M, et al. Conventional, conformal, and intensity-modulated radiation therapy treatment planning of external beam radiotherapy for cervical cancer: the impact of tumor regression. Int J Radiat Oncol Biol Phys. 2006;64:189–96.
2. Bol GH, Kotte ANTJ, Lagendijk JJW. "Volumetool" An image evaluation, registration, and delineation system for radiotherapy. Phys Med. 2003;19:80.
3. Jürgenliemk-Schulz IM, Tersteeg RJ, Roesink JM et al. MRI guided treatment planning optimisation in intracavitary or combined intracavitary/interstitial PDR brachytherapy using tandem ovoid applicators in locally advanced cervical cancers. Radiother Oncol. 2009;93:322–30.

21 USA: Dana-Farber/Brigham and Women's Cancer Center, Harvard Medical School, Boston

Akila N. Viswanathan, Jorgen Hansen, and Robert Cormack

Both low-dose-rate (LDR) and high-dose-rate (HDR) modalities are available for cervical cancer patients receiving brachytherapy treated at the Brigham and Women's Hospital (BWH). The majority of patients receive concurrent chemoradiation and have a dramatic response after 45 Gy of external beam radiation (EB); these patients subsequently proceed to HDR tandem and ovoid (T/O) or tandem and ring (T/R) therapy. LDR T/O is reserved for patients unable to return for five outpatient HDR treatments. A subset of patients who have a large amount of residual disease after EB, or those who had lower vaginal involvement at diagnosis with >5 mm of residual after EB, receive LDR interstitial therapy In 2002, CT simulation for cervical cancer began as part of routine practice. Beginning in 2004, a prospective protocol for real-time magnetic resonance (MR) image-guidance in interstitial gynecologic brachytherapy began in the BWH magnetic resonance therapy (MRT) unit [1]. In 2005 in addition to the MRT unit, a dedicated brachytherapy suite with a built-in CT scanner (CTS) opened, and all patients treated with all forms of gynecologic brachytherapy received CT simulation after insertion for treatment planning. Until 2007, most patients had a diagnostic MR within 1 week prior to the first implant, and this was used to aid in contouring the primary tumor following the GEC ESTRO guidelines. As of 2007, during the first fraction T/O or T/R the patient received an MRI after CT simulation while still under general anesthesia, and the images were fused to contour the primary target. Patients with residual disease receive an MRI while under anesthesia for their first fraction. A new MRT unit with MR, PET, and CT capabilities in an operating room environment will open in 2011.

At BWH, for LDR, the tandem and ovoid with or without shielding (non-CT compatible) is available. For HDR, the tandem and ovoid, tandem and ring, tandem and cylinder, and non-CT compatible tandem and ovoid applicators are available. For either HDR or LDR, interstitial catheters are inserted into a Syed-Neblett template.

A.N. Viswanathan (✉), J. Hansen, and R. Cormack
Department of Radiation Oncology, Brigham and Women's Hospital/
Dana-Farber Cancer Institute, 75 Francis Street L2, Boston, MA 02115, USA
e-mail: aviswanathan@lroc.harvard.edu

A.N. Viswanathan et al. (eds.), *Gynecologic Radiation Therapy*,
DOI: 10.1007/978-3-540-68958-4_21, © Springer-Verlag Berlin Heidelberg 2011

21.1 Insertion Techniques

21.1.1 Anesthesia

All patients receive anesthesia that commences prior to insertion and continues through applicator removal, with the majority choosing general endotracheal anesthesia; few patients receive spinal anesthesia. Intravenous conscious sedation is reserved for special cases based on the preference of the patient and the anesthesiologist with a contraindication to either general or spinal anesthesia, including bleeding risk, severe obesity, or other medical (primarily pulmonary) comorbidities. LDR or HDR interstitial patients undergo epidural anesthesia, which continues throughout the inpatient hospitalization.

21.1.2 Insertion

In the dedicated brachytherapy suite, the patient is placed in the dorsal lithotomy position in stirrups on a movable tabletop that is attached to the CT table covered with a foam mat and sheet. Approximately 40 cc of barium is inserted using a rectal tube into the sigmoid and rectum. The perineum is washed with betadine and draped with sterile towels. A Foley catheter is inserted in the bladder and 50/50 Hypaque contrast material is injected into the balloon. A sterile speculum is inserted into the vagina for adequate visual examination of the cervix. A bimanual exam is then performed, noting any residual nodularity, the cervix size, and the size of the fornices.

The uterine sound is inserted to the maximum amount feasible; the clamps are placed at the point where the sound enters the cervix; and the distance from where the sound was inserted to the point of the clamp is measured to determine the length of tandem required. If the sound does not enter the uterus easily, ultrasound is used. The bladder is filled with 200 cc of saline and an abdominal transducer is used to visualize the uterine canal. The sound is inserted, followed by the dilators. After serial dilation with Hegar dilators, the tandem is inserted, followed by either the ring or ovoids. The ring or a cylinder applicator is preferentially chosen for women who have narrowing of the upper vaginal vault after EB. One gauze pack is inserted with fingers posteriorly in order to move the anterior rectal wall as far as feasible from the applicator, and a second pack is placed anteriorly to distance the bladder from the applicator. Two gauze packs are used to ensure that the packing does not twist around the applicator, allowing for easy removal. For all cases, the bladder is then drained completely, the bladder catheter is clamped, and 60 cc of dilute Hypaque is placed into the bladder directly to provide contrast over the entire bladder. For LDR cases, a stitch sewn on the outer labia holds the applicator in place. Prior to imaging, radiopaque markers are placed into the applicator.

21.1.3
Imaging

Using a mobile table top, patients slide from lithotomy cranially toward the CT bore. We ensure that the patient's legs will fit through the bore by lowering them while still in stirrups. The patient's arms are strapped across their chest. During the scan and treatment, all vital signs are monitored on a slave screen set up outside of the procedure in the CT control room. A CT scan (General Electric Medical Systems, Milwaukee, WI) visualizes images from the top of the pelvic brim to approximately 3 cm below the most inferior aspect of the applicator. The CT scans are acquired using 140 KVp, 250 mA, with a slice thickness of 1.25 mm. If radiologically indicated, the packing is repositioned. Patients with large (>4cm) of residual tumor move while under general anesthesia to the diagnostic 1.5-T MRI for imaging with T2 axial and sagittal images.

21.1.4
Contouring

For patients who have an MR with the tandem in place, the MR images are fused with the CT images for contouring. Patients that have had a complete response after chemoradiation do not have an MR during brachytherapy and the CT images alone are used for contouring following CT based guidelines [2]. The entire cervix is contoured to the level of the anterior flexion and expansion of the uterus, as the cervix cones inward for an additional centimeter. For all cases, contours of the outer wall of the bladder, rectum, and sigmoid are generated. The rectum is contoured from 1 cm above the anus until the rectosigmoid flexure. The sigmoid contours end once the sigmoid crosses anteriorly to the pubic symphysis. The sigmoid is contoured for each fraction given the relationship between fractional tandem position and sigmoid dose [3]. In selected cases where the small bowel lies adjacent to the applicator, the bowel is also contoured and the small bowel dose will be recorded separately.

21.1.5
Treatment Planning MR Cases

In order to identify the radiopaque markers on MRI, the air gap distance is measured. For patients who have an MRI performed immediately before or during the insertion, the MR images are fused with the CT. Fusion entails importing the MRI images into the fusion element of AdvantageSim (GE), identifying suitable fusion points – the tip of the tandem and the ovoids, the sacral promontory, the femoral heads, and the pubic symphysis – and performing a rigid registration. The quality of the registration is assessed with priority on registration of the tissue surrounding the applicator. The fused images of the MR/CT composite data set, optimized for soft tissue delineation, are imported into the HDR planning system (Plato Nucletron). Source trains, evidenced by dummy radiopaque markers, are identified and a plan is generated. CT simulation images are transferred to a treatment planning system (LDR: Brachyvision version 6.5 build 7.3.10; HDR: Plato version 14.2). In 2009, we received a test version of the Oncentra Gyn software package from Nucletron. The first patient was parallel planned and a comparison between Plato and Oncentra Gyn was made. The Oncentra Gyn software reduced planning time by an average of 0.5 h, significantly reducing the required anesthesia time [4]. In addition, the clear delineation of the organ at risk (OAR) contours results in better optimization of the OAR and reduced dose to these normal tissues.

21.1.6 Treatment Planning All Cases

The standard dose and fractionation is 5.5 Gy × 5 fractions for patients that have received 45 Gy of pelvic external beam radiation with concurrent weekly cisplatin chemotherapy for 5–6 cycles. Fractions are administered under anesthesia two times per week with a minimum of 48 h between fractions. For T/O cases, standard configurations of dose points are placed with respect to the applicator to allow computer optimization to create an initial plan with prescription dose delivered to point A, and modifications of the individual dwell weights are made to ensure coverage of the target as visualized on CT and to minimize the OAR dose. From 2002 to 2005, the 5.5-Gy dose was always specified to point A. Thereafter, optimization of the isodose distribution to maximize target coverage and minimize OAR dose based on CT volumes would often change the dose to point A; nevertheless, the point A dose is always recorded in the chart.

All external beam and brachytherapy doses are reported as nominal doses. In order to facilitate comparisons with the literature, they are also converted into equivalent 2-Gy doses (EQD2) using the linear quadratic formula. The dose to 0.1 cc ($D_{0.1cc}$), D_{1cc}, and D_{2cc} for sigmoid, rectum, and bladder are calculated using dose–volume histograms. D_{2cc} < 70–75 Gy for sigmoid and rectum, and D_{2cc} < 90–95 Gy for bladder are the optimal dose–volume constraint parameters. The D90 and V100 for the target are also recorded.

21.1.7 Documentation

The physician dictates a standard template note for each applicator type (Fig. 21.1). Specifics related to the individual patient are dictated into the note. The chart must contain a current history and physical examination, a cervical tumor diagram, the written directive, a prescription, a pathology report signed by the physician, a simulation note, and photo identification of the patient prior to treatment initiation.

21.2 Quality Assurance/Avoidance of Errors

A computer file containing dwell times and positions is exported to the microSelectron Treatment Control System. The treatment plan is printed out on paper for check and

Operation: Placement of HDR Brachytherapy tandem and ring applicator

PHYSICIAN:
FELLOW/RESIDENT(s):
PHYSICIST:
THERAPIST:
NURSE:
ANESTHESIA:
INSERTION PERFORMED BY:
PROCEDURE, SIMULATION, AND TREATMENT IN DETAIL:

The patient's identity was confirmed, and a written consent for the procedure and separate consent for anesthesia were present in the chart. The patient was brought into the brachytherapy suite where anesthesia was administered.

The patient was placed supine and in the lithotomy position in the procedure room. The patient was prepped and sterilely draped in the usual fashion. A Foley catheter was inserted under sterile conditions into the bladder with 10cc of water with Hypaque contrast in the balloon. A supervised vaginal examination was performed. The cervical os was visualized. The uterine sound was used to measure the length of the uterus. The cervix was then serially dilated with the dilators. A tandem of the correct length was inserted into the uterus, with the flange flush against the cervix. The ring was assembled, coated with KY jelly, and placed over the tandem.

The brachytherapy board was attached to the applicator for immobilization. Two radiopaque markers were inserted to assist with visualization of the applicator under CT. A CT scan for simulation was then performed to confirm applicator placement and plan treatment. The attending physician evaluated the applicator placement and identified the structures of bladder and rectum, prescription points, and any dose optimization parameters on the CT scan. A physics consult was requested to create a graphic plan and perform complex computer-optimized dosimetry. The radiopaque markers were removed and cleaned. There were no complications as a result of the simulation.

Once a satisfactory treatment plan had been generated, the applicator was connected to the Nucletron Microselectron High Dose Rate brachytherapy apparatus via the transfer tubes. Channel one was connected to the ring and channel three to the tandem. The attending physician reviewed the dosimetry, treatment plan, channel assignments, and verification films prior to the administration of radiation. All safety checks were performed, including the room and patient radiation survey. Radiation was delivered to the prescribed isodose curve using high-dose-rate Iridium 192, prescribed to point A in 5-mm steps according to plan. The radiation oncologist and physicist as authorized users were in the immediate vicinity at all times while HDR brachytherapy was administered. The patient and the equipment were monitored by video and audio observation.

Following treatment, the room and patient were surveyed and were negative for radioactivity. The applicator was removed, and the patient was transferred to the recovery room in stable condition for anesthesia recovery and discharge. There were no complications.

PRIOR EXTERNAL BEAM RADIATION DOSE:
PLANNED TOTAL # FRACTIONS:
CURRENT FRACTION #:
APPLICATOR: CT compatible ____ Non-CT compatible ____
TANDEM LENGTH:
RING SIZE:
RADIOACTIVE SOURCE:
CURRENT SOURCE STRENGTH:
TOTAL TREATMENT TIME:
NUMBER OF DWELL POSITIONS:
PRESCRIPTION POINT:
DOSE TO PRESCRIPTION POINT:
CUMULATIVE BRACHYTHERAPY DOSE TO DATE:
RECTAL DOSE: (values for D0.1cc, D1cc, 2cc)
BLADDER DOSE: (values for D0.1cc, D1cc, 2cc)
TIME INTERVAL BETWEEN HDR FRACTIONS:
FOLLOW-UP:

I, _________, as the attending physician, attest that I was present with the patient in the brachytherapy suite during the examination, directly witnessed and supervised the placement of the applicator by the resident or fellow into the patient, and was present for all aspects of the treatment.

Fig. 21.1 For all cases, the physician calls up a templated note into the dictation system, then specifies the unfilled blanks. Separate dictations exist for cylinder, tandem and ovoid, interstitial, tandem and ring, and general treatments. The tandem and ring note is shown

signature by a physicist and an attending physician. In order to check the reconstruction of the applicator in the treatment planning system, the geometry of the applicator on the plan is checked against scout views from the CT scan.

Integrity of the dwell times is checked against a secondary treatment planning system. At BWH this is accomplished by choosing a number of points (depending on the complexity of the plan). The distances from each of these points to all the dwell positions are measured or calculated and the expected dose to the points is calculated. These values are expected to be within 3% of the treatment plan doses. Prior to treatment delivery, the pre-treatment plan is printed out. This printout is checked for accuracy of the HDR source and consistency of the product of total dwell time and source activity. This printout is signed by the therapist, the physicist, and the clinician.

The therapist connects the afterloaded connector cable to the applicator. The physician checks this connection immediately prior to treatment. Standard surveys of the patient immediately before and after the delivery of dose are performed by the medical physicist. The medical physicist and physician are present for all treatments the physician dictates while treatment is ongoing. The applicator is then removed and the patient is transferred to the recovery area. The majority of patients return for follow-up every 3 months for 2 years in order to ensure careful management of any potential side effects.

References

1. Viswanathan AN, Cormack R, Holloway CL et al. Magnetic resonance-guided interstitial therapy for vaginal recurrence of endometrial cancer. Int J Radiat Oncol Biol Phys 2006; 66(1):91–9.
2. Viswanathan AN, Dimopoulos J, Kirisits C, Berger D, Poetter R. CT- versus MR-based Contouring in Cervical Cancer Brachytherapy: Results of a Prospective Trial and Preliminary Guidelines for Standardized Contours. Int J Radiat Oncol Biol Phys 2007 Jun 1;68(2):491–8.
3. Holloway CL, Racine ML, Cormack, RA et al. Sigmoid dose using 3D imaging in cervical-cancer brachytherapy. Radiother Oncol 2009;93(2):307–10.
4. Hansen J, Viswanathan AN. Comparing oncentra gyn and plato: a time study. Brachytherapy. 2010;9:S25–6.

USA: Medical College of Wisconsin, Milwaukee

22

Jason Rownd and Beth E. Erickson

22.1 Introduction

CT-based dosimetry for every high-dose-rate (HDR) brachytherapy fraction was initiated at the Medical College of Wisconsin (MCW) in 2004. Normal organ point doses based on films often unreliably define doses to normal tissues, especially the circuitous sigmoid. Additionally, organs are deformed differently by each HDR insertion. Magnetic resonance imaging (MRI) at the time of fraction 1 was also initiated in 2004, since even though normal organ dose–volume relationships can be well-defined with computed tomography (CT), the tumor dose–volume relationships could not be due to poor soft tissue resolution. The Gyn GEC ESTRO Guidelines defined MRI-based targets and relevant dose specifications [1, 2]. The logistical and financial challenges of MRI with each HDR fraction made this impossible at MCW until 2008 when a 3-T MR unit was installed. We will describe CT-based planning for each of 5 HDR fractions and MRI-based planning for fraction 1.

22.2 Applicators

The usual applicator at MCW is the MRI/CT-compatible Nucletron 45/60-degree Tandem and Ring (Nucletron, Veenendaal, the Netherlands). The medium (40-mm outer diameter) and large rings (44-mm outer diameter) are used most frequently. If the patient's vagina is too narrow to accommodate a small ring (36-mm outer diameter), we use the Nucletron MRI/CT-compatible tandem and cylinder applicator. Typically, we treat only the upper vagina, using the domed portion of the applicator. The entire vagina is treated only if there is vaginal involvement. The MRI/CT-compatible Nucletron Fletcher-style ovoids are used

B.E. Erickson and J. Rownd (✉)
Department of Radiation Oncology, Medical College of Wisconsin Clinics,
Froedtert Hospital, 9200 W Wisconsin Ave., Milwaukee, WI 53266, USA
e-mail: berickson@mcw.edu and jrownd@mcw.edu

A.N. Viswanathan et al. (eds.), *Gynecologic Radiation Therapy*,
DOI: 10.1007/978-3-540-68958-4_22, © Springer-Verlag Berlin Heidelberg 2011

in patients with deep vaginal fornices or when the uterine tandem length cannot be accommodated by the fixed tandem lengths of 2, 4, or 6 cm, standard with the ring applicators. When patients require interstitial implantation, the Syed-Neblett intracavitary/interstitial system is utilized.

22.3 Insertion Techniques

Patients receive spinal anesthesia for the first fraction and monitored sedation for the remaining five fractions. After fraction 1, an endocervical stent maintains patency and reduces painful manipulation of the endocervical canal, allowing the use of IV sedation alone. The insertions take place in the Radiation Oncology brachytherapy suite. A bladder catheter is inserted by the assistant and a vaginal and perineal prep performed. A pelvic exam is performed under anesthesia. After sterile draping, the endocervical canal is dilated and the tandem is inserted. Ultrasound guidance is used if there is difficulty finding the canal or if there is concern regarding perforation. Gold seeds are placed into the anterior and posterior cervical lips. The largest ring that fits through the introitus and fills the upper vagina is chosen, threaded over the tandem, and carefully inserted obliquely through the introitus. The applicator is clamped together, avoiding pinching of the vaginal mucosa between the ring and tandem interlock system. Palpation of the interface between the ring and the cervix follows to assure close approximation, and the rectal retractor and saline/gadolinium-soaked bladder packing are inserted. C-arm fluoroscopy is available if there is concern over the position of the applicator relative to the cervix or other pelvic organs. A plastic perineal bar and strap system is used to fix the applicator in place, and a rectal catheter is inserted for contrast. The patient is moved from the dorsal lithotomy position to the legs-down position; the applicator is readjusted to ensure proximity to the cervix.

22.4 Imaging Protocol and Caveats

Patients are transferred using a sliding board on the mobile insertion table into the CT simulation room next to the brachytherapy suite. The bladder bag is brought to gravity and the catheter is clamped and 30 cc of dilute contrast (omnipaque) is injected into the bladder. A 30 cc of contrast (gastrograffin) is injected into the rectosigmoid with care not to distend the rectum. Dummy catheters are inserted into the applicator for visualization on the CT scout and for later dosimetric planning. The dummy catheters are visualized at the tip of the tandem and first dwell position in the ring. A pelvic scan protocol with metal is chosen from the CT options. On the CT scout, the ring must be flush with the gold seed–marked cervix, and the applicator must be midline in the pelvis. Adjustments may be accomplished on the CT table during sedation. Axial images with a slice thickness of 2.5 mm are reviewed to insure that there is no packing or air gap between the vaginal applicator and the cervix, and no need for a different applicator angle or additional bowel or bladder contrast. Copies of the CT scouts are made for the patient's chart.

Beginning in 2004, an MRI scan was obtained after the fraction 1 CT scan on a 1.5-T magnet. A phased array pelvic surface coil was strapped to the patient to improve the spatial resolution. To reduce time and cost, gadolinium was omitted, and only T2 images were obtained in the axial, sagittal, and coronal planes with a 24–28-cm field-of-view (FOV), 5-mm slice thickness with 1-mm gap, 16-kHz bandwidth, 256–521 × 256 matrix, and number of excitation (NEX) of 2. An echo train length (ETL) of 8 was used for the fast spin echo (FSE) T2 sequences. The bladder catheter was left on the patient's legs during the scan. Bowel motion was limited by fasting for 4–6 h prior to the study and absent medical contraindications, an anti-peristaltic agent (glucagon 1 mg IV or IM). In 2008, a 3-T MRI scanner was installed across from the CT simulator. Patients continue to have a CT scan for radiation planning prior to their 3-T MRI, but this will become unnecessary when dosimetry is generated directly from the MR scans. Patients are transferred from the CT table directly to the MR cart. Hollow plastic catheters (Best Medical part 536-30 and 536-35) filled with saline are inserted into the tandem and ring, and a pelvic coil is strapped to the patient. A 3D protocol has been piloted which has shown an excellent distinction of tumor and cervix from the saline-soaked vaginal packing as well as the vaginal applicator. Images are acquired on a Siemens 3T MAGNETOM Verio scanner (Siemens Healthcare, Erlangen, Germany) equipped with 45 mT/m (180 mT/m/ms) gradients. The body radiofrequency (RF) coil is used for signal transmission, and commercial flex and spine RF array coils are used for signal reception. Non-fat-suppressed, axial, T2-weighted images are acquired using a 3D slab-selective SPACE (Sampling Perfection with Application optimized Contrasts using different flip angle Evolutions) pulse sequence with the following parameters: FOV 384 mm; matrix 384 × 384; turbo factor 93; bandwidth 407 Hz/pixel; apparent echo time 79 ms; echo train duration 422 ms; repetition time 2,500 ms; average 1.4; and slice thickness 1 mm. Parameters are optimized to produce images with isotropic 1-mm cubic voxels, good signal-to-noise ratio and T2 contrast, and minimal respiratory artifacts. To reduce total acquisition time, partial Fourier encoding is employed in the slice direction, and parallel imaging is employed in the phase encode direction. Acquisition times are 12–16 min, depending on the required slice coverage. After imaging, the patient is returned to the brachytherapy suite for monitoring. Once the treatment fraction is delivered, the patient has the applicators removed while sedated and is then transferred to recovery for monitoring until discharge.

22.5 Contouring Protocol

The CT scans are transferred to the treatment planning system and contours of the opacified bladder, rectum, and sigmoid are performed. The bladder catheter bulb is also visible and is used for the ICRU bladder point calculations. Occasionally, it is difficult to separate sigmoid from small bowel, although sigmoid contrast makes this rare. Small bowel doses are occasionally tracked if there is a significant amount of bowel near the tandem. Treatment planning begins once the OAR have been contoured on the CT. The cervical anatomy as seen on MRI at fraction 1 is contoured based on the GEC ESTRO Guidelines after the first fraction and influences future insertions. The intermediate-risk clinical target volume (IR CTV) is contoured but is not used for treatment planning or alteration of dose. The greatest challenge with the 1.5-T images was separating tumor volume from parametrial vessels due to pixelation and defining the upper limits of the high-risk clinical target volume (HR CTV). On the 3-T images, it is easier to define the cervix as it interfaces with the vaginal packing and the ring and as it ascends into the uterine body. Axial images are used for contouring, and reconstructed sagittal and coronal images can help determine the boundaries of the HR CTV.

22.6 Treatment Planning

Axial images, either CT or MRI, are contoured on Nucletron's Oncentra Masterplan software version 3.1 and then transferred as DICOM objects to Nucletron's Plato system (version 14.3.5). Reconstructed planes (paracoronal, parasagittal, and para-axial) based on the original axial images identify the applicator for reconstruction. Nucletron X-ray markers are used for CT image-based planning. Saline-filled catheters in the tandem appear as white lines on the T2-weighted images and identify the source travel path inside the applicator (Fig. 22.1). A nominal offset from the end of the catheter determines dwell position 1. Based on the first several intercomparison plans (CT and MRI, same patient), dwell position 1 is placed 4–6 mm from the end of the white line on the reconstructed images. The positional accuracy of the Nucletron HDR source within a catheter is ±1 mm.

After applicator reconstruction, dose optimization points are placed along the tandem and the ring or vaginal cylinder surface. The dose optimization points for the tandem are defined in the paracoronal reconstructed view through the plane of the tandem and referenced from specific dwell positions with specific lateral distances. For instance, using a

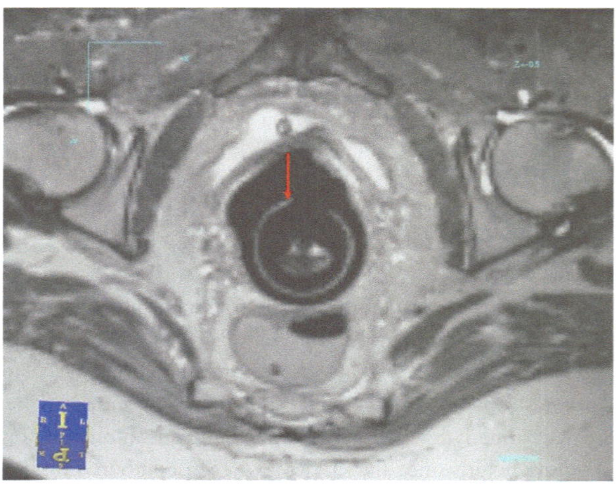

Fig. 22.1 A 3-T MRI scan in the plane of the ring (*red arrow*) demonstrating the saline-filled catheter identifying dwell position 1 for MRI- based planning

6-cm tandem, the dose optimization points are placed at 12 mm left and right of dwell position number 1, 14 mm left and right of dwell position number 2, 16 mm left and right of dwell position number 3, 18 mm left and right of dwell position number 4, 20 mm left and right of dwell position number 5, and this is continued down to the level of point A. These points help define the tapered portion of the pear-shaped dose distribution and are specifically weighted to 100% of the prescription dose. The optimization points for the ring surface are defined in the para-axial reconstructed plane. Four dwells on each side of the ring are activated for the small ring, five for the medium ring, and six for the large ring. Using only the active dwell positions (dwells are usually activated symmetrically on the left and right side of the ring, not the entire circumference), optimization points are placed on the ring surface using the –U axis of the planning system at 6 mm from the active dwell positions. These points help define the larger base of the pear-shaped dose distribution and are usually weighted to 160% of the prescription dose. If a vaginal cylinder is used, the dose optimization points are defined on the paracoronal plane and specifically placed at the surface of the vaginal cylinder using the active dwell positions, with the main portion of the vaginal cylinder as the reference points and the radius of the vaginal cylinder as the prescription distance for the dose optimization points. These points can be weighted anywhere from 100% to 120% of the dose prescription to avoid excessive doses to the bladder and rectum with the absence of packing and/or a rectal retractor inherent to this applicator.

Once all the dose optimization points have been placed, their weighted average is defined as the prescription dose, the tandem points are defined as 100% of the prescription dose, and the vaginal surface points (ring or cylinder) are defined to their respective prescription doses. There is usually a range of ~10% across the various dose optimization points because of the planning algorithm.

Using this dose distribution, the ICRU 38 rectal and bladder point doses and the bladder and rectosigmoid contrast points doses are defined. Dose–volume histogram (DVH) analysis identifies the D0.1cc, D1cc, and D2cc to these same normal organs.

22.7 Dose and Fractionation

The dose per fraction is usually 550 cGy and specified initially at point A. The vaginal surface receives 140–160% of the point A dose with the vaginal ring applicator or ovoids and 100% with the vaginal cylinder applicator. Adjustments are needed in some patients due to the doses to the OAR, which are evaluated with point doses, isodose curves, and DVH parameters. Dose points at the surrogate ICRU rectal and bladder points as well as select contrast points along the rectum (above the level of the vaginal applicator) and sigmoid closest to the tandem are chosen, and doses are calculated. The CT scans are carefully scrutinized for the proximity of the 80%, 90%, and 100% (point A) isodose curves to the walls of the OAR (Fig. 22.2). If the 90% or 100% or higher isodose curves intersect these OAR, the dose specification may be altered. This is usually done after the first 2–3 fractions rather than at fraction 1 or 2 unless the isodoses intersecting the OAR are very high (i.e., 110–120% the point A dose). Whole organ volumes are drawn for the rectum, sigmoid,

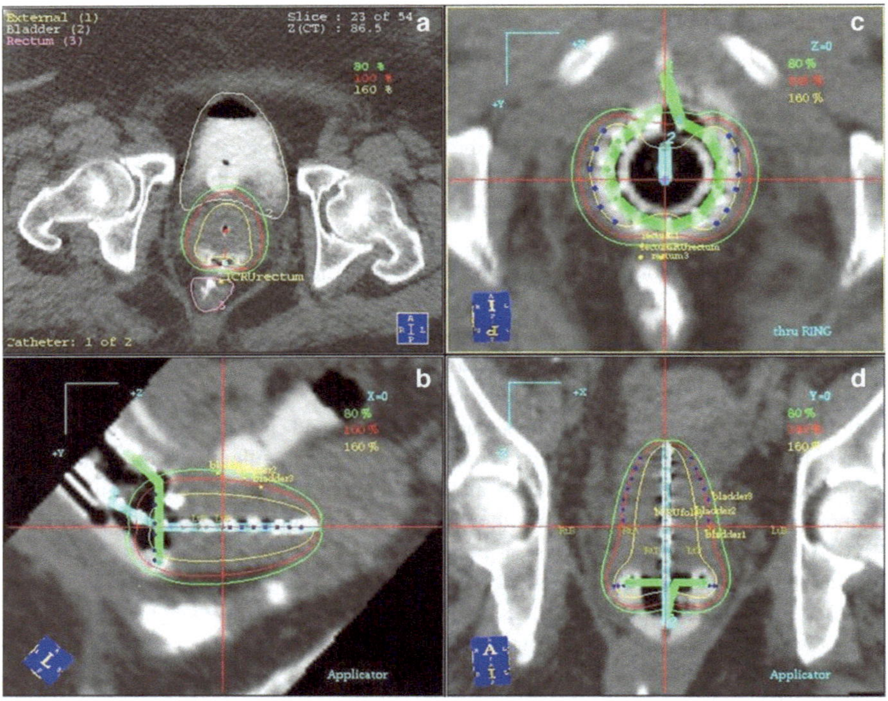

Fig. 22.2 Axial (**a**), sagittal (**b**), coronal (**c**), and ring plane (**d**) images at the level of point A following CT-based planning. Note the ICRU and rectal and bladder contrast points

and bladder, and doses received by 0.1 cc, 1 cc, and 2 cc are recorded from the DVH. The EQD2 worksheet D2cc doses are tracked along with the D90 and V100 from one fraction to the next. This volumetric analysis underscores the significance of high point doses or high isodoses intersecting the OAR. The MR at fraction 1 allows for the definition of the HR CTV and the assessment of coverage with the point A specified dose (Fig. 22.3). The isodose distribution can then be modified to better cover the HR CTV or exclude the OAR.

22.8 Documentation

An extrapolated response dose (ERD) worksheet is filled out by the physician for the physicists at the initiation of brachytherapy, documenting the total low dose rate (LDR) equivalent dose intended to point A, the external beam dose delivered, and the desired remaining LDR dose. This is then converted into the number of HDR fractions at a specified LDR (60 cGy/h at point A) to get to the HDR per fraction. A written directive including patient identification, applicator, dose per fraction, and specification points and dwell

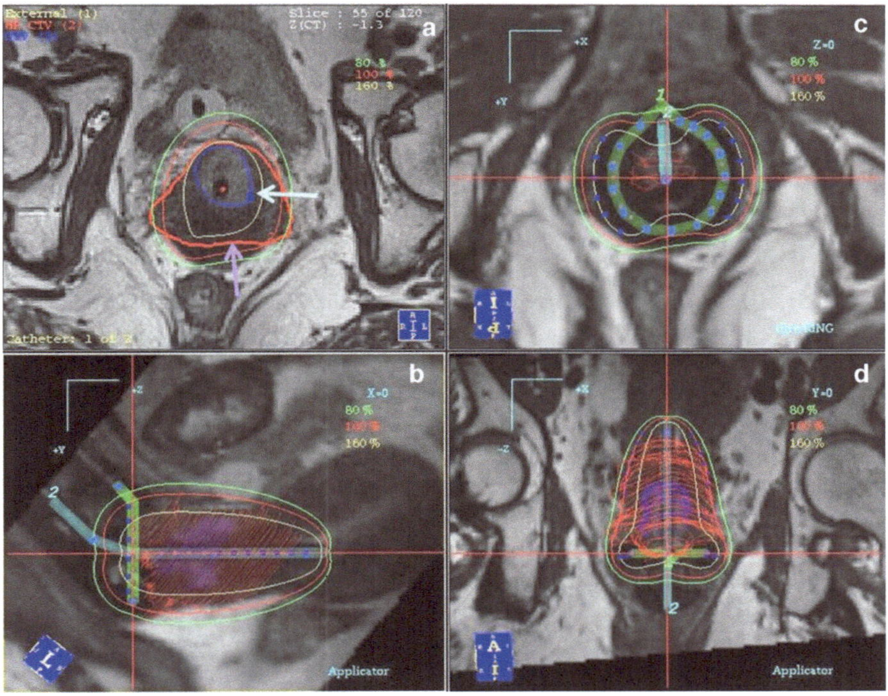

Fig. 22.3 A 3-T MRI of the same patient at the level of point A in axial (**a**), sagittal (**b**), coronal (**c**), and ring plane (**d**) views showing the high-risk clinical target volume (HR CTV) in *red* (*lavender arrow*), which extends outside of the 100% point A isodose. The gross tumor volume (GTV) is identified as the bright signal contoured in *blue* (*light blue arrow*)

positions is completed by the physician and reviewed by the physicists. The dosimetry is then generated and reviewed by the team and necessary modifications are made. Once approved by the physician, the quality assurance (QA) second check is made. A procedural note is dictated by the physician with all of the directive parameters as well as a detailed exam of the patient and other pertinent facts related to the insertion, dosimetry, and ultimate condition of the patient at the end of treatment. A paper copy as well as an electronic version of the written directive and physics data is signed by the physician prior to treatment.

22.9 Quality Assurance and Avoidance of Errors

QA for every treatment plan is done by an independent physicist. The applicator reconstruction and orientation is verified by the comparison of CT scout views and treatment plan printouts with applicator shape and dimensions. The printouts (text, plots, and screen captures) are verified against the physical dimensions of the applicators. The optimization and prescription are compared to the written directive. A QA dose point is calculated using a rudimentary point source model in an Excel spreadsheet for implants using one to three catheters, based on approximate (relative to QA point) dwell positions, exact dwell times, and exact source strengths. A separate spreadsheet for volume-based treatment plans checks the ratio of (dwell times × source activity/dose) and (treated volume) for consistency versus historic plans. Any discrepancies are reviewed and resolved (sometimes by generating a new plan) before treatment. Any differences in the QA dose point check beyond 5% are reviewed and resolved (often based on the exact applicator reconstruction and the spreadsheet approximations) before treatment.

The QA physicist reviews the entire process using information gathered by the planning physicist, including the review of scout films to understand the physical appearance and orientation of the applicator within the patient. It also involves comparing the complete dose distribution for distances and absolute doses against the written directive.

Errors are avoided by comparing the plan printout generated by the brachytherapy planning computer against the data received by the treatment delivery unit. Patient name, treatment date, activity, duration, catheters, and prescription dose are all checked for each fraction. In addition, at least two forms of patient identification are required. After treatment, a radiation survey meter is used to verify that the HDR brachytherapy source has been safely returned to the treatment delivery robot and that no radiation above background remains within the patient.

References

1. Haie-Meder C, Potter R, Van Limbergen E, et al. Recommendations for Gynecological (GYN) GEC-ESTRO Working Group (I): concepts and terms in 3D image-based 3D treatment planning in cervix cancer brachytherapy with emphasis on MRI assessment of GTV and CTV. Radiother Oncol. 2005;74:235–45.
2. Potter R, Haie-Meder C, Van Limbergen E, et al. Recommendations for Gynecological (GYN) GEC ESTRO Working Group (II): concepts and terms in 3D image-based treatment planning in cervix cancer brachytherapy- 3D volume parameters and aspects of 3D image-based anatomy, radiation physics radiobiology. Radiother Oncol. 2006;78:67–77.

Postoperative Vaginal Cylinder Brachytherapy in an Era of 3D Imaging

23

Caroline L. Holloway and Akila N. Viswanathan

23.1 Introduction

Postoperative adjuvant intravaginal brachytherapy (VBT), defined as the placement of a radiation source adjacent to the vaginal mucosa with the purpose of treating microscopic cancer, can be used alone or in conjunction with external-beam radiation therapy. The most frequent use is in the treatment of posthysterectomy endometrial cancer, though other indications include postoperative cervical cancer, or potential situations where gross disease is present such as vaginal or vulvar cancer, or palliative ovarian cancer management when vaginal metastases cause bleeding. The radioactive source runs through either a single channel plastic cylinder or two adjacent vaginal colpostats (Fig. 23.1). A single channel cylinder is the most common applicator utilized [1]. Traditionally, the dose has been delivered with either low dose-rate (LDR) cesium-137 or high dose-rate (HDR) iridium-192.

The clinical target volume ranges widely. The average treatment length in the United States (US) is the upper one-half to one-third (approximately 4–5 cm) of the vagina, with only 7% routinely treating the entire vaginal length [1]. The GEC ESTRO brachytherapy handbook recommends treatment to the vaginal cuff and upper one-third of the vagina for a mean target length of 3–5 cm [2]. Overall, the rates of distal vaginal recurrences are low [3] and treatment to the full length of the vagina may lead to increased vaginal morbidity. Some institutions will treat the full length of the vagina for high-risk features including clear cell or papillary serous histology, lymph vascular invasion, grade 3 or node positive disease [1].

Similarly, institutions differ on the prescription point, which may be either at the surface of the applicator or at a depth of 0.5 cm. There is also a wide variation on acceptable

C.L. Holloway
Radiation Oncology, BC Cancer Agency, Vancouver Island Centre,
2410 Lee Avenue, Victoria, BC V8R 6V5, Canada
e-mail: cholloway@bccancer.bc.ca

A.N. Viswanathan (✉)
Department of Radiation Oncology, Brigham and Women's Hospital/Dana-Farber Cancer Institute, 75 Francis St, L2, Boston MA, 02115, USA
e-mail: aviswanathan@lroc.harvard.edu

A.N. Viswanathan et al. (eds.), *Gynecologic Radiation Therapy*,
DOI: 10.1007/978-3-540-68958-4_23,

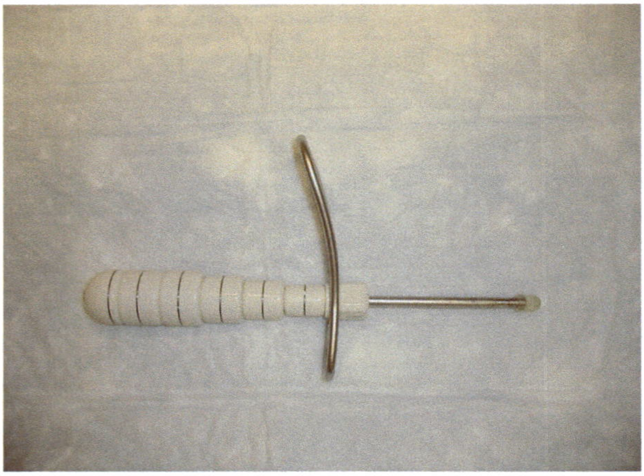

Fig. 23.1 An example of a low-dose-rate (LDR) vaginal cylinder with an attached perineal bar used to hold the applicator in place

HDR fractionation regimens [1, 2, 4–6] For LDR treatments, patients receive approximately 60 Gy when VBT is given alone [2].

The organs in the immediate vicinity of the brachytherapy dose include the bladder, rectum, sigmoid, urethra, perineal skin, and occasionally small bowel. Identification of these structures with 3D imaging is feasible. In contrast, 2D localization films allow verification of the applicator position, and may provide point bladder and rectal dose information if contrast has been placed into a Foley balloon and into the rectum.

Because the dose has a rapid fall-off that follows the inverse square rule ($1/r^2$), the placement of the apparatus is extremely important. The apparatus must be in apposition to the vaginal apex and walls. The greatest diameter cylinder that can be accommodated in the vagina should be selected. This allows for maximal dose penetration. The rapid dose fall-off results in lower doses to the organs at risk the dose to the organs at risk (OAR).

23.2 Imaging

Imaging is not performed by all institutions, but can provide useful information when available. Simulation enables verification and documentation of the size of the apparatus, apparatus placement, and dose to the OAR. In a survey by the American Brachytherapy Society, the most common method of imaging for simulation was with 2D films, with 18% using CT [1].

23.2.1 2D Imaging

2D imaging permits evaluation of several aspects of treatment. The proximity of the tip of the apparatus to the vaginal apex can be seen on 2D simulation films if clips are placed at the vaginal apex after surgery, and is also apparent on a CT scout film

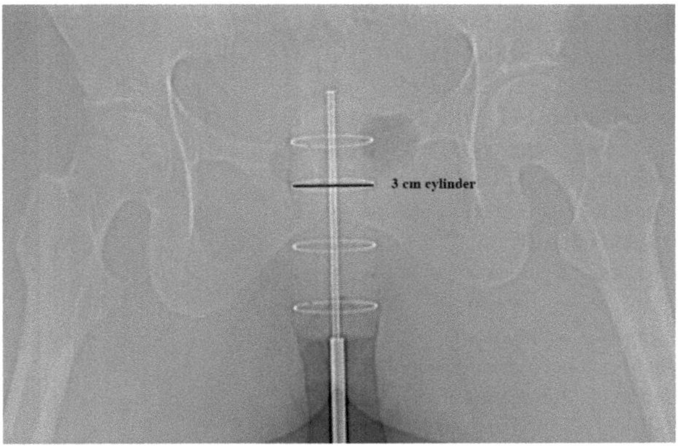

Fig. 23.2 A CT scout film can be used to verify the depth of placement of the cylinder and to confirm the width of the cylinder, shown here as 3 cm in diameter

(Fig. 23.2). The depth of insertion can also be appreciated on the simulation films by using the bony landmarks, and consistency between fractions can be obtained. The angle of the cylinder placement can be assessed with lateral films. Moving the cylinder to a horizontal plane from the natural angle of the vagina has been reported to decrease the dose to the rectum [7].

However, 2D films limit reporting to the OAR. Approximately 80% of oncologists record the dose to the OAR with VBT, 66% using rectal/bladder contrast to determine the dose on plain films [1]. The International Commission on Radiation Units and Measurements (ICRU) 38 recommended standardized dose reporting in gynecologic brachytherapy [8]. Limitations of the ICRU bladder and rectal dose points include underestimation of the dose delivered to the normal tissues [9–15]. In the case of VBT, the placement of a Foley catheter for the determination of the ICRU bladder point requires an additional invasive intervention that may result in unintended side effects such as a urinary tract infection. Another limitation of 2D imaging is that the apposition of the apparatus to the vaginal tissue cannot be assessed.

23.2.2 3D Imaging

CT simulation is the most common type of 3D imaging used for postoperative VBT. CT scans permit assessment of the placement of the cylinder, including the position in relation to the apex of the vagina, the conformity of the vaginal tissue with the apparatus, the depth of insertion, the angulation of the cylinder, and the location of the OAR.

The placement of the cylinder at the apex of the vagina can be assessed on both axial and sagittal CT images. The length of the vagina can be assessed with the cylinder in place in the sagittal view (Fig. 23.3). Individualization of the treatment length can then be achieved while sparing the vaginal introitus.

The 3D imaging can show air gaps at the apex of the vagina or along the length of the cylinder. A recently published paper did not find clinically significant air gaps in 25 patients who underwent CT simulation with the dose prescribed at 0.5 cm [16].

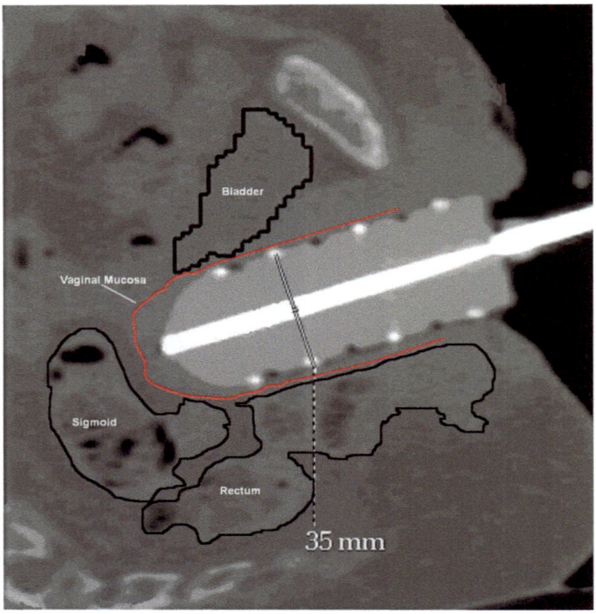

Fig. 23.3 Sagittal projection of a high-dose-rate (HDR) cylinder (35 mm diameter) as seen after reconstruction of CT images taken on a CT simulator in a dedicated brachytherapy suite at the Brigham and Women's Hospital. Organs at risk contoured include the sigmoid, rectum, and bladder. The vaginal mucosa (target) is delineated in *red* to illustrate the irregularities in the volume. In this instance, vaginal thickening is seen at the apex of the cylinder

Perhaps the areas where 3D imaging has the greatest advantage over 2D imaging are in dose optimization and the quantification of dose to the OAR.

Dose optimization for single-line cylinders has been evaluated. Gore et al. [17] evaluated the dose distributions between HDR and LDR vaginal cylinders and the parameters needed to produce a "uniform" dose distribution for HDR cylinder brachytherapy. They found the maximum dose uniformity in HDR cylinders when both the apex of the cylinder and curvature of the dome were taken into account. The HDR dose distributions were more uniform than LDR and there were fewer variations as a function of cylinder size with HDR cylinders. These dose distributions, however, do not apply for dose points prescribed at a distance from the cylinder. Li et al. further evaluated dose distributions both at the cylinder surface and at a 0.5-cm distance from the cylinder. They concluded that anisotropic dose calculations were required to avoid a 30% underdosage at the vaginal apex; however, anisotropic dose calculations increase the dose to the vaginal mucosa. They also found that it was impossible to acquire a uniform dose at a depth from the vaginal cylinder with the current design of the cylinder [18]. Dose homogeneity at a depth becomes more feasible with multichannel catheters, as well multichannel catheters allow for irregular clinical target volumes. The vaginal wall itself can have a varying thickness, especially at the vaginal cuff where there is an irregular surface and shape after surgery.

Target points can be placed to delineate the target, but one must always keep in mind the vicinity of the bowel and rectum. In a dose study of single-line versus multichannel catheters, the multichannel catheter was capable of dose sculpting around the rectum and bladder [19]. The decreased dose to the OAR is balanced by the decreased vaginal mucosal dose. Dose sculpting may also be used for irregular clinical target volumes.

Dose–volume histograms (DVH) which allow for a noninvasive evaluation of the dose to the OAR can be created, after bladder, rectum, and sigmoid contouring. The dose parameters to record with 3D evaluation of gynecologic brachytherapy are being evaluated [9, 10, 20–22]. The impact of bladder filling on bladder dose has been evaluated with 3D imaging [23, 24]. Hoskin and Vidler [24] conclude that the bladder volume does not affect the dosimetry to the bladder; however, with a full bladder the dose to the small bowel was decreased. This study did not use 3D evaluation of dose to the OAR. Stewart et al. [23] evaluated both DVH and dose–surface histograms, concluding that bladder dose was in fact higher in patients with full bladders, and advocated that patients be treated with an empty bladder. One question that arises is with what frequency the dose to the OAR needs to be recorded. A recently published article reviewing 2D simulation found that there was a wide range of doses recorded to the bladder at simulation but few genitourinary toxicities and that the simulation did not result in altering treatments [25]. A retrospective review of DVHs of the OAR with each fraction of VBT did not find sufficient variation in dose to the rectum and bladder to warrant recording dose to the OAR with each fraction. Predictors of dose to the OAR included the cylinder size, and the dose to the rectum increased with the increased vaginal treatment length [26]. Construction of DVHs in the clinic can be time-consuming. A maximal bladder point, which is described as the point of intersection of the bladder contour and the maximal isodose line on a midline-reconstructed sagittal CT image, has been found to correlate with the bladder DVH [23] and can be used in the clinic to record dose to the bladder.

23.3 Conclusion

Imaging in VBT in the US most commonly employs radiographs, which provide sufficient information regarding the size of the cylinder placed, but lacks information regarding proper placement or information regarding the OAR. 3D imaging allows for evaluation of dose to the OAR in a noninvasive manner, but whether this is of clinical benefit is not known. 3D imaging and new applicators also permit dose sculpting to ensure that the clinical target volume is covered for patients with gross disease present or for modification of the isodose lines to spare the OAR in complex cases such as vaginal cancer. However, in standard postoperative endometrial cancer cases, 3D simulation has not been shown to be required for each fraction of VBT.

References

1. Small Jr W, Du Bois A, Bhatnagar S, Reed N, Pignata S, Potter R, et al. Practice patterns of radiotherapy in endometrial cancer among member groups of the gynecologic cancer intergroup. Int J Gynecol Cancer. 2009;19(3):395–9.
2. The GEC ESTRO Handbook of Brachytherapy. http://www.estro-education.org/publications/Documents/GECESTROHandbookofBrachytherapy.html

3. Creutzberg CL, van Putten WL, Koper PC, Lybeert ML, Jobsen JJ, Warlam-Rodenhuis CC, et al. Survival after relapse in patients with endometrial cancer: results from a randomized trial. Gynecol Oncol. 2003;89(2):201–9.
4. Nag S, Erickson B, Thomadsen B, et al. The American brachytherapy society recommendations for high dose rate brachytherapy for carcinoma of the cervix. Int J Radiat Oncol Biol Phys. 2000;48(1):201–11.
5. Sorbe B, Straumits A, Karlsson L. Intravaginal high-dose-rate brachytherapy for stage I endometrial cancer: a randomized study of two dose-per-fraction levels. Int J Rad Oncol Biol Phys. 2005;62(5):1385–9.
6. Racine ML, Viswanathan AN. Adjuvant high-dose-rate brachytherapy alone for stage I/II endometrial adenocarcinoma using 4-gray versus 6-gray fractionation scheme. Int J Rad Oncol Biol Phys. 2008;72(1):S362.
7. Hoskin PJ, Bownes P, Summers A. The influence of applicator angle on dosimetry in vaginal vault brachytherapy. Br J of Radiol. 2002;75:234–7.
8. International Commission on Radiation Units and Measurements (ICRU). Dose and volume specifications for reporting intracavitary therapy in gynecology. ICRU report 38. Bethesda. MD. 1985.
9. Schoeppel SL, LaVigne ML, Martel MK, McShan DL, Fraass BA, Roberts JA. Three-dimensional treatment planning of intracavitary gynecologic implants: analysis of ten cases and implications for dose specification. Int J Radiat Oncol Biol Phys. 1994;28(1):277–83.
10. Pelloski CE, Palmer M, Chronowski GM, Jhingran A, Horton J, Eifel PJ. Comparison between CT-based volumetric calculations and ICRU reference-point estimates of radiation doses delivered to bladder and rectum during intracavitary radiotherapy for cervical cancer. Int J Radiat Oncol Biol Phys. 2005;62(1):131–7.
11. Ling CC, Schell MC, Working KR, Jentzsch K, Harisiadis L, Carabell S, et al. CT-assisted assessment of bladder and rectum dose in gynecological implants. Int J Radiat Oncol Biol Phys. 1987;13(10):1577–82.
12. Kim RY, Pareek P. Radiography-based treatment planning compared with computed tomography (CT)-based treatment planning for intracavitary brachytherapy in cancer of the cervix: analysis of dose-volume histograms. Brachytherapy. 2003;2(4):200–6.
13. Katz A, Eifel PJ. Quantification of intracavitary brachytherapy parameters and correlation with outcome in patients with carcinoma of the cervix. Int J Radiat Oncol Biol Phys. 2000;48(5):1417–25.
14. Kapp KS, Stuecklschweiger GF, Kapp DS, Hackl AG. Dosimetry of intracavitary placements for uterine and cervical carcinoma: results of orthogonal film, TLD, and CT-assisted techniques. Radiother Oncol. 1992;24(3):137–46.
15. Fellner C, Potter R, Knocke TH, Wambersie A. Comparison of radiography- and computed tomography-based treatment planning in cervix cancer in brachytherapy with specific attention to some quality assurance aspects. Radiother Oncol. 2001;58(1):53–62.
16. Cameron AL, Cornes P, Al-Booz H. Brachytherapy in endometrial cancer: quantification of air gaps around a vaginal cylinder. Brachytherapy. 2008;7:355–8.
17. Gore E, Gillin MT, Albano K, Erickson B. Comparison of high dose-rate and low dose-rate dose distributions for vaginal cylinders. Int J Radiat Oncol Biol Phys. 1995;31(1):165–70.
18. Li Z, Liu C, Palta JR. Optimized dose distribution of a high dose rate vaginal cylinder. Int J Radiat Oncol Biol Phys. 1998;41(1):239–44.
19. Tanderup K, Lindegaard JC. Multi-channel intracavitary vaginal brachytherapy using three-dimensional optimization of source geometry. Radiother Oncol. 2004;70(1):81–5.
20. Koom WS, Sohn DK, Kim JY, Kim JW, Shin KH, Yoon SM, et al. Computed tomography-based high-dose-rate intracavitary brachytherapy for uterine cervical cancer: Preliminary demonstration of correlation between dose–volume parameters and rectal mucosal changes observed by flexible sigmoidoscopy. Int J Rad Oncol Biol Phys. 2007;68:1446–54.

21. Wachter-Gerstner N, Wachter S, Reinstadler E, Fellner C, Knocke TH, Wambersie A, et al. Bladder and rectum dose defined from MRI based treatment planning for cervix cancer brachytherapy: comparison of dose-volume histograms for organ contours and organ wall, comparison with ICRU rectum and bladder reference point. Rad and Oncol. 2003;68:269–76.
22. Potter R, Haie-Meder C, Van Limbergen E, Barillot I, De Brabandere M, Dimopoulos J, et al. Recommendations from gynaecological (GYN) GEC ESTRO working group (II): concepts and terms in 3D image-based treatment planning in cervix cancer brachytherapy-3D dose volume parameters and aspects of 3D image-based anatomy, radiation physics, radiobiology. Radiother Oncol. 2006;78(1):67–77.
23. Stewart AJ, Cormack RA, Lee H, Xiong L, Hansen JL, O'Farrell DA, et al. Prospective clinical trial of bladder filling and three-dimensional dosimetry in high-dose-rate vaginal cuff brachytherapy. Int J Radiat Oncol Biol Phys. 2008;72:843–8.
24. Hoskin PJ, Vidler K. Vaginal vault brachytherapy: the effect of varying bladder volumes on normal tissue dosimetry. Br J Radiol. 2000;73:864–6.
25. Barney BM, MacDonald OK, Lee CM, Rankin J, Gaffney DK. An analysis of simulation for adjuvant intracavitary high-dose-rate brachytherapy in early-stage endometrial cancer. Brachytherapy. 2007;6(3):201–6.
26. Holloway CL, Macklin EA, Cormack R, Viswanathan A. Should the organs at risk be contoured in vaginal cuff brachytherapy? An analysis of within-patient variance. Brachytherapy. 2008;7(2):147–8.

Image-Based Approaches to Interstitial Brachytherapy

24

Akila N. Viswanathan, Beth E. Erickson, and Jason Rownd

24.1 Introduction

Brachytherapy, the placement of radioactive isotopes in close proximity to the tumor, provides a method of conformal dose escalation after external beam radiation so the tumor receives a high dose in comparison to the surrounding normal tissues. Interstitial brachytherapy refers to the placement of hollow needles or catheters directly into tumor-bearing tissues. The most common gynecologic cancers treated with interstitial brachytherapy include large locally advanced cancers of the cervix with extension into the paracervical, para-uterine tissues, the lower third of the vagina [1], or those invading the bladder or rectum; vaginal cancers invading into the paravaginal tissues or covering a large surface area of the vagina; large vulvar carcinomas, particularly those with vaginal extension; or recurrent gynecologic malignancies in the vagina, most commonly involving the vaginal apex or urethral region. These interstitial needles typically hold a single strand of seeds of one particular radiation source or are loaded using a remote afterloading mechanism. Though the technique was originally proposed using Radium 226 [2], physicians now prefer Iridium 192 given its shorter half-life [1]. Either high-dose rate (HDR) or low-dose rate (LDR) radiation may be administered using Ir-192 seeds on a strand inserted through the interstitial catheters. In general, treatment commences as soon after the completion of external beam radiation as possible.

All patients with localized cervical cancer should receive brachytherapy after external beam radiation (EBRT), as EBRT alone is far less likely to be curative [3]. EBRT, including dose escalation with intensity modulated radiation therapy (IMRT), runs the risk of

A.N. Viswanathan (✉)
Department of Radiation Oncology, Brigham and Women's Hospital/Dana-Farber Cancer Institute, 75 Francis Street L2, Boston, MA 02115, USA
e-mail: aviswanathan@lroc.harvard.edu

B.E. Erickson and J. Rownd
Department of Radiation Oncology, Medical College of Wisconsin Clinics, Froedtert Hospital, 9200 W Wisconsin Ave., Milwaukee, WI 53266, USA
e-mail: berickson@mcw.edu; jrownd@mcw.edu

A.N. Viswanathan et al. (eds.), *Gynecologic Radiation Therapy*,
DOI: 10.1007/978-3-540-68958-4_24,

insufficient internal tumor/cervical dose resulting in a high rate of pelvic relapse (see Chap. 12). The high dose provided by brachytherapy within the cervix allows conformal dose escalation with tissue sparing not feasible with IMRT. If possible, all patients with an intact uterus should have a tandem placed, whether using intracavitary or interstitial techniques, to adequately dose escalate the central region of the tumor while also providing dose to the nodal regions and the parametrium [4, 5].

24.2 Image Guidance

Image guidance, either during or after the insertion of a brachytherapy applicator, allows careful assessment of the planned dose of radiation in relation to the tumor and normal tissues. With 3D imaging during the insertion (image-guided brachytherapy, IGBT), the physician may determine the depth of insertion and avoid insertion into the bowel, may reposition a misdirected catheter, or may immediately pull a catheter out of an OAR. With 3D images obtained from a scan after insertion is complete (image-planned brachytherapy, IPBT), the dose distribution may be altered to conform to the tumor volume and avoid the OAR. Both IGBT and IPBT result in the optimal number of needles placed and/or treated, and consequently in an optimal dose distribution.

The use of 3D image guidance with CT, MRI, or PET may be difficult in some countries. In general, ultrasound is more easily available worldwide. For patients with significant anatomical distortion of the endocervical canal, ultrasound guidance enables identification of an os through which an intrauterine tandem can be placed. Only patients who have had a prior total or radical hysterectomy and have suffered a vaginal cuff recurrence should be candidates for interstitial brachytherapy alone. Also, if the endocervical canal is so distorted that it cannot be negotiated by a tandem, those patients may also be considered for interstitial brachytherapy alone. An ultrasound probe may be placed into the rectum to visualize the depth of needle insertion and the placement of the needles in the cervix/parametria, but this method has limited utility for anterior vaginal lesions. An abdominal ultrasound may help visualize the tandem and the insertion of needles into the uterus/cervix and prevent inadvertent bladder penetration. In some institutions, surgical laparotomy or laparoscopy allows for palpation and visualization of the catheter tips internally.

Incorporation of imaging requires close collaboration with radiology to schedule the patient on the appropriate scanner, to determine the algorithm necessary for image acquisition, and to encompass the tumor in entirety. Interpretation of the images by a radiologist can aid in proper delineation of the tumor target and adjacent structures. Pre-implant MR imaging assists with contouring proper volumes for each patient if an MR is not feasible at the time of brachytherapy. Compared with MRI, CT images of cervical cancer do not show tumor enhancement, vaginal involvement, or the superior extent of the cervix as clearly as MR, and CT images often overestimate the lateral extension of the cervix [6]. PET scans depict diffuse uptake in the primary tumor as well as in lymph nodes and distant metastatic sites; PET may assist with tumor volume measurements but, as with CT, the images are less specific and the borders less clearly defined than MRI for primary tumor assessment. CT should be undertaken when MRI is not available. CT images, when taken after a standardized protocol of bladder filling and rectal emptying, with the patient supine, and with minimal time between scans, adequately visualize the organs at risk (OAR), but may overestimate the tumor volume [6].

24.3 Brachytherapy Procedure

24.3.1 Patient Preparation

Patients receive information about interstitial brachytherapy during the external beam component of treatment. Nurses provide instructions on bowel cleanse preparation (initiated 24 h prior to admission) and information regarding the inpatient stay, skin care, and diet management prior to admission. Those patients selected by the radiation oncologist for brachytherapy must meet with an anesthesiologist approximately 1 week before the procedure for routine preoperative assessment. Patients with a prior laminectomy, significant degenerative disease, or labile blood pressure may not be optimum candidates for epidural anesthesia. In addition, patients receiving anticoagulation with Warfarin must switch to low-molecular weight (LMW) heparin (Enoxaparin) approximately 1 week prior to the planned procedure date. LMW Heparin administration should stop 24 h prior to the insertion time and should be withheld throughout the duration of the implant while the patient receives subcutaneous heparin.

Upon the patient's arrival in the clinic, the nurse or anesthesiologist places an intravenous (IV) and ensures that all signed consent forms have been completed. At Brigham and Women's Hospital (BWH), before the procedure begins an epidural catheter is inserted and may be initiated during the procedure, but in some cases may not be initiated until after the procedure, once the patient has been released to the postanesthesia care unit. At the Medical College of Wisconsin (MCW), the epidural is placed, activated, and assessed for efficacy prior to general anesthesia but is used primarily beginning in the recovery room. Epidural anesthesia allows for patient-controlled pelvic analgesia (PCA) for the duration of the inpatient hospitalization without resulting in the systemic effects, somnolence, and mental status changes that may occur with a peripheral PCA. Once the patient enters the operating room or brachytherapy suite, the anesthesiologist initiates general endotracheal anesthesia; spinal anesthesia is available for patients who have a contraindication to general anesthesia. The anesthesiologist remains present for the duration of the case. If MR imaging is planned, an MR-compatible epidural catheter should be chosen.

Once the patient is under anesthesia, the legs are raised to the lithotomy position using padded stirrups to prevent nerve or soft tissue injury. The legs should be in a neutral rather than a retracted position so that needles are not displaced significantly when the legs are lowered back to the supine position. The speculum examination reveals the extent of vaginal disease. The digital examination allows the assessment of vaginal width, the tumor size and location, the amount and thickness of residual parametrial or paravaginal disease, and the presence of a fistula. Radiopaque markers may be placed to define the tumor borders.

24.3.2 Applicator Selection

To cover the tumor and target volumes appropriately, selection of the most suitable applicator is essential. For patients who have had a complete response to external beam radiation for vaginal lesions (i.e., residual <5 mm), vaginal cylinder brachytherapy may suffice; for those with residual vaginal wall thickening or mass (≥5 mm) interstitial brachytherapy is necessary. Interstitial brachytherapy can either be inserted through a template or free hand [7]. The Syed–Neblett template, which has a circular formation, is useful for vaginal cancer or cervical cancer cases with extensive vaginal involvement, as the catheters can follow the oblong configuration of the vaginal mucosal surface (Fig. 24.1) [8]. The Martinez (MUPIT) applicator has angled insertion openings, designed to enhance parametrial tissue coverage [9]. The plastic template for both the Syed–Neblett and Martinez applicators rests on the perineal surface and requires suturing of the template to the perineal skin. The Vienna applicator allows for the insertion of short needles through a ring applicator at the level of the cervix to cover parametrial or parauterine extension of disease but does not cover extensive mid-to distal-vaginal disease [10]. No external template is required for the Vienna applicator, the Utrecht customized needles through ovoids, or the Mount Vernon system of needles with a tandem and ring applicator (Chap. 9). Custom-designed applicators include vaginal obturators with customized insertion sites for needles, templates, or freehand insertion of needles without a template or obturator. With freehand insertion, the equal spacing of catheters necessary to achieve a homogeneous dose distribution may be difficult; freehand techniques are best reserved for tumors in the lower vagina, where the mass can be palpated or visualized. Regardless of the type of applicator selected, the risk of insertion of a needle into the bladder or rectum is higher without 3D visualization used during or after insertion to correct misplacement.

3D image guidance requires CT- or MRI-compatible applicators, made of either titanium or solid, non-deformable plastic catheters (Fig. 24.1). Stainless-steel needles with sharp or blunt tips used with CT may cause streak artifacts. Scanning with radiopaque markers instead of metal obturators and careful adjustment of the window and level settings can reduce these artifacts. The use of titanium needles in higher-strength 3 Tesla magnets should be approached with caution given the potential for heating the tissues around the needles, and for imaging artifacts. Plastic flexible needles instead of metal needles may be inserted with rigid internal obturators to prevent internal bending; nevertheless, needles may deviate if fibrotic tumor or the pubic bone impedes insertion. Imaging during needle placement shows the trajectory and ultimate location of the needles; however, besides the Brigham and Women's Hospital, few institutions have access to real-time image guidance. Instead, most institutions scan patients with an MRI or CT scan after insertion. Inappropriately placed needles may be reinserted or removed prior to treatment, or the catheters may be left in place but must not be loaded with radioactive sources.

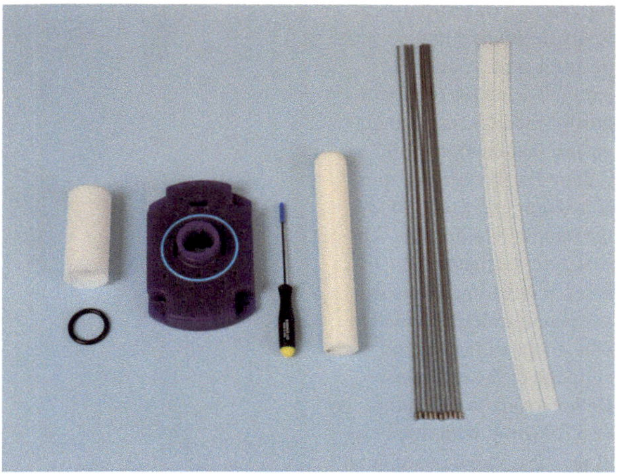

Fig. 24.1 Set up for an interstitial implant requires a vaginal obturator and template. Shown in this figure is a disposable Syed–Neblett template with plastic flexible catheters inserted with metal trocars placed through the center for stability. The plastic catheters have a sharp point to aid with insertion through the skin

24.3.3 Insertion Technique

For insertion, a sterile setup including a modified dilation and curettage (D & C) kit and sterile applicator are necessary. After a Betadine vaginal and perineal prep, a Foley catheter is inserted into the bladder. The vaginal apex or cervix and the most distal extension of tumor down the vaginal walls may be marked with gold seeds. A stitch may be placed at the apex of the vagina for retraction to ensure contact between the obturator and the vaginal apex during the insertion process. The obturator is placed in the vagina with the template sutured to the perineal skin either before or after needle insertion (Fig. 24.2).

The needles are inserted into the obturator tracks and the template holes. Imaging is performed either simultaneously or immediately after insertion. If there is no bladder or rectal invasion, the template holes nearest the bladder and rectum are avoided. The depth of needle insertion is typically quite uniform throughout the template, though the obturator needles can be inserted to the same depth as the tandem if they reside within the uterus. Small bowel and pelvic blood vessels can be at risk if the template needles are advanced too deeply into the pelvis. The ureters may be very close to the lateral needles and in some patients may be identified by stents if there is disease-associated hydronephosis. At BWH, the first needle is inserted to a specified depth. Thereafter, the patient is advanced into the MR or CT scanner, and the needle depth is adjusted to the maximum permissible depth without entering the bowel. Subsequently, a number of needles are inserted, then the patient is brought again into the MR or CT scanner for a scan; after assessment of the coverage of the tumor by the needles on the images, any adjustments to existing needles are made, or new needles are inserted. The process is reiterated until all needles cover the entire target volume; a final CT simulation is performed and imported into the planning software. At the Medical College of Wisconsin, there is no MR or CT scanner in the operating room suite, so the needles are placed with guidance via laparoscopy or laparotomy as well as fluoroscopy or ultrasound to confirm depth of insertion. Divergent and convergent

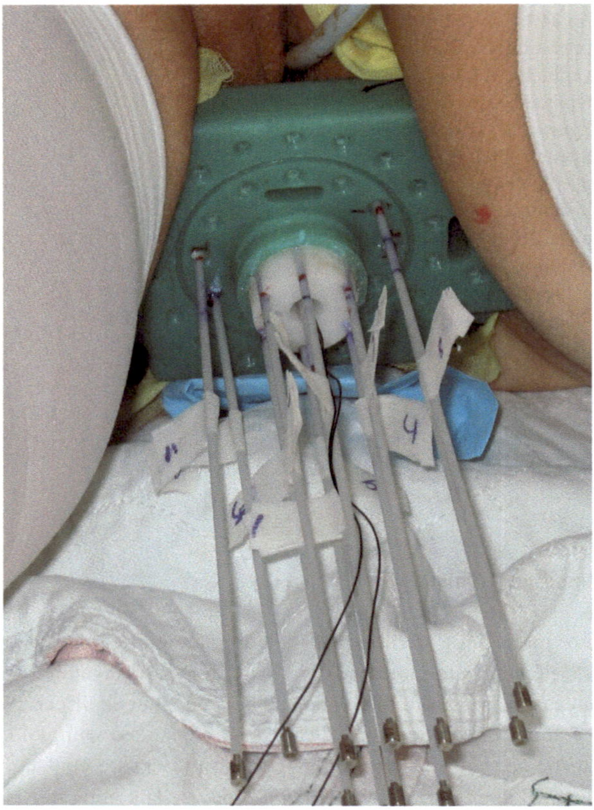

Fig. 24.2 An interstitial template sutured to the perineal skin. A central suture is used for retraction during catheter insertion to ensure that the obturator remains at the vaginal apex. Xerofoam gauze surrounds the template to prevent skin irritation. Catheters are marked with a permanent ink pen in order to visualize placement and ensure no slippage of the catheters. Catheters are numbered in order starting with number 1 at the 12-o'clock position on the ring and working in concentric circles outward. All catheters are attached to the template with adhesive glue. The patient will keep the Foley catheter, the TEDS stockings and pneumoboots in place while on bedrest throughout the hospitalization

needles can be identified and replaced after visualization with fluoroscopy. The position of the needles relative to the cervical and vaginal markers can also be assessed and adjusted. Laparoscopy and laparotomy are especially helpful in the post-hysterectomy state for institutions where in-operating room image guidance is not available to avoid needle insertion through the small bowel and sigmoid. At MCW, after the insertion is completed and the patient is discharged from the recovery room, the patient undergoes a CT scan. The depth of needle insertion is assessed, and minor adjustments can be made with the aid of ongoing epidural anesthesia.

24.3.4 Imaging Protocol

The Foley bag is placed below the patient, pressure is manually placed on the bladder to ensure complete emptying, and then the Foley catheter is clamped above the instillation opening. Dilute Hypaque contrast (10 cc Hypaque, 40 cc saline) is injected into the bladder.

A total of 50 cc of barium is introduced into the rectosigmoid using a rectal tube that is removed prior to the CT scan. CT slices of 1.25–2.5 mm are used. Gold seeds that mark the upper vagina, the cervix, and the most distal spread of tumor are identified if inserted. A margin is added to the distance between these radiopaque markers to determine the length of source activation in each needle.

24.3.5 Post-Imaging Protocol

After the final adjustments, the template is sutured to the skin in the position that causes the least amount of skin retraction. At least 1 cm is left between the template and the suture tie in order to allow for edema of the perineal skin. The catheters are numbered in sequential order starting at the 12-o'clock position using steri-strips or plastic numbered ties (Fig. 24.2). For patients who have plastic template and needles, strong bond adhesive glue attaches the needles to the template; some templates also come with screws that tighten the obturator to the template.

Given the complexities of these cases, special consideration to medical issues must be taken. All patients receive subcutaneous heparin; TED stockings and pneumoboots (triple prophylaxis) placed prior to placing the patient in lithotomy and continued throughout the inpatient hospitalization to decrease the risk of a thromboembolic event. All patients are preferably placed on an air mattress to decrease the risk of a decubitus ulcer, with Xeroform gauze around the template edge and a soft-formed pillow between their legs to decrease any chafing by the applicator. Patients must be isolated if they are receiving LDR. A low-residue diet and scheduled around-the-clock antidiarrheals can help to prevent bowel movements; the Foley catheter remains in place throughout the implant. During the procedure, IV antibiotics are initiated, and followed by a 7-day course of oral antibiotics. Diligent perineal care is important after the implant is completed. Peak normal tissue reactions occur between 1 and 2 weeks post-implant and patients need close follow-up during the recovery period. All patients need appropriate aftercare, sometimes including physical therapy or a rehabilitation program in order to regain mobility.

24.3.6 Contouring

Proper scanning of the appropriate volume is necessary; the sequence, slice thickness, and region to scan must be carefully selected. The primary mass is scanned and contoured based on information from the pre-implant imaging; however, if the anatomy is distorted by the applicator, an approximation of tumor extension is required. Interstitial cases imaged by CT may benefit from an MRI from the time of diagnosis or immediately prior to implantation in order to aid contouring. The entire tumor and extent of disease at the time of brachytherapy resembles that of the HR CTV (high risk-CTV) for cervical cancer based on the GEC-ESTRO nomenclature, and this nomenclature may be extrapolated to other sites such as vaginal or recurrent cancers. For vaginal cancers, the tumor volume marked by radiopaque markers is contoured as the HR CTV. For all cases, the entire vagina is contoured as well as the disease extension at diagnosis in order to define an IR CTV (intermediate-risk CTV) (Fig. 24.3). If patients have a CT scan instead of an MRI, the primary volume contoured is the HR CTV. Parameters to describe tumor volumes are D90, D100,V100, V150, and V200. The organs at risk (OAR), are contoured (Fig. 24.4) after needle insertion and the D_{2cc} and $D_{0.1cc}$ for the bladder, rectum, and sigmoid reported [11].

24.4 Treatment Planning

In the early years of interstitial brachytherapy, no information on dose distribution or normal tissue constraints was available and rates of complications and local failure were high [1]. Subsequently, the Paris and the Manchester (Paterson–Parker) systems developed, taking into account the source strengths, geometry, and method of application in order to

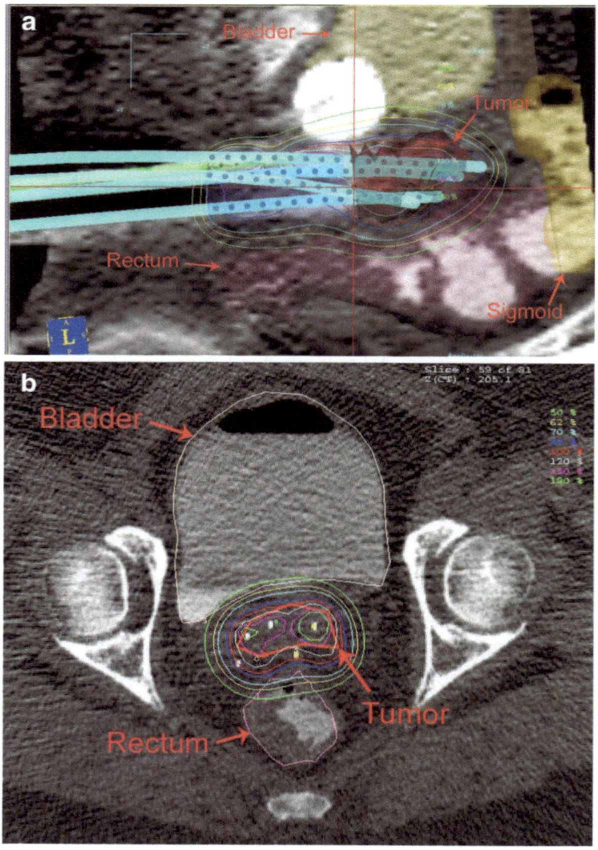

Fig. 24.3 (**a**) The entire vagina is contoured and treated with a boost given to the residual mass. (**b**) Imaging with contrast in the bladder and rectum on CT allow clear visualization and contouring of the organs at risk (OAR)

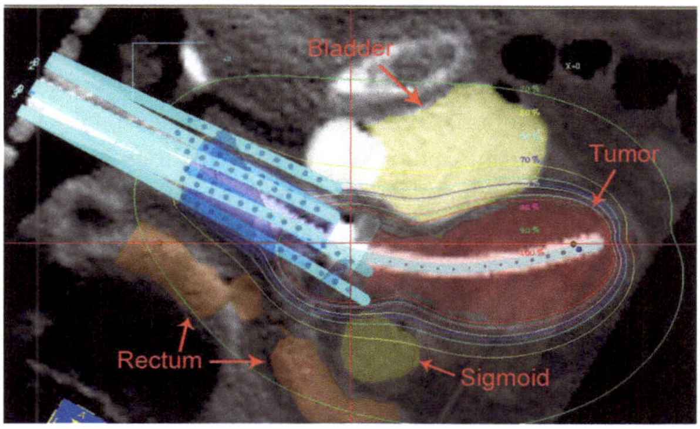

Fig. 24.4 Interstitial catheters placed around a central tandem for a patient with vaginal and parametrial residual disease after chemoradiation for cervical cancer

obtain suitable dose distributions over the volumes treated. The large volume implants of the pelvis defy these rules, as needle and source placement are defined by the template holes, without the ability to cross sources and with few guidelines for selection of source activity, dose rate, and total dose constraints. With the advent of computerized dosimetry, these volume implants can be evaluated in three dimensions and a better understanding of the ability to alter the implant to obtain better dose distributions and reduce normal tissue doses has been achieved [1]. Conceptually, interstitial implants have been viewed as volume implants with core sources and peripheral sources. When using LDR techniques, low-activity Ir-192 sources are used. The core sources may have one half to one third the strength of the peripheral sources, or may be of equal strength depending on the size and dimensions of the tumor. To avoid a central cold spot, the vaginal obturator surface and the tandem are loaded with Iridum-192 and the tandem is loaded with Cesium 137. A reference point A dose rate of 60–80 cGy/h is the goal with 80–100 cGy/h at the obturator surface, giving careful attention to the location and dimensions of any hot spots.

At the Medical College of Wisconsin, the CT-based HDR interstitial volume receives 100% of the dose and the obturator surface receives 120–130% of the reference dose. Hot spots of up to 150% of the reference dose are allowed only around individual needles. The normal tissue doses should be minimized to 80% or less of the reference dose. Optimization techniques are used to reduce hot and cold spots, improve coverage, and decrease doses to the normal tissues. The shortfall of CT-based dosimetry is poor soft tissue resolution and the potential for artifact when using metal needles. MR-based brachytherapy has been used to better define the tumor and its extensions to guide needle insertion and dose distribution optimization. At BWH, all interstitial cases, regardless of LDR or HDR, have a volume-based approach with an individualized, optimized plan based on tumor coverage [12]. For LDR, sources of equal activity are loaded, and needles are placed preferentially through the core of the visible tumor. Isodose distributions are visualized on the 3D image, and dose-volume histogram (DVH) analysis is performed for the bladder, rectum, and sigmoid, and, when necessary, small bowel.

A good implant can be achieved by using the traditional rules such as ICRU 58 to determine the number and placement of needles needed to cover the target appropriately. Dose homogeneity should be evaluated by parameters used for conventional interstitial implants such as the size and spatial distribution of the V150, V200, or by parameters describing the dose-nonuniformity or a conformal index [13]. An important issue remains the spatial dose distribution; therefore, one must visually inspect the dose distribution, especially for high-dose regions. The total doses to target structures and organs at risk can be calculated using radiobiological calculations such as the EQD2. Similarly, criteria recommended for intracavitary cervix cancer brachytherapy, with maximum EQD2 D_{2cc} values of 70–75 Gy for rectum and sigmoid and 90 Gy for the bladder, may be applied for interstitial brachytherapy. Interstitial implants may cause considerable dose to other organs at risk including the vagina, the urethra, and other adjacent tissues such as connective or fatty tissue, which may be more vulnerable than the radioresistant muscular uterus. Because data is lacking to dictate the necessary dose volume parameters and the risk of late effects, the dose distribution should be compared to traditional implant geometries and source loading patterns. Based on such standards, fine-tuning the dose distribution may be performed with appropriate dwell time optimization.

24.5 Prescription

If using 3D-based planning, the dose to the contoured targets may be specified in terms of the D90 in EQD2. For cervical cancer, the dose to the HR CTV of at least 85 Gy and to the IR CTV of at least 60 Gy, including the external beam dose, remains standard. For vaginal cancer cases with gross residual disease at the time of brachytherapy, a dose of 70–90 Gy may be prescribed to the gross disease with 60 Gy to the entire, vaginal surface, and special caution used during optimization for patients with bowel in close proximity to the tumor. At the MCW for CT-based implants, a central and peripheral dose may be more appropriate as it is very difficult to accurately define the HR CTV with the poor soft tissue resolution of CT, especially in the setting of metal needle-induced artifacts. In this setting, a central or core dose of 80–85 Gy can be achieved with a peripheral dose of 70–75 Gy given the proximity of the OARS. Additionally, the D90 dose distributions for intracavitary versus interstitial implants often differ quite substantially. That is, an equivalent D90 for an intracavitary implant and an equivalent D90 for an interstitial implant typically have a different dose distribution pattern and volume of tissue receiving that dose. Intracavitary implants have much higher doses in the vicinity of the interuterine source compared to potentially more homogeneity with interstitial implants. Comparisons between different approaches are difficult and should account for the dose to the GTV (D90, D100) and high-dose volume parameters (e.g., D50). The combined intracavitary/interstitial approaches require special attention. When using the ring or ovoids with needles, similar dose distributions as with pure intracavitary implants may be achieved if the interstitial needles are inserted in the proximity of the intrauterine tandem. These dose distributions, however, are very different from those obtained with the challenging combination of intracavitary and interstitial sources when using the tandem and multiple template needles; these often result in a central high region of dose around the cervix and paracervical tissues and a more homogenous but lower dose more laterally, achieved with the optimum distribution of sources or dwell times. Careful dose specification and optimization can lead to an acceptable implant even when dealing with many needles, while avoiding excessive high-dose regions. It is always important to remember that the high central dose achieved with use of a tandem is often pivotal in curing cervical cancer [5]. This is a different situation than when dealing with a vaginal cuff recurrence [12] where a more homogeneous, lower dose is acceptable.

For patients treated with HDR interstitial at BWH, we perform the implant on Monday and treat twice a day (BID) for nine to ten fractions of between 200 and 300 cGy per fraction at least 6 h between fractions; we do not perform a second interstitial implant. At the Medical College of Wisconsin, patients are also treated with one insertion of needles rather than two and are treated with fraction sizes ranging from 450 to 650 cGy twice a day, a minimum of 6 h apart, in three to six fractions.

24.6 Follow-up

Prior to discharge, after implant removal, patients are checked to ensure that a decubitus ulcer has not developed, particularly for thin, elderly patients. Patients are typically seen 2 to 4 weeks after the implant has been removed for a skin check, then in 3-month intervals for 1 year, then every 6 months to ensure that no side effects result from treatment. If patients develop tissue necrosis, a dilute hydrogen peroxide douching regimen is initiated. If a malodorous discharge accompanies the necrosis, antibiotics (metronidazole) are recommended.

24.7 Outcomes with 3D Interstitial Therapy

Syed et al., reported an approximately 10% toxicity rate with long-term follow-up [14] without IPBT; fluoroscopic [15] or ultrasound-guided [16], laparoscopic, open laparotomy, or closed procedures have been reported. An approximate 11% rate of bowel insertion and a long-term fistula rate of 4–10% results from using CT for planning [17, 18].

The BWH report of real-time MR guidance during interstitial gynecologic therapy for recurrent endometrial cancer of the vaginal apex [12] to date recorded one sigmoid-vaginal fistula where the vaginal apex tumor was adherent to the sigmoid, and regression of the tumor resulted in opening of a previously unknown fistula tract. No inadvertent insertions of the bowel or bladder were detected in any of the 25 patients treated to date with MR-guided therapy, regardless of diagnosis [19]. A report on the use of the Vienna applicator for cervical cancer described clinical outcomes in 22 patients followed for a median of 20 months; no grade 3 or 4 toxicities were noted, and one patient had a local recurrence [20]. Dose optimization with either PDR or HDR may improve the normal tissue doses for interstitial therapy for some patients.

24.8 Limitations

3D imaging is helpful in very difficult cases, including tumors that are adjacent to the pubic symphysis, in the perivaginal regions, or close to the rectum. However, increased anesthesia and procedure time, as well physician and physicist effort are required. The number of needles inserted may be decreased, and if a needle is inserted into an OAR, it may not be loaded with radiation resulting in potentially fewer side effects for patients.

24.9 Conclusion

Interstitial therapy requires close collaboration with anesthesiologists, radiologists, medical and surgical oncologists, physicists, and nurses. Challenges to broader use of 3D-guided interstitial therapy include access to the appropriate imaging equipment, treatment planning using standardized contours and systems, and the need for publications showing definitive outcome results. Recent nomenclature standardizing the description of proper DVH parameters for gynecologic brachytherapy can be applied to interstitial treatments, thereby improving communication between centers. Though we may assume that accurate visualization and reporting of the dose to the tumor and normal tissues will improve outcomes, long-term follow-up is necessary.

References

1. Erickson B, Gillin M. Interstitial implantation of gynecologic malignancies. Armonk: Futura; 1997.
2. Abbe R. The use of radium in malignant disease. Lancet. 1913;2:524–7.
3. Lanciano RM, Martz K, et al. Tumor and treatment factors improving outcome in stage III-B cervix cancer. Int J Radiat Oncol Biol Phys. 1991;20:95–100.
4. Lee LJ, Sadow CA, et al. Correlation of point B and lymph node dose in 3D-planned high-dose-rate cervical cancer brachytherapy. Int J Radiat Oncol Biol Phys. 2009;75(3):803–9.
5. Viswanathan AN, Cormack R, et al. Increasing brachytherapy dose predicts survival for interstitial and tandem-based radiation for stage IIIB cervical cancer. Int J Gynecol Cancer. 2009;19(8):1402–6.
6. Viswanathan AN, Dimopoulos J, et al. Computed tomography versus magnetic resonance imaging-based contouring in cervical cancer brachytherapy: results of a prospective trial and preliminary guidelines for standardized contours. Int J Radiat Oncol Biol Phys. 2007; 68(2):491–8.
7. Viswanathan AN, Petereit D. Gynecologic brachytherapy. Philadelphia: Lippincott; 2007.
8. Fleming P, Nisar Syed AM, et al. Description of an afterloading 192Ir interstitial-intracavitary technique in the treatment of carcinoma of the vagina. Obstet Gynecol. 1980;55(4):525–30.

9. Martinez A, Edmundson GK, et al. Combination of external beam irradiation and multiple-site perineal applicator (MUPIT) for treatment of locally advanced or recurrent prostatic, anorectal, and gynecologic malignancies. Int J Radiat Oncol Biol Phys. 1985;11(2):391–8.
10. Kirisits C, Lang S, et al. The Vienna applicator for combined intracavitary and interstitial brachytherapy of cervical cancer: design, application, treatment planning, and dosimetric results. Int J Radiat Oncol Biol Phys. 2006;65(2):624–30.
11. Kirisits C, Potter R, et al. Dose and volume parameters for MRI-based treatment planning in intracavitary brachytherapy for cervical cancer. Int J Radiat Oncol Biol Phys. 2005; 2(3):901–11.
12. Viswanathan AN, Cormack R, et al. Magnetic resonance-guided interstitial therapy for vaginal recurrence of endometrial cancer. Int J Radiat Oncol Biol Phys. 2006;66(1):91–9.
13. Baltas D, Kolotas C, et al. A conformal index (COIN) to evaluate implant quality and dose specification in brachytherapy. Int J Radiat Oncol Biol Phys. 1998;40(2):515–24.
14. Syed AM, Puthawala AA, et al. Long-term results of low-dose-rate interstitial-intracavitary brachytherapy in the treatment of carcinoma of the cervix. Int J Radiat Oncol Biol Phys. 2002;54(1):67–78.
15. Nag S, Martinez-Monge R, et al. The use of fluoroscopy to guide needle placement in interstitial gynecological brachytherapy. Int J Radiat Oncol Biol Phys. 1998;40(2):415–20.
16. Stock RG, Chan K, et al. A new technique for performing Syed-Neblett template interstitial implants for gynecologic malignancies using transrectal-ultrasound guidance. Int J Radiat Oncol Biol Phys. 1997;37(4):819–25.
17. Eisbruch A, Johnston CM, et al. Customized gynecologic interstitial implants: CT-based planning, dose evaluation, and optimization aided by laparotomy. Int J Radiat Oncol Biol Phys. 1998;40(5):1087–93.
18. Erickson B, Albano K, et al. CT-guided interstitial implantation of gynecologic malignancies. Int J Radiat Oncol Biol Phys. 1996;36(3):699–709.
19. Viswanathan AN, Racine ML, et al. Final results of a prospective study of MR-based interstitial gynecologic brachytherapy. *Brachytherapy* 2008; 7(2):148.
20. Dimopoulos JC, Kirisits C, et al. The Vienna applicator for combined intracavitary and interstitial brachytherapy of cervical cancer: clinical feasibility and preliminary results. Int J Radiat Oncol Biol Phys. 2006;66(1):83–90.

Part V

Clinical Outcomes of 3D Based External Beam Radiation and Image-Guided Brachytherapy

Outcomes Related to the Disease and the Use of 3D-Based External Beam Radiation and Image-Guided Brachytherapy

25

Alina Sturdza and Richard Pötter

25.1 Introduction

Brachytherapy is an essential component of the radical radiation treatment of patients with gynecological malignancies, especially locally advanced cervical cancer, endometrial, and vaginal cancer. Until recently, brachytherapy for locally advanced cervical cancer was delivered in a standard fashion, using a standard X-ray–based technique with the dose prescribed to a standard point (point A). In the last decade, with the advent of IGRT, the focus of research and development has shifted toward finding more accurate methods for delivering radiation treatment to these patients, and magnetic resonance imaging (MRI)/computed tomography (CT)/ultrasound (US)–guided brachytherapy for patients with locally advanced cervical cancer have been implemented in some centers. Based on the experience with cervical cancer, IGRT is now also being used in the treatment of vaginal cancer and in cases of definitive therapy for endometrial cancer as well as for any recurrent disease.

Image-guided adaptive brachytherapy (IGABT) is currently gaining momentum as this emerging technique has been shown to provide major improvements in dose-volume parameters and also in clinical outcome, primarily due to a high precision of the dose delivered by gynecological IGABT [28]. The advancement of this technique is primarily based on the use of repetitive MRIs performed at brachytherapy and has been described in detail in this book. Other imaging modalities such as CT and US and functional imaging are also under evaluation but so far only very limited data are available [24, 30, 31]. In the last few years, outcome data on MRI-guided BT in patients with cervical cancer has matured and there is now literature available on the results of this new technique from two centers: Medical University of Vienna [26] and Institut Gustave Roussy, Villejuif, France [3]. Additional data, partially published, with MRI- and/or CT-guided brachytherapy in gynecological malignancies is available from the Brigham and Women's Hospital/Dana-Farber Cancer Institute [33], and personal communication form Tata Memorial. Data on US-guided BT combined with MRI findings is available from Peter MacCallum Cancer Centre,

A. Sturdza (✉) and R. Pötter
Department of Radiotherapy, Vienna General Hospital,
Medical University of Vienna, Währinger Gürtel 18-20, 1090 Vienna, Austria
e-mail: alina.sturdza@akhwien.at

A.N. Viswanathan et al. (eds.), *Gynecologic Radiation Therapy*,
DOI: 10.1007/978-3-540-68958-4_25, © Springer-Verlag Berlin Heidelberg 2011

Melbourne, Australia [24]. Outcome data on CT-guided BT for cervical cancer patients is available on a small number of large tumors treated at the University of Pittsburgh Cancer Institute, Pittsburgh, USA [2], and from Addenbrooke's Hospital [30], UK.

Some preliminary outcome data is also available on small series of patients treated with MRI- or US-guided brachytherapy for vaginal and endometrial cancer primary treatment or recurrence from the Medical University of Vienna [6, 34, 35]. In order to facilitate the understanding and comparison of data, all physical doses to the target and organs at risk (OARs) reported in this chapter were re-calculated in EQD2 according to the linear-quadratic (LQ) model, applying an α/β value of 10 Gy for tumor effects and 3 Gy for effects at OARs [20].

25.2 Cervical Cancer

25.2.1 Definitive Treatment Using IGBT

25.2.1.1 Locally Advanced Cervical Cancer

The delivery of optimal brachytherapy as part of a complex treatment in patients with locally advanced cervical cancer requires careful consideration and integration of several specific critical treatment decisions. These include the determination of the appropriate target volume dependent on disease extent at diagnosis and the response to radiochemotherapy, the choice of applicator type in order to achieve appropriate target coverage (dose-volume adaptation) with sparing of OARs, quality assurance methods, total dose to be delivered, and overall duration of treatment. Recently published data on the use of image-guided brachytherapy (IGBT) show that most of the shortcomings associated with classical 2D brachytherapy delivery can nowadays be overcome, and better outcome results are to be expected. Currently, there are three major types of IGBT used for cervical cancer: MRI, CT, and US.

MRI-Guided Brachytherapy

A reasonable number of institutions in Europe and few in North America and India have already implemented MRI-guided BT for locally advanced cervical cancer. Outcome data is available thus far from two centers: Vienna and Paris on approximately 200 patients.

Vienna Experience

This is the first retrospective series with outcome results of MRI-guided brachytherapy for cervical cancer published in 2007 [26]. From 1998 to 2003, a total of 145 patients with cervical cancer stages IB–IVA were treated with MRI-guided brachytherapy in addition to concurrent chemoradiation or radiation alone. Data on patients with a median follow-up of 40 months was reported. All patients were treated with whole pelvis 3D conformal external beam radiotherapy (EBRT) on a linear accelerator with 25-MV photons using a four-field treatment box with individual blocks based on CT-assisted 3D treatment planning following an in-house protocol [13]. Dose prescribed was 45 Gy (25 fractions of 1.8 Gy) at the international commission on radiation units and measurements (ICRU) point for patients receiving concomitant cisplatin-based chemotherapy and 50.4 Gy (28 fractions of 1.8 Gy) for patients without chemotherapy. Intracavitary brachytherapy (ICBT) with Ir 192 with a tandem ring applicator (Nucletron) and individual packing was completed in all patients [29]. In 29 patients a combined interstitial and intracavitary brachytherapy approach was used due to an unfavorable spread of residual disease at the time of brachytherapy. A 3D computer-assisted treatment planning for brachytherapy based on MRI and thorough clinical examination was performed in 142 of 145 patients (patients with pacemaker, hip implant, or extreme obesity were excluded) with a total of 420 MRI examinations and 3D treatment planning procedures. Between 1998 and 2000 (learning period), 73 patients were treated using dose adaptation mainly based on the visual inspection of the isodose lines and dose changes to point A. In the period 2001–2003, a systematic MRI-guided planning was applied for each fraction with prospective contouring of GTV and high-risk clinical target volume (HR CTV), OAR (rectum, sigmoid, bladder, bowel), optimization of dwell time and position, and prospective evaluation of dose-volume parameters for HR CTV and OARs, applying the LQ model [16, 27, 17]. The treatment planning procedure always started with a standard plan normalized to point A. In this treatment period (72 patients) manual dwell time optimization was based on the contoured HR CTV and control of dose volume histogram (DVH) parameters [17]. Prescribed dose for the HR CTV was 4×7 Gy at high dose rate (HDR) in advanced disease and $5–6 \times 7$ Gy at HDR in limited disease, corresponding to a prescribed dose of 80–85-Gy EQD2. In case of insufficient coverage, combined intracavitary and interstitial brachytherapy has been systematically applied since 2001. The dose to OARs was first estimated by using ICRU points and visual control of the dose distribution on the MRI. DVH constraints were implemented step by step first for the rectum and later for bladder, sigmoid, and HR CTV (D90). Dose to HR CTV was evaluated in terms of dose covering 90% of the HR CTV (D90). A minimum D90 of 85 Gy was aimed at. Dose-volume constraints for OAR were 75-Gy EQD2 as minimum dose in the most exposed tissue (2 cm^3) of rectum and sigmoid and only later during this period 90-Gy EQD2 in 2 cm^3 of the bladder [27]. No dose-volume constraints were applied for the vagina. Dose and target coverage were adapted according to dose-volume constraints for OARs. If appropriate and feasible, dose was escalated, particularly in advanced disease. For limited disease, dose de-escalation was not performed in case of high D90 doses in the HR CTV (>90 Gy).

Dose-volume adaptation was performed in 130 of 145 patients (90%). The mean D90 ± 1SD during the whole period was 86 Gy ± 16 Gy, with a mean D90 of 81 Gy ± 16 Gy during the first period and a mean D90 of 90 Gy ± 15 Gy during the second period ($p = 0.0007$). For intracavitary treatment alone the mean dose to point A during the whole period was 79 Gy ± 11 Gy, during the first period 78 Gy ± 10 Gy and during the second period 82 Gy ± 9 Gy (Table 25.2).

Complete remission was achieved in 138 patients (95%). Seven patients showed locally persistent and progressive disease in the central ($n = 5$) and non-central ($n = 2$) pelvis. Two could be salvaged by hysterectomy, one of whom was showing no evidence of disease at 2 years. Pelvic recurrence occurred in 21 patients (14.5%) during the whole follow-up period, 18 in true pelvis (ten central, eight non-central), 14 during the first 3 years, and 3 in the regional lymph nodes, all within 3 years. Central pelvic recurrences were in the cervix (5), in the uterine corpus (1), and in the adjacent (1) and the remote (3) vagina. Noncentral recurrences were in the proximal ($n = 6$) and distal ($n = 2$) parametria. Recurrent lymph node regions in the pelvis were obturator (1) and iliac (2 (one external, one internal)).

A detailed description of the different outcome parameters is given in Table 25.1. Overall PFS in true pelvis (local control) was 85% at 3 years. For 1998–2000 progress free survival (PFS) in the true pelvis was 82% and for 2001–2003 it was 89%. For the periods 1998–2000 and 2001–2003, PFS in the true pelvis for tumors 2–5 cm was 100% and 96%, and for tumors >5 cm 64% and 82% ($p = 0.09$), respectively. Overall continuous complete remission (CCR) for true pelvis at 3 years was 88%. CCR for true pelvis was 83% for 1998–2000 compared with 93% for 2001–2003. For tumors of 2–5 cm CCR for true pelvis was 96% for both treatment periods. For tumors >5 cm, the CCR in true pelvis was 71% for 1998–2000 and 90% for 2001–2003 ($p = 0.05$). Distant metastases were 32 overall with 26 occurring at 3 years with a PFS of 80% for distant metastasis (Table 25.1). There is no difference between the treatment periods at 3 years; with 13 events in the period 1998–2000 versus 13 events in the period 2001–2003. Para-aortic lymph node

Table 25.1 Combined data from Vienna and Paris on absolute local and distant recurrence as absolute numbers and crude rates. Postradiotherapy surgery was performed for the Paris series in 26 of 35 patients with stage I/II disease. Failure rate overall: 64/190: 34%, Pelvic recurrence alone: 17/190: 9%, Overall local control: 91% at median follow up of 26 months (Paris) and 51 months (Vienna)

Stage	Number of patients		Local recurrence		Distant recurrence alone*		Overall failure	
	Vienna	Paris	Vienna	Paris	Vienna	Paris	Vienna	Paris
IA	1	NA	–	NA	–	NA	–	NA
IB	13	14	1	–	1	2	2	2
IIA	6	2	–	–	1	7	1	8
IIB	81	21	8	–	9		21	
IIIA	4	1	–	–	2	2	2	4
IIIB	33	5	7	–	10		19	
IVA	7	2	1	–	3		5	
Total	145	45	17	–	26	11	50**	14
Total combined	190		17 (9%)		37 (19%)**		64 (34%)	

*Including Para-aortic node recurrences

failure was observed in 7 of 32 patients with distant failure. Overall Survival (OS) was 58% at 3 years. OS was 53% and 64% for 1998–2000 and 2001–2003, respectively. For tumors >5 cm OS was 28% in the first period and 58% in the second period (p = 0.003). Cancer-specific survival (CSS) was 68% at 3 years. For tumors >5 cm CSS was 40% in the first period and 62% in the second period (p = 0.07). No impact of chemotherapy on PFS in the true pelvis was found with 82% in the first period and 85% in the second period. Actuarial late morbidity rate (LENT SOMA, grades 3 and 4) at 3 years was gastrointestinal 4%, urinary 4%, and vaginal 5% (stage IIA/IIIA). Gastrointestinal and urinary late morbidity (G3, G4) was 10% in 1998–2000 and 2% in 2001–2003. Types and frequencies of side effects are described in detail in the subchapter on morbidity.

Institut Gustave Roussy Experience

The group from Institut Gustave Roussy, Villejuif, France, recently reported clinical results from patients with locally advanced cervical cancer after MRI-guided BT with a median follow-up of 26 months [3]. A total of 45 consecutive patients with primary locally advanced cervical carcinoma were treated between February 2004 and October 2006 with pulse dose rate brachytherapy (PDR-BT) after initial concurrent chemo-EBRT. Most patients presented with stage IB2-II disease (82%). Of the 45 patients, 23 (51.1%) and 4 (8.9%) had radiologic pelvic and para-aortic nodal involvement, respectively (based on CT and PET imaging). Analysis of the data on all patients revealed a median tumor cervical volume of 64.0 cm^3 (range, 3–178). Of the 45 patients, 24 (53%) had histologic and/or radiologic pelvic involvement. After EBRT, the PDR-BT boost was delivered using the PDR Selectron (Nucletron, Veenendaal, the Netherlands). In this series, no patient underwent interstitial BT, and all BT procedures were delivered during a single hospitalization. In the case of pelvic or para-aortic nodal involvement, a radiation boost was performed, unilaterally or bilaterally (6 and 12 patients, respectively), at a median dose of 9 Gy (range, 8–10) for the pelvic nodes, taking into account the dose contribution of BT to reach a minimum of 60 Gy to the involved pelvic or para-aortic nodes. BT consisted of the vaginal mold technique; for each patient, a customized vaginal mold was made, with one intrauterine and two vaginal catheters, from a vaginal impression. The length and positions of the vaginal catheters were determined from the patient's vaginal anatomy and adapted to the tumor shape, size, and extent. A 3D computer-assisted treatment planning for BT using MRI was performed in all patients. Normalized doses were calculated using an α/β 10 Gy for the target doses and α/β 3 Gy for the OARs. A dose of ≥15 Gy was prescribed to the intermediate-risk CTV (IR CTV). The dose to the HR CTV was aimed at reaching 250% of the dose to the IR CTV (i.e., a dose of 80 Gy to the HR CTV). The dose and target coverage were adapted according to the dose-volume constraints for the OARs, which were derived from the maximal total dose acceptable for each OAR.

Surgery was chosen for FIGO stage IB, IIA, and IIB tumors if tumor persistence was suspected 6 weeks after the BT procedure on clinical examination or MRI. Surgery was also suggested to patients with a complete clinical and radiologic response 6–8 weeks after BT within the frame of a randomized trial. For 26 patients, surgery was performed and consisted of radical vaginal hysterectomy (n = 3) or extrafascial hysterectomy (n = 23). Para-aortic lymph node dissection (n = 20) or pelvic lymph node dissection (n = 3) was performed at the hysterectomy. Exclusive para-aortic lymph node dissection (without hysterectomy) was performed in three other patients. One patient underwent metastasectomy associated with para-aortic lymph node dissection after perioperative discovery of a liver metastasis. Of these 26 patients, one underwent postoperative para-aortic EBRT because of histologic nodal involvement. The 2-year overall survival (OS) rate and disease-free survival rate in this group were 78% and 73%, respectively. At the last follow-up visit, the disease of all patients remained locally controlled (Table 25.1). Adding EBRT and PDR using the LQ model, the median doses received by 100% and 90% of the target were 54-Gy EQD2 and 64-Gy EQD2 for the IR CTV and 62-Gy EQD2 and 75-Gy EQD2 for the HR CTV, respectively (Table 25.2). Of the 45 patients, 23 and 2 developed acute grade 1–2 and grade 3 complications, respectively; 21 patients presented with delayed

Table 25.2 Dose-volume histogram parameters related to primary tumor target and critical organs and comparison with previously published reports on MRI-guided BT for locally advanced cervical cancer

Variable	Chargari et al. [3]	Lindegaard et al. [23]	De Brabandere et al. [6]	Dimopoulos et al. [7] Georg et al. [12] Kirisits et al. [19]
Patients (*n*)	45	21	16	141
Point A dose (Gyα/β10)	71.4 ± 6	81 ± 5	79 ± 5	79 ± 10
HR CTV				
Volume (cm³)	36.3 ± 35	34 ± 12	48 ± 19	36 ± 23
D100 (Gyα/β10)	61.66 ± 7	76 ± 5	64 ± 6	65 ± 19
D90 (Gyα/β10)	74.85 ±10	91 − 8	79 ± 7	86 ± 16
Urinary bladder				
$D_{0.1cc}$ (Gyα/β3)	87.6 ± 12	86 ± 12	100 ± 12	162 ± 75
D_{1cc} (Gyα/β3)	75.9 ± 7	77 ± 8	86 ± 7	108 ± 31
D_{2cc} (Gyα/β3)	71.7 ± 6	73 ± 6	82 ± 6	95 ± 22
ICRU (Gyα/β3)	63.7 ± 9	67 ± 8	74 ±15	72 ±15
Rectum				
$D_{0.1cc}$ (Gyα/β3)	70.6 ± 11	74 ± 9	68 ± 7	86 ± 27
D_{1cc} (Gyα/β3)	63.3 ± 7	69 ± 6	64 ± 5	69 ± 14
D_{2cc} (Gyα/β3)	60.5	67 ± 6	62 ± 4	65 ± 12
ICRU (Gyα/β3)	67.3 ± 8	71 ± 7	66 ± 9	67 ± 13
Sigmoid				
$D_{0.1cc}$ (Gyα/β3)	72.7 ± 18	79 ± 10	82 ± 13	84 ± 32
D_{1cc} (Gyα/β3)	63.6 ± 7	72 ± 7	72 ± 9	67 ± 14
D_{2cc} (Gyα/β3)	60.6 ± 6	69 ± 6	68 ± 7	62 ± 12

grade 1–2 complications. One other patient presented with grade 3 vesicovaginal fistula. No grade 4 or greater complications, whether acute or delayed, were observed.

Combined outcome data from Vienna [26] and Paris [3] are presented in Table 25.1. The crude rate of local failure alone after 2–3 years is 17/190 (9%); the overall crude failure rate is 64/190 (34%). For stage IB local control is 26/27 (96%), for IIB it is 94/102 (94%), and for IIIB it is 31/38 (82%).

Brigham and Women's Hospital/Dana-Farber Cancer Institute Experience

The first prospective phase II trial of MRI-guided brachytherapy recruited 25 patients from 2004 to 2006 with gynecologic cancer to the Brigham and Women's Hospital/Dana-Farber Cancer Institute, Boston, MA, United States (BWH/DFCI); the first ten enrolled from 2004 to 2005 with recurrent endometrial cancer utilized interstitial catheters alone [32]. One-year outcome and toxicity results of this real-time intraoperative MRI-guided interstitial approach to gynecologic cancer using the Syed-Neblett template for all the 25 patients enrolled were presented in abstract form [33]. The final group included cervical cancer – 3 patients with stage IIIB, 1 with IVA, and 1 with IVB; vaginal cancer – 1 patient for each of the following stages: I, IIB, IVA; a total of 17 patients with recurrences – 14 from endometrial cancer and 1 of each of the following malignancies: cervical, vulvar, and ovarian. MR-guided insertion was followed by a CT simulation with MR fusion and CT-based treatment planning. All patients had a minimum of 1-year follow-up. Reported values included median volume, 76.2 cc; V100, 52.9 cc; V150, 29.4 cc; V200, 14.7 cc; and a median brachytherapy dose of D90, 28.4 Gy, and D100, 12.5 Gy. DVH of OARs showed the following median D_{2cc} brachytherapy doses: bladder, 24 Gy; rectum, 29 Gy; and sigmoid, 15.8 Gy. Persistent disease was noted in one vaginal cancer patient and in one cervical cancer patient. Other relapses included either regional-nodal ($n = 2$) or distant metastases ($n = 4$). No patients suffered a local relapse during a minimum of 1-year follow-up for all surviving patients.

To date, 85 patients with cervical cancer have been treated with HDR using 5.5–6 Gy per fraction for 5 fractions after concurrent chemoradiation at the same center in dedicated CT simulator with CT-based treatment planning (personal communication with A. Viswanathan). For the first 23, prescription was to point A and the optimization was purely to the OAR. For all subsequent patients the optimization encompassed the cervix as seen on CT and therefore shifted the prescription either lateral or medial to a standard point A at 2 cm. The median follow-up at this time is 33 months. Of 11 patients who have relapsed, 2 have a component of local relapse concurrent with distant relapse, 8 have a distant recurrence alone, and 1 has nodal and distant relapse. No grade 3 or 4 GI or GU toxicities have occurred.

Tata Memorial Experience

The data set of 24 patients (stage IB2: 1, stage IIA: 1, stage IIB: 10, and stage IIIB: 12) with high dose rate intracavitary (ICA-HDR) applications in biopsy-proven cases of cervical cancers (squamous cell carcinoma) was analyzed. With a median follow-up of 12 months [5] (mean, 12 months; range, 4–29 months), 2 patients had local failures, 1 had PET-CT and biopsy-proven right external iliac nodal failure, and 1 patient had cytology-proven left supraclavicular nodal failure that was locally controlled. All patients received radical radiation therapy with/without concomitant cisplatin chemotherapy. The calculated mean HR CTV was 45.2 ± 15.8 cc. The mean point A dose was 73.4 ± 4.5 Gy, while mean D90 doses were

70.9 ± 10.6 Gy. The mean ICRU rectal and bladder points were 63.5 ± 8.1 Gy and 80.4 ± 34.4 Gy, respectively. The $D_{0.1cc}$ and D_{2cc} for rectum were 66.0 ± 9.9 Gy and 57.8 ± 7.7 Gy, for bladder were 139.1 Gy and 93.4 Gy, and for sigmoid were 109.4 Gy and 74.6 Gy.

CT-Based Brachytherapy

Addenbrooke Experience

A single institution experience of 28 patients (7 IB1, 3 IB2, 2 IIA, 12 IIB, and 4 IIIB) with a median follow-up of 23 months, who received initial EBRT followed by HDR CT-guided brachytherapy (planned dose 21 Gy to point A in 3 fractions over 8 days) was reported [30]. For each insertion, a CT scan was obtained with the brachytherapy applicator (tandem-ring) in situ. The cervix, uterus, and OARs were contoured on the CT images (software: Pro-Soma v.3.1, Medcom, Germany) which were then transferred to the BT planning software (PLATO v.14.3.5, Nucletron, the Netherlands) to create an individualized dosimetry plan (new plan for each insertion). The standard loading pattern used was as recommended by the Vienna group [12]. The Addenbrooke's group protocol stated that the aim is to cover the tumor and cervix with the 100% isodose while limiting the minimum dose in the most exposed 2-cm^3 volume (D_{2cc}) of rectum to 5 Gy per fraction [30]. If this could not be achieved using the standard loading pattern, manual optimization of source positions and dwell times was carried out to try and improve the dosimetry.

The *D*90, *V*100, and the minimum dose in the most exposed 2-cm^3 volume (D_{2cc}) of rectum, bladder, and bowel were recorded. The equivalent dose in 2-Gy fractions delivered by EBRT and brachytherapy was calculated.

The 3-year actuarial CSS in this group was 81%, with a pelvic control rate of 96%: 5 of 28 patients were dead of para-aortic or other distant disease, one of them being the only one with local recurrence (LR) presenting a malignant vesicovaginal fistula. In 24 patients, a $D90 \geq 74\ Gy_{\alpha/\beta 10}$ was achieved. The only patient with LR had a *D*90 of 63.8 $Gy_{\alpha/\beta 10}$. Seventeen patients had satisfactory OAR doses using the standard loading pattern. Seven patients needed modifications to reduce the risk of toxicity, whereas two had modifications to improve the tumor dose. Comparison with a previous cohort of patients treated with chemoradiotherapy and a conventionally planned low dose rate triple source brachytherapy technique showed an improvement in local pelvic control of 20% ($p = 0.04$).

University of Pittsburgh Cancer Institute Experience

A small series of 16 patients treated with interstitial CT-guided brachytherapy and a median follow-up of 25 months is available from the University of Pittsburgh Cancer Institute, Pittsburgh, USA [2]. These patients were treated between 1998 and 2004 due to unsuitability for ICBT because of distorted anatomy or extensive vaginal disease. There were 11 patients with carcinoma of the cervix FIGO stage IIA (1), IIB (3), IIIA (1), IIIB (5), and IVA (1), and 5 patients with vaginal cancer (FIGO stage II (4) and IVA (1)). Median pretreatment tumor size was 6.5 cm. All patients received whole pelvis EBRT followed by interstitial implantation. The median whole pelvis external beam dose was 45 Gy (range,

39.6–50.4 Gy) with 11 patients receiving parametrial boost to a median dose of 9 Gy. Of these patients, 12 (75%) received concurrent cisplatin-based chemotherapy during EBRT. All patients received a single HDR BT procedure performed in the operating room under general anesthesia using a modified Syede-Neblett template (a total of 5 fractions of 3.5 Gy each at at least 6-h interval). A CT scan was performed postimplant for needle placement verification and treatment planning purposes. The clinical target volume was contoured based on radiographic and clinical examination. Nucletron PLATO Brachytherapy Planning Software Version 14.2 (Nucletron B.V., Veenendaal, the Netherlands) was used for treatment planning. The dose was prescribed to this clinical target volume. The acceptable value was 90% of the volume getting the prescription dose. Optimization modes (geometric and graphical) were used according to the criteria described by Erickson et al [10] and included in this book, to ensure adequate coverage of the target volume and to constrain the dose to nearby critical structures, bladder, and rectum. In contrast to what the authors describe, the dose is here given as EQD2 (see introduction [20]). Dose as re-calculated according to the reported physical data to the target volume ranged from 64- to 73-Gy EQD2 with a median of 68 Gy, which represented the majority of patients (62.5%). Median cumulative doses for the rectum and bladder were 60- and 58-Gy EQD2, respectively. Complete response was achieved in 13 of 16 (81%) patients and 3 patients had persistent disease (none could be salvaged). Out of 13 patients with complete response, 5 developed recurrent disease (distant in 4 and combined local and distant in 1) at a median time of 14 months (6–48 months). The 5-year local control and cause-specific survival were 75% and 64%, respectively. In subset analysis, the 5-year actuarial local control was 63% for cervical cancer patients and 100% for vaginal cancer patients. No patient had treatment-related acute grade 3 or 4 complications. No patient had acute grade 3 or 4 morbidity. Grade 3 or 4 delayed morbidity resulting from treatment occurred in 1 patient with a 5-year actuarial rate of 7%. Three patients had late grade 2 rectal morbidity and one patient had grade 2 small bowel morbidity.

Preliminary Results of the STIC 2004

Preliminary results were recently reported from the French trial: STIC 2004 [4]; 2D versus 3D planning are compared in three different treatment groups according to their clinical stage: (1) preoperative brachytherapy (BT), (2) pre-operative EBRT plus BT, and (3) definitive EBRT plus BT. In both 2D and 3D arms, doses to point A, ICRU bladder, and rectal points were defined. In the 3D group, dose-volume histograms (DVH) were determined for the HR CTV, IR CTV, bladder, and rectum and sigmoid. By August 2008, 708 patients were available for preliminary analysis and results were reported in abstract form. In the 3D arm, the dose delivered to volumes was as shown for group 1, 2, 3, respectively: HR CTV D90: 74.4 $EQD2Gy_{10}$, 63.4 $EQD2Gy_{10}$, 75.1 $EQD2Gy_{10}$; IR CTV D90: 57.3 $EQD2Gy_{10}$, 55 $EQD2Gy_{10}$, 63.8 $EQD2Gy_{10}$.

With a median follow-up of 17 months, local control was lower in the 2D versus 3D arm in group 1 ($p = 0.04$) and 2 ($p = 0.05$). Higher doses were delivered in the 3D arm, mainly in group 3 (definitive radiotherapy). Local control seems to be higher in 3D arm in this interim analysis. Severe digestive complications rate was comparable between 2D and 3D arms, but urinary toxicity was lower in the 3D arm for group 1 and 3. Definitive results are still pending publication.

US-Guided Brachytherapy

Peter MacCallum Cancer Centre Experience

A report on outcome data on US-guided brachytherapy for cervical cancer has been recently published [24]. Data on 127 patients who were treated in Peter MacCallum Cancer Centre, between January 1999 and May 2006, with curative intent was analyzed. These patients were treated by EBRT 40 Gy in 20 fractions to pelvis and a small boost of 6–10 Gy to involved nodes, and conformal high dose rate (HDRc) ICBT 5 fractions of 6 Gy each. These data were compared to 90 patients treated with LDR brachytherapy planning and treatment which was performed using conventional orthogonal film-based planning and standard Manchester–based loading pattern; therefore these patients are excluded from our current analysis. All patients had pretreatment MRI and fluorodeoxyglucose positron emission tomography (FDG-PET) scan for nodal staging. MRI and PET information were not used to change clinical FIGO staging. There were 41, 20, 42, 1, 22, and 1 FIGO stage IB, IIA, IIB, IIIA, IIIB, and IVA, respectively. Eighty-five percent of patients had Squamous Cell Carcinom (SCC) histology. The median tumor diameter was 4.5 cm and the median tumor volume was 35.3 cc. Nodal disease was identified in 48% and was used to guide EBRT fields. Patients without nodal metastasis and those with metastatic nodes confined to the pelvis were treated with pelvic radiotherapy using concurrent weekly cisplatin 40 mg/m^2 for four doses only. The patients with upper common iliac or para-aortic nodes were treated with four-field extended field radiotherapy (EFRT). Involved nodes received small anteroposterior–posteroanterior (AP–PA) rectangular boosts of 6–10 Gy in 2-Gy fractions in between the ICBT which was given always at the completion of EBRT. ICRT consisted of 30 Gy in 5 fractions or 28 Gy in 4 fractions, given twice weekly. Mostly, standard CT/MRI compatible, Nucletron (Veenendaal, the Netherlands) tandem and ovoids were used. Occasionally, if gross tumor was present in the middle or lower vagina at the time of ICBT then a tandem and vaginal cylinder were used. At the first treatment, the applicator was inserted under transabdominal US guidance. Brachytherapy target was mapped by vertical measurements from tandem to the surface of the tumor containing cervix and the body of uterus and recorded on a graph paper. This defined the target volume in the sagittal plane. A plan using the given tandem and ovoid combination was retrieved from the planning computer library. The displayed isodose distribution was adjusted to conform to the US-derived target measurements. Intent was to treat residual disease, cervix, and uterus (as defined by US) to a total dose of 80 Gy_{10}, including the EBRT radiation dose. Individual HDRc fractions were calculated using a table described by Nag and Gupta [22] which is in accordance with what it is used for this book chapter [19]. First treatment was then given, based on the US conformal treatment plan. Following treatment, the patient was sent to the MRI suite for a planning MRI with applicators in situ. Following the MRI the applicator was removed and the patient was sent home. Planning MRI images were imported into the treatment planning system (Plato, Nucletron) and the treatment plan isodose pattern used in the first treatment was assessed and the sagittal plane superimposed over MRI images and, if required, isodose was adjusted. Subsequent treatments were given using the MRI adjusted treatment plan. Transabdominal US was always used to reproduce the positioning of the tandem within the uterus and the position of the uterus in relation to bladder balloon and the bony sacrum. Radiation dose at the target surface (prescription dose) and point A doses were recorded in 2-Gy equivalent doses using early tumor response α/β_{10} and ICRU bladder and rectal point doses were recorded using late tissue response α/β_3.

All follow-up data was prospectively collected at the time of patient's routine appointments.

The 5-year OS rate was 60% (SE = 4%). The 5-year RFS rate was 67% (SE = 3%). There were 13, 18, 25, and 30 failures at primary, pelvis, para-aortic (nodal), and distant, respectively. The patients were further divided into two groups using the median point A dose as a divider. Patients who received <72.8 Gy_{10} EQD2 to point A (group 1) had smaller brachytherapy target than those who received >72.8 Gy_{10} to point A (group 2). Doses at ICRU rectal and bladder points were 54 Gy and 56 Gy (44–80), respectively. Thirty-four patients failed. Sites of failure were local (cervix and/or uterus) (13), pelvic (18), abdominal (nodal) (25), and distant sites (30). Most patients failed at multiple sites at first failure.

Sixty-eight percent (87/127) of patients treated by HDRc remained free from only bowel and bladder symptoms following treatment. Only two patients developed grade 3 and 4 bladder and bowel toxicity. No grade 3 or 4 rectal toxicity was observed.

25.2.1.2 Limited Stage Cervical Cancer (IA, IB, IIA) Treated with EBRT ± Chemotherapy and IGBT (± Surgery)

Twenty patients with stage IA, IB, IIA in Vienna were treated with definitive (chemo)-radiation including MRI-guided BT. In Paris, 16 patients diagnosed with these stages underwent the same treatment, however a major part of these undergoing also limited surgery (extrafascial hysterectomy). Of these patients, none had LR, one from Vienna had a pelvic recurrence in the Lymph Nodes (LN), and a total of five had distant recurrence.

Of the 28 patients treated at Addenbrooke's with CT-guided BT [30], 12 were actually limited stage (7 IB1, 3 IB2, 2 IIA), none of these experiencing LR. One patient with stage 1B2 developed distant metastasis.

Based on this limited experience for this patient population we may conclude that by using 3D image-guided brachytherapy we are able to achieve a local control rate of 100%.

The outcome data on US-guided brachytherapy for cervical cancer [24] included data on 61 stage IB, IIA patients treated with HDRc which were compared to 42 patients treated with LDR, 2D BT. The 5-year overall local failure was similar, 12% and 14% in the two groups. However, there is no information available in regard to stage-related local control.

In a large population cohort of 2,997 patients from MD Anderson Hospital in Houston with stage I–II SCC of the cervix (including 709 stage IIB) treated with 2D conformal RT, 245 patients had a central recurrence, the majority within the first 3 years of follow-up. The actuarial risks of central recurrence in this population were 6.8%, 7.8%, 8.8%, 9.6%, and 10.9% at 5, 10, 15, 20, and 25 years, respectively [9].

25.2.1.3 Correlation of DVH Parameters and Local Control

There is a large variation of dose-volume parameters in regard to dose in the CTV, which applies for both HR CTV and IR CTV (Table 25.2) [3,26]. This is also striking in regard to dose variation between limited and advanced disease [21]. The 2D tradition of prescription (e.g., point A and the Institute Gustave Roussy (IGR) volume approach) has resulted in very high doses for limited disease (e.g., D90 > 90 Gy for HR CTV) and rather low doses for advanced disease (e.g., D90 < 75 Gy for HR CTV). This paradox is putting the classical paradigm for radiotherapy prescription upside down: the larger the tumor, the more the radiation dose is needed for ultimate complete cell kill in order to achieve local control. This paradox of 2D cervix cancer radiotherapy can only be explained by the fact that until now 3D image-based dose prescription for the 3D target has been mainly performed following the respective 2D tradition with dose prescription in a particular center.

Little clinical evidence has been provided thus far about a correlation between certain dose-volume parameters for the target and disease outcome, which is primarily central and true pelvis control and secondly any parameters related to non–true pelvis survival. This can be understood by the small amount of clinical data provided thus far for disease outcome within the 3D image-based framework. There is furthermore no clear terminology which correlates dose-volume parameters to local outcome. The classical clinical terms for local outcome assessment in the 2D era have been true pelvis recurrence and/or central and lateral pelvic recurrence [9], whereas for pelvic recurrence nodal disease is usually included. Central recurrence was defined clearly in regard to the central pelvic structures which are the uterus, the adjacent proximal parametria, and the vagina. Lateral pelvic recurrence is not clearly defined as this may involve distal parametrial or pelvic sidewall tumor recurrence as well as lymph node recurrence [26]. In a recent article discussing clinical outcome in the 3D framework, these outcome parameters are evaluated in regard to the 3D topography and the 3D dose distribution, and suggestions for appropriate assessment are put forward [7].

Altogether, looking at the few different series providing clinical disease outcome data, as summarized in the preceding paragraphs, it has to be stated that a large variation of doses has been reported for HR CTV and IR CTV together with a low rate of LR (~10%) after a mean observation period of 2–3 years. However, the clinical conditions at present seem to be rather heterogenous. This low incidence of true pelvis recurrence is in agreement with reports from a recent workshop of the Gyn GEC ESTRO network (Leuven 03/2009), where similar findings were reported for six more centers (on approximately 200 patients) that had not published their results thus far: Aarhus, Leuven, Tata Memorial, Utrecht in addition to a selected group from Vienna. There is evaluation work under development (RetroEMBRACE) which aims to systematically assess the outcome in patients treated with image-guided (MRI/CT) brachytherapy until data of the EMBRACE study matures (applying the same parameters evaluated by this inquiry).

In the following paragraphs, the focus is on presenting the largest series provided thus far and the reported correlation between dose-volume parameters and disease outcome from Vienna.

A significant dependence of local control was found using the dose-volume histogram parameters D100 and D90 in the HR CTV for cervix cancer [8]. This analysis was done on the 141 patients from Vienna (stages IB-IVA) treated with 45–50.4 Gy EBRT ± cisplatin plus 4 × 7 Gy IGBT as described in the paragraph on the Vienna results [26]. Gross tumor volume (GTV), HR CTV, and IR CTV) were delineated and DVH parameters (D90, D100) were assessed. Doses were converted to the equivalent dose in 2 Gy (EQD2) according to the LQ model using $\alpha/\beta = 10$ Gy. Results of DVH analysis were presented for the total patient population, the subgroups of patients treated within the two study periods (learning: 1998–2000, application: 2001–2003) and the patients ± LRs. In a further analysis the patients were stratified into four groups according to the maximum diameter of the GTV at diagnosis (GTVD) and of the HR CTV at time of brachytherapy:

(1) Tumors 2–5 cm at diagnosis (2–5 cmDIAG); (2) Tumors > 5 cm at diagnosis (>5 cmDIAG) divided as follows: (2a) Tumors > 5 cm at diagnosis and HR CTV 2–5 cm at time of brachytherapy (>5 cmDIAG 2–5 cmBT) and (2b) Tumors > 5 cm at diagnosis and HR CTV > 5 cm at time of brachytherapy (>5 cmDIAG >5 cmBT). Eighteen LRs in the true pelvis were observed. The mean D90 and D100 for HR CTV were 86 ± 16 Gy and 65 ± 10 Gy, respectively. D90 for HR CTV of >87 Gy resulted in an LR incidence of 4% (3/68) compared with 20% (15/73) for D90 < 87 Gy. The effect was most pronounced in the group of patients with poor response **(2b)**. This analysis demonstrated an increase for local control in IGBT of cervical cancer with the dose delivered, which can be expressed by the D90 and D100 for HR CTV. Local control rates of >95% can be achieved if the D90 (EQD2) for HR CTV is ≥87 Gy. No effect was assessable for limited disease.

A further detailed analysis of dose effects was performed on the same patient population (including the subgroup division as above). LR was used as the quantal endpoint. Dose-response dependence for LR in the true pelvis was evaluated by logit analysis [8]. This revealed EDxx values, i.e., doses at which a response is expected in xx% of the patients treated, and their confidence intervals (SAS institute). Also, *p*-values for the effect of dose on the recurrence rate were calculated, based on the slope of the probit regression line. A *p*-value <0.05 was considered statistically significant (Fig. 25.1).

The γ-value represents the normalized dose-response gradient [1], which is a measure of the steepness of the dose-response curves, describing the increase in response in percentage points for a 1% increase in dose (at the level of ED50).

For the total patient population, a statistically significant effect of dose on local control was found only for the D90 and D100 for the HR CTV ($p = 0.005/0.02$), and a statistical trend for the D90 of the IR CTV ($p = 0.08$).

For small tumors, no statistically significant dependence of local control rates on any of the DVH parameters was found. In contrast, for large tumors, D90 as well as D100 for IR CTV and HR CTV were significantly correlated with LR rates. The latter was – at least for the HR CTV – dominated by the dose response of the tumor subgroup without a major volume response during EBRT.

The ED50-values for tumor control were 33 ± 15 Gy (D100) and 45 ± 19 Gy (D90). ED90-values were 86 Gy for D90 HR CTV and 67 Gy for D100 HR CTV, respectively. Tumor control rates of >90% can be expected at doses >67 Gy for HR CTV D100 and of 86 Gy for HR CTV D90.

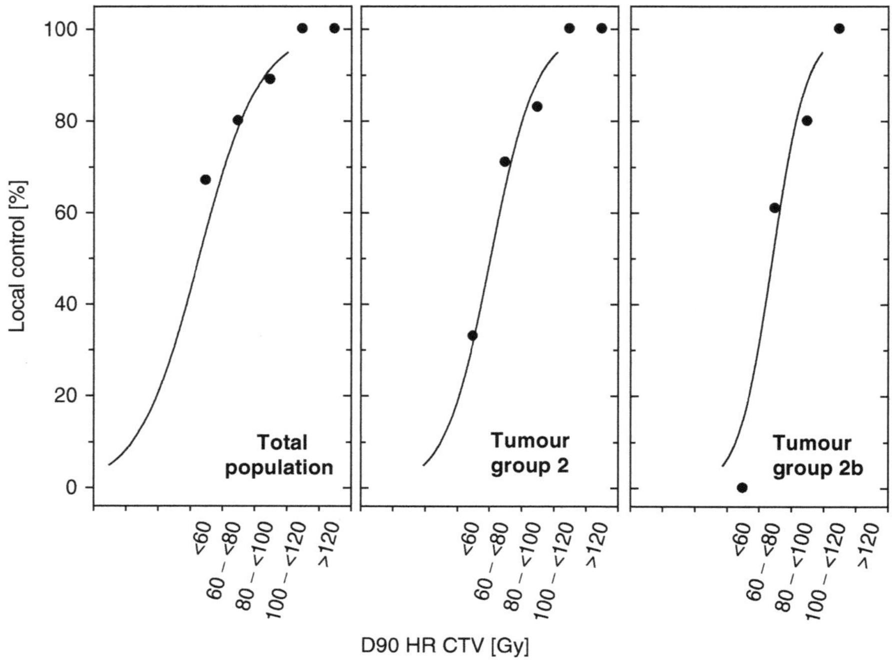

Fig. 25.1 Dose effect curves [8] depicting local control in the entire population, in tumors >5cm (tumor group 2) and for large non-responding tumors (tumor group 2b). Adapted from Dimopoulos et al [8]

25.2.1.4 Early Stage Cervical Treated by Preoperative MRI-Guided BT and Surgery

The Institut Gustave Roussy, Villejuif, France, Experience

Although the role of MRI-guided BT combined with external beam radiochemotherapy in locally advanced cervical cancer is clearly established, the place of radiotherapy in limited stage cancer in combination with surgery is not fully clarified. Preoperative intracavitary uterovaginal BT in patients with limited stage cervical carcinoma has been in use in some centers since long [11,12].

Very recently, data on outcome of MRI-guided BT in the preoperative setting was published [15]. Thirty-nine patients with primary early cervical carcinoma (stage distribution not published) were treated with preoperative MRI-based LDR BT, consisting of utero-vaginal BT to a total dose of 60 Gy to the IR CTV, followed 6 weeks later by bilateral salpingo-oophorectomy and extrafascial hysterectomy plus pelvic node dissection. Adjuvant chemoradiation was delivered to patients with pelvic lymph node involvement.

With a median follow-up of 4.4 years (range, 2.6–6.6 years), there was no central recurrence; one LR occurred in the lateral pelvis (2.6%). The 4-year actuarial OS and disease-free survival were 94% (95%CI, 82–98) and 86% (95%CI, 67–95), respectively. The 2- and 4-year actuarial local relapse-free survival were 94 (95%CI, 86–100) and 91% (95%CI, 81–100), respectively. For central recurrence, this is not given by the authors, but it would be 100%.

For IR CTV (CTV for dose prescription), median D100 and D90 were respectively 43 Gy EQD2 and 75 Gy EQD2. For HR CTV, the median D100 and D90 were 69 Gy EQD2 (range, 24–137) and 109 Gy EQD2 (range, 37–198), respectively. These doses seem to be significantly higher compared to doses as applied for more advanced disease (see preceding paragraph).

Twenty grade 1–2 late complications were observed in 13 patients (33%): 10 urinary bladder, 3 ureteral, 1 rectal, 1 small bowel, 1 vaginal, 1 pelvic fibrosis, 1 peripheral nerve, and 2 others. No grade 3 or 4 complication occurred. This small series shows that MRI-guided brachytherapy following the traditional adaptation of time duration and/or the length of each radioactive source as having been practiced at IGR since long allows for both, almost 100% local control and a low toxicity in the combined radiosurgical treatment of early stage cervical cancer.

It has to be taken into account that these results are not superior to those achieved with definitive radiotherapy including external beam and IGBT (see preceding paragraph).

One of the arms of the recently published STIC 2004 trial [4] included patients treated with preoperative BT comparing 2D planning and 3D planning. A second arm included preoperative EBRT and BT comparing the same two modalities of planning. Demographic data is not yet available on these patients. Doses delivered to HR CTV in these two groups achieved mean levels of D90: 74.4 EQD2Gy10 and 63.4 EQD2Gy10, respectively. Local control was lower in the 2D arm. Severe G3 urinary toxicities were lower in the 3D arm in the first group, but not in the second group.

25.3 Vaginal Cancer

One of the most important therapeutic goals for locally advanced vaginal cancer is local control. The local failure rates reported in the literature for FIGO stage II–IVA usually range between 20% and 60%, even in recent series.

25.3.1 MRI-Guided Brachytherapy, Vienna Preliminary Data

A pilot study was designed in Vienna, based on the experience with cervical cancer and along the traditional LDR and HDR experience with vaginal cancer, in order to investigate the clinical feasibility and to report about the first treatment outcomes of MRI IGBT in vaginal cancer patients [6]. Out of 40 patients with locally advanced vaginal cancer treated between 1999 and 2006, 13 received IGBT based on a prospective protocol and met the inclusion criteria for this study. FIGO stage distribution was as follows: stage II = 4, stage III = 5, stage IV = 4. Five patients had positive pelvic lymph nodes and in seven patients, tumor size was >5 cm. All patients received external beam irradiation (40–50 Gy) and 11 patients received concomitant chemotherapy (9 patients – cisplatin; and 2 patients – 5-FU and mitomycin C). IGBT dose prescription was either 4 × 7 Gy (HDR) or 35–40 Gy PDR with 0.5–0.8 Gy per pulse to the HR CTV, adding to a total dose of 75–85 Gy EQD2. In ten cases a combined intravaginal/interstitial application technique was used. Following the recent developments in the treatment of cervical cancer patients with IGBT (Gyn GEC ESTRO Recommendations I and II), systematic concepts for assessment of HR CTV and OARs, for biological modeling, and for dose-volume-histogram analysis were applied for these patients with vaginal cancer. Dose-volume-adaptation (D90, D_{2cc}) and dose escalation, respectively, were integrated into the treatment (planning) of all these patients. Doses were converted to the equivalent dose in 2 Gy per fraction (EQD2) applying the LQ model (α/β of 10 for tumor and 3 for OARs). Clinical results were calculated using the Kaplan–Meier method. In this group, the spatial relations between the vaginal cylinder +/− needle applicators, HR CTV, and OARs were clearly visible on MRI in all cases. The mean D90 for the HR CTV was 86 Gy EQD2 (1SD ± 13 Gy). For OARs the following mean D_{2cc} were documented (all EQD2): 80 Gy (1SD ± 20 Gy) for the bladder, 76 Gy (1SD ± 16 Gy) for the urethra, 70 Gy (1SD ± 9 Gy) for the rectum, and 60 Gy (1SD ± 9 Gy) for the sigmoid colon.

All patients achieved complete remission at 3 months. Median follow-up was 43 months (range, 19–87 months). A total of three recurrences were documented: one LR in a patient with FIGO stage III and two distant metastases. All these patients had positive pelvic lymph nodes. The actuarial local control rate at 3 years was 92%. The actuarial OS and actuarial CSS at 3 years were 85%. For the FIGO stages II, III, and IV they were 100%, 80% and 75%, respectively.

Two patients experienced fistula (one vesicovaginal, one rectovaginal) caused by tumor necrosis in stage IVA disease involving the urinary bladder and rectum, respectively. In one patient with involvement of the distal vagina, complete obliteration of the organ was observed.

The dosimetric and clinical results of this first clinical experience with IGBT for locally advanced vaginal cancer are promising. Local control and survival in this small patient population seem to be significantly higher than in previous reports with conventional X-ray–based brachytherapy, associated at the same time with acceptable morbidity. However, further prospective multicenter studies with more patients are needed to confirm these results.

25.4 Endometrial Cancer

Definitive brachytherapy treatment for endometrial cancer has been not infrequent in the past [18,29]; however, due to major progress in anesthesia and less invasive surgery, it is nowadays reserved for a limited number of patients with very major comorbidities that preclude them definitely from undergoing surgery. There is some amount of clinical data on the outcome of definitive radiation treatment for endometrial cancer, mainly brachytherapy, which has shown good results in the majority of patients treated in large series [25] with local control rates between 60% and 80%. IGBT with sufficient follow-up for this particular group of patients has been described previously [35].

25.4.1 MRI-Guided Brachytherapy, the Vienna Experience

Data on 16 patients are presented in this study with 14 newly diagnosed locally confined endometrial carcinoma [35]. These patients were treated between 1997 and 2001 and had a median follow-up of 47 months. Work-up included CT, MRI, US, and hysteroscopy, as appropriate. Heyman packing was performed with a mean of 11 Norman-Simon applicators. Three-dimensional treatment planning based on CT in 29 applications or MRI in 18 applications was done in all patients with contouring of GTV, CTV, and OARs. Dose-volume adaptation was achieved by dwell location and dwell time variation. Twelve patients treated with curative intent received 5–7 fractions of HDR brachytherapy (7 Gy per fraction) corresponding to a total dose of mean 60 Gy EQD2 (2 Gy per fraction and α/β ratio 10 Gy) to the CTV, which was chosen to be the whole uterus. Four patients had additional EBRT (range, 10–40 Gy). One patient had salvage brachytherapy and three patients were treated with palliative intent.

A dose-volume-histogram analysis was performed in all patients. On average, 68% of the CTV and 92% of the GTV were encompassed by the 60 Gy EQD2 reference volume. After a D90 > 68 Gy EQD2 in the GTV no patient recurred.

All patients treated with curative intent had complete remission (12/12). Five patients were alive without tumor at the time of analysis. Seven patients died without tumor from intercurrent disease after a median of 22 months. The patient with salvage treatment had a second LR after 27 months and died of endometrial carcinoma after 57 months. In patients treated with palliative intent, symptom relief was achieved. No severe acute and late side effects (grade 3/4) were observed.

25.5 Concluding Remarks

The clinical impact of IGABT in gynecological malignancies in general and locally advanced cervical cancer in particular is increasingly demonstrated by the establishment of this advanced treatment approach in a growing number of centers in Europe, the USA, Canada, and worldwide. Clinical evidence is gradually showing that this advanced radiotherapy approach results in excellent treatment results, approaching 100% local control in limited disease, >90% in stage IIB, and 80–90% in stage IIIB. First correlations have been reported between target-related DVH parameters and true pelvis control, in particular for far advanced disease not responding well to EBRT +/− chemotherapy.

Similarly, favorable treatment results can be expected for image-guided approaches for vaginal cancer, for vaginal recurrent disease after primary surgery, and for inoperable endometrium cancer.

These favorable results seem to be reproducible under different conditions at various treatment centers worldwide and are now prospectively evaluated in a large-scale prospective international multicenter study in cervical cancer (IntErnational study on MRI-guided BRAchytherapy in locally advanced CErvical cancer [EMBRACE]).

References

1. Bentzen SM. Randomized controlled trials in health technology assessment: overkill or overdue? Radiother Oncol. 2008;86(2):142–7.
2. Beriwal S, Gan GN, et al. Early clinical outcome with concurrent chemotherapy and extended-field, intensity-modulated radiotherapy for cervical cancer. Int J Radiat Oncol Biol Phys. 2007;68(1):166–71.
3. Chargari C, Magne N, et al. Physics contributions and clinical outcome with 3D-MRI-based pulsed-dose-rate intracavitary brachytherapy in cervical cancer patients. Int J Radiat Oncol Biol Phys. 2008;74:133–9.
4. Charra-Brunaud C. Preliminary results of a French prospective multicentric study of 3D pulsed dose-rate brachytherapy for cervix carcinoma. Cancer Radiothér. 2008; 12(6–7):527–31.
5. Cozzi L, Dinshaw KA, et al. A treatment planning study comparing volumetric arc modulation with RapidArc and fixed field IMRT for cervix uteri radiotherapy. Radiother Oncol. 2008;89(2):180–91.
6. DeBrabandere M et al. Potential of dose optimisation in MRI based PDR brachytherapy of cervix carcinoma. Radiother Oncol. 2008;88(2):217–26.
7. Dimopoulos J, Schmid M Treatment of locally advanced vaginal cancer with radio-chemotherapy and MRI-guided brachytherapy: clinical feasibility and first results Brachytherapy. 2009;
8. Dimopoulos J, Lang S, et al. Dose-volume histogram parameters and local tumor control in MR image-guided cervical cancer brachytherapy. Int J Radiat Oncol Biol Phys. 2009; 75(1):56–63.
9. Dimopoulos J, Lang S, et al. Dose-effect relationship for local control of cervical cancer by magnetic resonance image-guided brachytherapy. Radiother Oncol. 2009;93(2):311–5.
10. Eifel PJ, Jhingran A, et al. Time course and outcome of central recurrence after radiation therapy for carcinoma of the cervix. Int J Gynecol Cancer. 2006;16(3):1106–11.
11. Erickson B, Albano K, et al. CT-guided interstitial implantation of gynecologic malignancies. Int J Radiat Oncol Biol Phys. 1996;36(3):699–709.
12. Georg P et al. Correlation of dose-volume parameters, endoscopic and clinical rectal side effects in cervix cancer patients treated with definitive radiotherapy including MRI-based brachytherapy. Radiother Oncol. 2009;91(2):173–80.
13. Gerbaulet A, Potter R, et al. Cervix cancer. In: Gerbaulet A, editor. GEC ESTRO handbook of brachytherapy. Brussels: ESTRO; 2002. p. 301–63.
14. Gerbaulet A, Pötter R, et al. The GEC ESTRO handbook of brachytherapy. Brussels: ESTRO; 2002.
15. Gerstner N, Wachter S, et al. The benefit of Beam's eye view based 3D treatment planning for cervical cancer. Radiother Oncol. 1999;51(1):71–8.
16. Grigsby PW. Role of PET in gynecologic malignancy. Curr Opin Oncol. 2009;21(5):420–4.
17. Haie-Meder C. DVH parameters and outcome for patients with early-stage cervical cancer treated with preoperative MRI-based low dose rate brachytherapy followed by surgery. Radiother Oncol. 2009;93(2):316–21.

18. Haie-Meder C, Potter R, et al. Recommendations from Gynaecological (GYN) GEC-ESTRO Working Group (I): concepts and terms in 3D image based 3D treatment planning in cervix cancer brachytherapy with emphasis on MRI assessment of GTV and CTV. Radiother Oncol. 2005;74(3):235–45.
19. Kirisits C, Potter R, et al. Dose and volume parameters for MRI-based treatment planning in intracavitary brachytherapy for cervical cancer. Int J Radiat Oncol Biol Phys. 2005; 62(3):901–11.
20. Knocke TH. Primary treatment of endometrial carcinoma with high-dose-rate brachytherapy: results of 12 years of experience with 280 patients. Int J Radiat Oncol Biol Phys. 1997; 37(2):359–65.
21. Lang S, Kirisits C, et al. Treatment planning for MRI assisted brachytherapy of gynecologic malignancies based on total dose constraints. Int J Radiat Oncol Biol Phys. 2007; 69(2):619–27.
22. Lang S, Nulens A, et al. Intercomparison of treatment concepts for MR image assisted brachytherapy of cervical carcinoma based on GYN GEC-ESTRO recommendations. Radiother Oncol. 2006;78(2):185–93.
23. Lindegaard JC, Tanderup K, et al. MRI-guided 3D optimization significantly improves DVH parameters of pulsed-dose-rate brachytherapy in locally advanced cervical cancer. Int J Radiat Oncol Biol Phys. 2008;71(3):756–64.
24. Nag S, Erickson B, et al. The American Brachytherapy Society recommendations for high-dose-rate brachytherapy for carcinoma of the cervix. Int J Radiat Oncol Biol Phys. 2000;48(1):201–11.
25. Narayan K, Fisher R. Patterns of failure and prognostic factor analyses in locally advanced cervical cancer patients staged by positron emission tomography and treated with curative intent. Int J Gynecol Cancer. 2009;19(5):912–8.
26. Narayan K, van Dyk S. Comparative study of LDR (mancester system) and HDR image-guided conformal brachytherapy of cervical cancer: patterns of failure, late complications and survival. Int J Radiat Oncol Biol Phys. 2009;74(5):1529–35.
27. Potter R. Modern imaging in brachytherapy. In: Gerbaulet A, Potter R, Mazeron JJ, Meertens H, Van LE. The GEC ESTRO handbook of brachytherapy. 2002; p. 123–151.
28. Potter R, Dimopoulos J, et al. Clinical impact of MRI assisted dose volume adaptation and dose escalation in brachytherapy of locally advanced cervix cancer. Radiother Oncol. 2007;83(2):148–55.
29. Potter R, Haie-Meder C, et al. Recommendations from gynaecological (GYN) GEC ESTRO working group (II): concepts and terms in 3D image-based treatment planning in cervix cancer brachytherapy-3D dose volume parameters and aspects of 3D image-based anatomy, radiation physics, radiobiology. Radiother Oncol. 2006;78(1):67–77.
30. Potter R, Kirisits C, et al. Present status and future of high-precision image-guided adaptive brachytherapy for cervix carcinoma. Acta Oncol. 2008;47(7):1325–36.
31. Potter R, Knocke TH, et al. Definitive radiotherapy based on HDR brachytherapy with iridium 192 in uterine cervix carcinoma: report on the Vienna University Hospital findings (1993-1997) compared to the preceding period in the context of ICRU 38 recommendations. Cancer Radiothér. 2000;4(2):159–72.
32. Tan LT, Coles CE, et al. Clinical impact of computed tomography-based image-guided brachytherapy for cervix cancer using the tandem-ring applicator – the Addenbrooke's experience. Clin Oncol (R Coll Radiol). 2009;21(3):175–82.
33. Van Dyk S, Narayan K, et al. Conformal brachytherapy planning for cervical cancer using transabdominal ultrasound. Int J Radiat Oncol Biol Phys. 2009;75(1):64–70.
34. Viswanathan AN, Cormack R, et al. MR-guided interstitial brachytherapy for recurrent endometrial cancer. Int J Radiat Oncol Biol Phys. 2006;66(1):91–9.

35. Viswanathan AN, Racine ML, et al. Final results of a prospective study of MR-based interstitial gynecologic brachytherapy. Brachytherapy. 2008;7(2):148.
36. Weitmann HD, Knocke TH, et al. Ultrasound-guided interstitial brachytherapy in the treatment of advanced vaginal recurrences from cervical and endometrial carcinoma. Strahlenther Onkol. 2006;182(2):86–95.
37. Weitmann HD, Potter R, et al. Pilot study in the treatment of endometrial carcinoma with 3D image-based high-dose-rate brachytherapy using modified Heyman packing: clinical experience and dose-volume histogram analysis. Int J Radiat Oncol Biol Phys. 2005;62(2):468–78.

Morbidity Related to the Use of 3D-Based External Beam Radiation and Image-Guided Brachytherapy

26

Alina Sturdza, Carey Shenfield, and Richard Pötter

Radiation-related side effects, particularly with regard to brachytherapy, are an important potential consequence of the treatment of various cancers.

To date, several publications have reported toxicity rates related to standard brachytherapy techniques for cervical cancer. For three-dimensional image-guided brachytherapy (3D IGBT), due to its relatively recent introduction into clinical practice, reports on side effects are limited. This section will focus primarily on 3D IGBT-related side effects as well as refer to standard BT-related side effects in cervical cancer.

A number of toxicity grading systems have developed over the years, including the WHO, RTOG/EORTC, LENT-SOMA, French-Italian glossary, and CTC systems [1, 2]. All of these systems incorporate toxicities resulting from the sum of the external beam radiotherapy (EBRT) and the brachytherapy dose. There is some, but not complete, overlap of the grading system, which makes comparison more difficult. The difference between these scoring systems may have consequences for the reporting of late side effects. The most recent system used in publications is the National Cancer Institute's Common Terminology Criteria for Adverse Events or CTCAE v3.0; version 4.0 was released on October 1, 2009 [1, 3]. This system enables a detailed definition of the gastrointestinal and genitourinary side effects compared to the previously existing ones. In addition, physician-based quantification of side effects may be perceived and consequently ranked differently by patients. A recent paper from Norway [4] compared physician-assessed morbidity with patient-rated symptoms more than 5 years after pelvic radiotherapy in cervical cancer survivors (CCS). The 5-year Kaplan–Meier estimates of physician-assessed Grade 3–4 intestinal, bladder, and vaginal morbidity were 15%, 13%, and 23%, respectively. The prevalence of patient-rated severe symptoms was much higher with bowel 45%, bladder 23%, and

A. Sturdza (✉) and R. Pötter
Department of Radiotherapy, General Hospital of Vienna,
Medical University of Vienna, Währinger Gürtel 18-20, 1090 Vienna, Austria
e-mail: alina.sturdza@akhwien.at

C. Shenfield
Department of Radiation Oncology, Kingston Regional Cancer Centre, Queen's University,
25 King Street West, Kingston, Ontario, K7L5P9, Edmonton, AB, Canada

A.N. Viswanathan et al. (eds.), *Gynecologic Radiation Therapy*,
DOI: 10.1007/978-3-540-68958-4_26,

vaginal discomfort among sexually active 58%. Stress incontinence, diarrhea, nausea, and sexual problems were significantly ($p < 0.001$) more prevalent when compared with a control sample from the general female population. This chapter indicates that physicians underreport patients' symptoms. In the future, it will be important to incorporate patient-reported outcomes in the evaluation of treatment-related morbidity.

26.1 3D-Conformal EBRT for Gynecological Malignancies

In the era of 3D-guided BT, most centers that have implemented IGBT deliver external beam radiation therapy (EBRT) using 3D-conformal techniques. The issue of organ at risk (OAR) sparing by way of intensity-modulated radiotherapy (IMRT) to the pelvis is controversial. Moreover, differentiating chemotherapy-related side effects from radiation-related side effects may be challenging.

With IGBT, there is a trend toward decreasing dose to OARs and subsequently radiation-related late side effects. Nevertheless, existing data must mature in order to reach definitive conclusions. The literature on the side effects of 3D-conformal EBRT combined with 3D IGBT is very limited. We will address both acute and late radiation effects, with a greater focus on late morbidity. Key OARs include the rectum, bladder, sigmoid colon, vagina, and small bowel.

26.1.1 3D Conformal/IMRT to the Pelvis

One of the earliest randomized control trial (RCT) comparing conformal versus conventional treatment of the pelvis was carried out at Royal Marsden NHS Trust and Institute of Cancer Research [5]. Although this study did not include cervical cancer patients it randomized 266 patients that required EBRT to pelvis (mainly for bladder and prostate cancer). The primary end point was the quantification of acute side effects in both arms according to patients' appreciation (self-reported questionnaires). Although substantial differences in normal tissue volumes (rectum, bladder) were achieved, the median high-dose volume was 689 cm^3 for the conformal technique versus 792 cm^3 for the conventional technique; a very extensive analysis has not revealed any statistically significant differences between the two arms in level of symptoms, nor in medication prescribed. However, the proportions of patients experiencing symptoms with conformal treatment were consistently lower compared with those treated conventionally, 9% in perception of mild symptoms and 7% for severe symptoms.

With the advent of IMRT as technique of EBRT, it is logical to compare the outcome of this modality in terms of acute and late toxicity on the pelvis with older 3–4 field techniques. Many publications show a large reduction (50–67%) in the volume of small bowel irradiated to more than 45 Gy with IMRT when compared to the traditional 4-field box [3]. Mutic et al. [6] used IMRT to escalate the dose to 59.4 Gy to positive para-aortic lymph nodes identified by positron emission tomography (PET), and to 50.4 Gy to the para-aortic area while treating the pelvis with conventional methods. Estehappan et al. [6] described a more aggressive technique allowing dose escalation to para-aortic lymph nodes (PAN) by means of PET/CT-guided IMRT planned to deliver 60.0 Gy to the PET – positive PAN and 50.0 Gy to the PAN and pelvic lymph node bed while sparing the kidneys and small bowel. Similar results were achieved with arc IMRT in Japan [7]. While these papers address the issue of simulation, planning, and target delineation for IMRT delivery, others describe the clinical results of these sophisticated techniques; however, most of them have limited follow-up.

One of the first publications on the outcome of intensity-modulated whole pelvic radiotherapy (IM-WPRT) in women with gynecological malignancies comes from Mundt et al. [8]. Forty gynecological patients underwent customized immobilization and contrast-enhanced CT. A clinical target volume (CTV) was contoured consisting of the upper vagina, parametria, uterus (if present), and presacral and pelvic lymph node regions. The CTV was expanded by 1 cm to create a planning target volume (PTV). Using commercially available software, 7- or 9-field, 6-MV, coplanar IM-WPRT plans were generated for all the patients. The worst acute gastrointestinal and genitourinary toxicity during treatment was scored on a 4-point scale: 0, none; 1, mild, no medications required; 2, moderate, medications required; and 3, severe, treatment breaks or cessation, hospitalization. As a comparison, acute toxicities in 35 previously treated conventional WPRT patients were analyzed. No significant differences were noted in the clinicopathological and treatment factors between the two groups. IM-WPRT plans provided excellent PTV coverage, with considerable sparing of the surrounding normal tissues. On average, 98.1% of the PTV received the prescription dose. The average percentage of the PTV receiving 110% and 115% of the prescription dose was 9.8% and 0.2%, respectively. IM-WPRT was well tolerated, with no patient developing Grade 3 toxicity. Grade 2 acute gastrointestinal toxicity was less common in the IM-WPRT group (60% vs. 91%, $p = 0.002$) than in the conventional WPRT group. Moreover, the percentage of IM-WPRT and WPRT patients requiring no or only infrequent antidiarrheal medications were 75% and 34%, respectively ($p = 0.001$). Although less Grade 2 genitourinary toxicity was seen in the IM-WPRT group (10% vs. 20%), this difference was not statistically significant ($p = 0.22$). In this study IMRT planning resulted in excellent PTV coverage, with considerable sparing of normal tissues. Treatment was well tolerated and associated with less acute gastrointestinal sequelae than conventional WPRT.

In another paper, Brixey et al. [9] assessed hematological toxicities (HT) associated with concurrent chemoradiation to the pelvis and explored ways of improving clinical outcome. They compared 36 patients with gynecological malignancies that underwent whole pelvis IMRT (IM-WPRT) with 88 gynecological cancer patients treated to the same target volume and total dose (45 Gy) with a conventional 4-field technique. Significant HT was infrequent in women treated with radiotherapy (RT) alone and was comparable in the two groups. In contrast, patients treated with whole pelvis RT and chemotherapy (WPRT–CTX) experienced more Grade 2 or greater white blood count (WBC) toxicity (60% vs. 31.2%, $p = 0.08$) and developed lower median WBC (2.8 vs. 3.6 g/dL, $p = 0.05$) than did IM-WPRT–CTX patients. Moreover, CTX was held more often in the WPRT group secondary to HT (40% vs. 12.5%, $p = 0.06$). Although Grade 2 or greater absolute neutrophil count (ANC) (23.5% vs. 15.3%) and hemoglobin (Hgb) (35.2% vs. 15.2%) toxicity were lower in the IM-WPRT–CTX group, these differences did not reach statistical significance ($p = 0.58$ and 0.22, respectively). The comparison of pelvic bone marrow (PBM) dose–volume histograms (DVH) revealed that IM-WPRT planning resulted in significantly less BM volume being irradiated compared with WPRT planning, particularly within the iliac crests. This study showed that IM-WPRT has a favorable impact on the risk of acute HT in gynecological patients, particularly in those receiving CTX. The same group published [10] data from seven cervical cancer patients treated with concurrent chemotherapy and IMRT without bone marrow sparing (BMS), compared with data using 4-field and anteroposterior–posteroanterior (AP–PA) techniques. All plans were normalized to cover the PTV with the 99% isodose line. The CTV consisted of the pelvic and presacral lymph nodes, uterus and cervix, upper vagina, and parametrial tissue. Normal tissues included bowel, bladder, and PBM, which comprised the lumbosacral spine and ileum and the ischium, pubis, and proximal femora (lower PBM). DVHs for the PTV and normal tissues were compared for BMS-IMRT versus 4-field box and AP–PA plans. BMS-IMRT was superior to the 4-field technique in reducing the dose to the PBM, small bowel, rectum, and bladder. Compared with AP–PA plans, BMS-IMRT reduced the PBM volume receiving a dose >16.4 Gy. BMS-IMRT reduced the volume of ileum, lower PBM, and bowel receiving a dose >27.7 Gy, >18.7 Gy, and >21.1 Gy, respectively, but increased dose below these thresholds compared with the AP–PA plans. BMS-IMRT reduced the volume of lumbosacral spine bone marrow, rectum, small bowel, and bladder at all dose levels in all the seven patients. This small series showed that BMS-IMRT reduced irradiation of PBM compared with the 4-field box technique. Compared with the AP–PA technique, BMS-IMRT reduced lumbosacral spine bone marrow irradiation and reduced the volume of PBM irradiated to high doses. Therefore BMS-IMRT might reduce acute HT compared with conventional techniques.

In the setting of postoperative EBRT concurrent with cisplatin, Chen et al. [11] showed in 33 patients that IMRT provided similar local tumor control compared with 4F RT and significantly improved the tolerance to adjuvant chemoradiotherapy. The actuarial 1-year locoregional control for patients in the IMRT and 4F-RT groups was 93% and 94%, respectively. IMRT was well tolerated, with significant reduction in acute gastrointestinal (GI) and genitourinary (GU) toxicities compared with the 4F-RT group (GI 36 vs. 80%, $p = 0.00012$; GU 30 vs. 60%, $p = 0.022$). Furthermore, the IMRT group had lower rates of chronic GI and GU toxicities than the 4F-RT patients (GI 6 vs. 34%, $p = 0.002$; GU 9 vs. 23%, $p = 0.23$).

26.1.2 3D Conformal/IMRT to an Extended Para-Aortic Nodal Field

Prospective Phase II cooperative group trials have reported 49% Grade 3–4 acute bowel toxicity [6, 12] with the delivery of concomitant chemotherapy and extended-field radiotherapy in patients with PAN metastases. With the traditional AP–PA fields to the PAN area, generous portions of the small bowel have been included in the treatment field, causing significantly increased toxicities. As a means of reducing toxicity, IMRT has been shown to decrease the incidence of acute and late gastrointestinal toxicities as already mentioned above [13, 14].

At the University of Pittsburgh Cancer Institute extended-field IMRT (EF-IMRT) with concurrent chemotherapy for cervical cancer has been routinely performed since

January 2001. A preliminary report on the outcome data with this technique on 36 patients was published [14]. The pelvic lymph nodes were involved in 19 patients, 10 of them also having para-aortic nodal disease. The treatment volume included the cervix, uterus, parametria, presacral space, upper vagina, and pelvic, common iliac and para-aortic nodes to the superior border of L1. Patients were assessed for acute toxicities according to the NCI–CTCAE, v3.0.

All late toxicities were scored with the Radiation Therapy Oncology Group (RTOG) late toxicity score. All patients completed the prescribed course of EF-IMRT. All but two patients received brachytherapy. Median length of treatment was 53 days. The median follow-up was 18 months. Acute Grade >3 gastrointestinal, genitourinary, and myelotoxicities were seen in 1, 1, and 10 patients, respectively. Thirty-four patients had complete response to treatment. Of these 34 patients, 11 developed recurrences. The first site of recurrence was in-field in two patients (pelvis in one, pelvis and para-aortic in one) and distant in nine patients. The 2-year actuarial locoregional control, disease-free survival, overall survival, and Grade >3 toxicity rates for the entire cohort were 80%, 51%, 65%, and 10%, respectively. This study showed that EF-IMRT with concurrent chemotherapy was tolerated well, with acceptable acute and early late toxicities. The locoregional control rate was good, with distant metastases being the predominant mode of failure.

A smaller series of 13 patients with gynecological malignancies treated with EF-IMRT was published from the University of Chicago [15]. With a median follow-up of 11 months, 2 patients were found to have had experienced Grade 3 or higher toxicity. Both patients were treated with concurrent cisplatin-based chemotherapy. Neither patient was planned with BMS. Eleven patients had no evidence of late toxicity. One patient with multiple previous surgeries experienced a bowel obstruction. One patient with bilateral, grossly involved and unresectable common iliac nodes experienced bilateral lymphedema.

In conclusion of these papers, EF-IMRT is safe and effective with a low incidence of acute toxicity. Longer follow-up of these studies is needed to assess chronic toxicity, although early results are promising.

26.1.3 3D Conformal/IMRT/EBRT Boost as a Replacement for Brachytherapy

Although most studies of IMRT for patients with cervical cancer have focused on IMRT as a replacement for locoregional treatment, IMRT and other conformal methods have also been proposed as a replacement for brachytherapy; for example, as a sequential boost after external pelvic irradiation.

A recently published study from Christie Hospital, Manchester, United Kingdom, described outcome data on 44 patients with cervical cancer that could not receive BT for various reasons [16]. A total radiation dose of 54–70 Gy was delivered to these patients by way of EBRT plus a 3D conformal EBRT boost in most cases. The median follow-up was 2.3 years. Recurrent disease was seen in 48%, with a median time to recurrence of 2.3 years. Central recurrence was seen in 16 of the 21 patients with recurrent disease. The 5-year overall survival rate was 49.3%. The 3-year cancer-specific survival rate by stage was 100%, 70%, and 42% for Stages I, II, and III, respectively. Late Grades 1 and 2 bowel, bladder, and vaginal toxicity were seen in 41%. Late Grade 3 toxicity was seen in 2%. These results are inferior to those obtained by the use of IGBT [17, 18], but are comparable to standard BT results [19–21], indicating that IMRT is not an acceptable alternative to brachytherapy when feasible.

A group from Princess Margaret Hospital, Toronto, analyzed dosimetric and toxicity information on 12 patients with cervical (8), endometrial (2), or vaginal (2) cancer previously treated with external beam pelvic radiotherapy and conformal radiotherapy (CRT) boost [22]. Optimized IMRT boost treatment plans were developed for each of the 12 patients and compared to CRT and 4-field (4F) plans. The plans were compared in terms of dose conformality and critical normal tissue avoidance. The median PTV was 151 cm^3 (range, 58–512 cm^3). The median overlap of the contoured rectum with the PTV was 15% (1–56%), and 11% (4–35%) for the bladder. Two of the 12 patients, both with large PTVs and large overlaps of the contoured rectum and PTV, developed Grade 3 rectal bleeding. The dose conformity was significantly improved with IMRT over CRT and 4 field box (4FB) ($p \leq 0.001$ for both). IMRT also yielded an overall improvement in the rectal and bladder dose–volume distributions relative to CRT and 4FB. The volume of rectum that received the highest doses (>66% of the prescription) was reduced by 22% ($p < 0.001$) with IMRT relative to 4FB, and the bladder volume was reduced by 19% ($p < 0.001$). This was at the expense of an increase in the volume of these organs receiving doses in the lowest range (<33%).

In contrast to this paper which compares three different EBRT boost techniques, but no brachytherapy, a different paper looks at inversely planned EBRT with photons (IMRT) and protons (IMPT) compared to 3D magnetic resonance imaging (MRI)-guided BT [23].

Gross tumor volume, high-risk CTV (HR CTV), intermediate-risk CTV (IR CTV), bladder, rectum, and sigmoid were delineated. Magnetic resonance (MR)-guided BT planning was manually optimized with respect to organ dose limits. Margins (3 and 5 mm) were added to BT CTVs to construct PTVs for EBRT. EBRT was challenged to deliver the highest possible doses to PTVs while respecting D_{1cc} and D_{2cc} limits from BT, assuming the same fractionation (4 × 7 Gy). The D90 for target structures and normal tissue volumes receiving fractionated doses between 3 and 7 Gy were compared. This study showed that HR CTV dose depends on the clinical situation and radiation quality. If IMRT was limited to D_{2cc} and DD_{1cc} from BT, the D90 for high-risk PTV and intermediate-risk PTV was lower. Volumes receiving 60 Gy (in equivalent dose in 2-Gy fractions) were approximately twice as large for IMRT compared with BT. For IMPT, this volume ratio was lower. PTV doses of IMPT plans with 3-mm margins were comparable to those with BT. Gross tumor volume doses were mostly lower for both IMRT and IMPT. This finding led to the conclusion that for cervix cancer boost treatments, both IMRT and IMPT seem to be inferior to the advanced BT (MRI-guided BT).

In addition, when planning EBRT delivery by way of IMRT for patients receiving chemoradiation for cervical cancer, cervix regression and internal organ motion should be taken into account as they contribute to marked interfraction variations in the intrapelvic position of the cervical target as revealed by various studies [24–26]. A study from MD Anderson Cancer Center quantified this movement [27]. Mean maximum changes in the center of mass of the cervix were 2.1, 1.6, and 0.82 cm in the superior–inferior, anterior–posterior, and right–left lateral dimensions, respectively. Mean maximum changes in the perimeter of the cervix were 2.3 and 1.3 cm in the superior and inferior, 1.7 and 1.8 cm in the anterior and posterior, and 0.76 and 0.94 cm in the right and left lateral directions, respectively.

In summary, IMRT is a useful tool that is particularly beneficial in the treatment of patients with cervical cancer undergoing concurrent chemoradiation therapy, especially when EFRT is necessary. To a very limited extent, IMRT seems to be helpful in the treatment of gross disease that is not amenable to brachytherapy, especially in less experienced BT hands. However, this technology must be used wisely taking into account that the cervix undergoes dramatic and unpredictable changes in size, shape, and location during the course of treatment.

26.2 3D IGBT

The main OARs in cervix cancer brachytherapy are rectum, bladder, sigmoid, vagina, and relevant parts of the bowel loops adjacent to the target volumes. For the reporting of dose–volume parameters, the GEC ESTRO Working Group has recommended that $D_{0.1cc}$, D_{1cc}, and D_{2cc} be reported for the OAR and that D_{5cc} and D_{10cc} be reported as well if contouring of organ walls is performed [28]. Specific dose–volume constraints were not reported.

The outcome data on 3D IGBT published thus far and described in detail with regard to local control, overall survival, cause-specific survival in the first section show promising results with a small number of Grade 3–4 toxicities.

26.2.1 Institutional Experiences

26.2.1.1 Vienna Experience with MRI-Guided BT

In this group of 145 patients with a median follow-up of 40 months, adverse late side effects were prospectively assessed using the LENT SOMA score [17]. Late side effects were defined as events occurring more than 91 days after the end of treatment.

Seven patients experienced Grade 3–4 genitourinary or gastrointestinal late side effects: six in the period 1998–2000 and one bladder G3 in the period 2001–2003. Two patients underwent surgical intervention with permanent colostomies, for G4 complete obstruction of the rectosigmoid junction occurred (G4). Two patients suffered from G3 persistent rectal bleeding and required blood transfusions. Two patients developed G4 severe late adverse effects in the urinary bladder 3–4 years after treatment with a refractory cystitis and excruciating dysuria, and consequently both underwent cystectomy [29]. One patient experienced G3 incontinence with 1–2-h interval urinary frequency, which started during treatment. The actuarial 3-year morbidity rate (LENT SOMA, G3/G4) for the whole period was gastrointestinal 4% (4 events) and urinary 4% (3 events). For the initial (learning) period 1998–2000, the overall actuarial toxicity rate, including gastrointestinal and urinary events, was 10% (6 events) and for the "systematic" period 2001–2003 it was 2% (1 event). The vast majority of G1–G2 late vaginal effects were asymptomatic or when symptomatic, patients presented with dryness and atrophy of the vaginal epithelium, or partial synechiae and stenosis of the upper vagina (114 cases). Five patients experienced G3 coaptation of the vagina (G3) (three patients with Stage IIA and two patients with Stage IIIA cervical cancer).

26.2.1.2 The Institut Gustave Roussy Experience

In this group of 45 patients with a median follow-up of 26 months, adverse acute and late side effects were prospectively graded using the RTOG late radiation morbidity scoring system [18]. Of note, a hysterectomy was recommended to patients with a complete clinical and radiologic response 6–8 weeks after BT in the context of a randomized trial. Twenty-six patients underwent surgery and this should be taken into consideration when looking at the toxicity profile.

Of 23 patients, the acute Grade 1–2 complications related to CC-EBRT included diarrhea in 16, vulvitis in 15, epidermitis in 5, cystitis in 2, and vaginal epithelitis in 1 patient. Acute Grade 3 complications developed in two patients and included vulvitis in two, dermatitis in one, and vaginal epithelitis in one. All acute side effects ceased by 3 months. Late toxicity was defined as any toxicity occurring >6 months after BT completion. Of the 45 patients, 21 presented with delayed Grade 1–2 complications, including moderate pelvic fibrosis in 8, hematuria and/or incontinence in 8, dyspareunia in 5, proctitis in 2, lymphedema in 2, and perineal pain in 1 patient. Of these 21 patients, 4 had Grade 1–2 late vaginal effects (symptomatic vaginal dryness/atrophy in 2 patients). One 75–year-old patient had a Grade 3 vesicovaginal fistula. The ICRU bladder point was 74 Gy, the radiation doses delivered to 0.1, 1, and 2 cm^3 of the bladder were 109, 93, and 87 Gy, respectively. No Grade 4 or greater toxicity was observed. After surgery, the acute complication rate was 15.4% (4 of 26) and consisted of lymphocele ($n = 3$) and pelvic abscess ($n = 1$). No statistically significant increase in delayed toxicities (Grade 1–2) was observed when stratified by surgical procedure (54% vs. 50%, for hysterectomy vs. no hysterectomy, respectively).

26.2.1.3 Brigham and Women's Hospital/Dana-Farber Cancer Institute Experience

All 25 patients with varied gynecological malignancies treated at Brigham and Women's Hospital/Dana-Farber Cancer Institute, Boston, MA, United States, with real-time intraoperative MR image-guided interstitial approach experienced either a Grade 1 or 2 acute toxicity related to the radiation [30]. With a minimum of 1 year follow-up, two Grade 4 recto/sigmoid-vaginal fistulas occurred in patients with recurrent endometrial cancer and one vaginal cancer patient developed Grade 3 proctitis. Considering the advanced disease stage in these patients and the fact that 17 cases were recurrent cancers (see previous chapter on outcome [25]), it could be concluded that this approach results in limited toxicity.

26.2.1.4
Tata Memorial Experience

Of the 24 patients treated with MRI-guided HDR BT in this institution and for whom the median follow-up was 12 months (range, 4–29 months), none developed G3 toxicity to the date of the report [31].

26.2.1.5
US-Guided Brachytherapy Peter MacCallum Cancer Centre Experience

A recently published paper by the gynecological group at Peter MacCallum compares outcome data of 127 patients treated with conformal ultrasound (US)-guided HDR BT with the 1 of 90 patients treated with 2D LDR BT [32]. In this study, toxicities were scored according to modified WHO/RTOG criteria. Only three categories of toxicities consisting of bladder, small and large bowel, and vagina have been included in this study (Table 3); the median follow-up period was 5 years. The largest difference between the LDR and HDR brachytherapy was the number of asymptomatic patients in the HDR group. Sixty-eight percent (87/127) of patients treated by HDR remained asymptomatic, whereas 42% (38/90) patients were asymptomatic from the bowel and bladder symptoms after treatment with 2D LDR. Statistically significant differences could be noticed for Grade 2 bowel and vaginal complications in those who received HDR compared to LDR.

26.2.1.6
CT-Guided Brachytherapy

Recently, Tan et al. [33] reported on morbidity in the setting of CT-guided brachytherapy for Stage IB–IIIB cervix cancer in 28 patients. Their overall actuarial 3-year serious late morbidity rate was 14%, as 3 patients were affected, 2 with Grade 3 abdominal pain and 1 with a colovaginal fistula. There were 3 (11%) patients with Grade 3 or 4 complications in the study group, resulting in a 3-year actuarial risk of serious late morbidity of 14%. Two patients had Grade 3 abdominal pain, but in both patients, pain was graded as 3 on only one assessment. In one patient, her pain resolved after 6 months and she has no permanent toxicity. In the other patient, her pain also resolved but she has residual Grade 2 diarrhea. The third patient developed a radiation-induced colovaginal fistula; however, this patient is unusual as she was the only patient who did not receive chemotherapy, suggesting that an underlying biologic sensitivity may predispose her to severe complications.

26.2.2
Preliminary Results of the STIC 2004

In recently reported preliminary results from the French STIC 2004 trial [34] comparing 2D vs. 3D planning, three different treatment groups were included according to their clinical stage: (1) preoperative brachytherapy (BT), (2) preoperative external beam radiation therapy (EBRT) plus BT, and (3) definitive EBRT plus BT. In both 2D and 3D arms, dose to point A, ICRU bladder and rectal points were defined. In the 3D group, DVH were determined for the HR CTV, IR CTV, bladder, rectum, and sigmoid. Toxicities were assessed using the CTCAE, v3.0 scale. By August 2008, 708 patients were available for preliminary analysis and results were reported. In the 3D arm, the dose delivered to volumes were as shown for group 1, 2, 3 respectively: bladder D_{2cc}: 69.5 $EQD2Gy_3$, 60.2 $EQD2Gy_3$, 72.3 $EQD2Gy_3$; rectum D_{2cc}: 34.1 $EQD2Gy_3$, 54.1 $EQD2Gy_3$, 62.9 $EQD2Gy_3$; and sigmoid D_{2cc}: 44.2 $EQD2Gy_3$, 53.5 $EQD2Gy_3$, 59.7 $EQD2Gy_3$. There was a difference in the rate of severe (Grade ≥ 3) toxicities between the 2D and 3D arm for urinary toxicities in group 1 (3.8% vs. 0% $p = 0.02$), but not in group 2 (4.8% vs. 5.8%, $p = 0.76$) or group 3 (5.9% vs. 1.7% $p = 0.08$); for digestive toxicities no differences were seen between 2D and 3D arms. Up to the date of the analysis, no difference in the mean DVH was seen between patients who presented with complications versus patients without complications. Higher doses were delivered in the 3D arm, mainly in group 3 (definitive radiotherapy). Severe gastrointestinal complications were comparable between 2D and 3D arms, but urinary toxicity was lower in the 3D arm for group 1 and 3. These results should be interpreted with caution, as in the 3D arm, doses delivered to the tumor were lower than those reported previously in the literature. Definitive analysis is still pending at the time of this publication.

26.3 Dose Constraints for OARs in the Modern Era of 3D IGBT: The Predictive Value of Dose–Volume Parameters for Late Adverse Side Effects

In clinical practice, the minimum dose to the most exposed 2 cc tissue volume (D_{2cc}) is the primary parameter used for treatment plan optimization. The dose–effect relationship for the rectum using the ICRU 38 reference point was reported and mean values for the ICRU 38 dose and the D_{2cc} seem to be comparable [35–39]. For the sigmoid, rectal dose constraints were applied. For the bladder, dose constraints were determined based on the current and traditional clinical practice [35, 39]. For the vagina, no dose–volume parameters and constraints have been recommended.

In an attempt to test the predictive value of dose–volume parameters for late effects of the rectum, sigmoid colon, and bladder, Georg et al. [46] calculated dose–volume parameters (DVH) for 2, 1 and 0.1 cm^3 (D_{2cc}, D_{1cc}, $D_{0.1cc}$) of these three OARs for the 141 cervical cancer patients from Vienna treated with 3D EBRT and MRI-guided BT (median follow-up, 51 months). The mean D_{2cc} for bladder, rectum, and sigmoid were 95 ± 22 Gy, 65 ± 12 Gy, and 62 ± 12 Gy respectively. For the rectum and sigmoid, there were 3 G1, 7 G2, 2 G3, and 2 G4 patients with late adverse side effects. For the bladder, there were 9 G1, 11 G2, 1 G3, and 2 G4 patients with late adverse side effects. The 5-year G3–4 actuarial late toxicity rates were 4% for bladder, 2% for rectum, and 2% for sigmoid, G1 and G2 late toxicity rates were 19% for bladder, 10% for rectum, and 1% for sigmoid (Fig. 26.1). Statistically significant G0–G1 versus G2–G4 side effects were noted for D_{2cc} of the bladder, rectum, and sigmoid. This study confirmed that D_{2cc} was a predictor of late toxicity for the rectum and bladder.

Fig. 26.1 The 5-year actuarial rates for late adverse side effects (G1–4) of the rectum, bladder, and sigmoid. Adapted from Georg et al. [46]

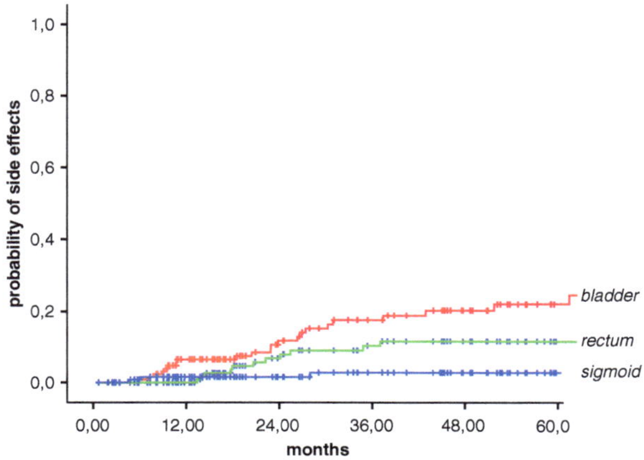

Further research is needed in order to determine the appropriate dose constraints and factors necessary for clinical practice.

26.4 Additional Studies

Rectum. Koom et al. showed that patients with a higher D_{2cc} had significantly more severe rectal side effects (endoscopy score >2) [40]. Seventy-one patients with FIGO Stage IB–IIIB uterine cervical cancer underwent CT-based high-dose-rate intracavitary brachytherapy; flexible sigmoidoscopy with the 6-scale scoring system evaluated recto-sigmoid mucosal changes. The total dose (EBRT plus intracavitary brachytherapy) to the International Commission of Radiation Units and Measurements rectal point (ICRURP) and DVH parameters for rectosigmoid colon were calculated using the equivalent dose in 2-Gy fractions (α/β = 3 Gy) [41]. The mean values of the DVH parameters and ICRURP were significantly greater in patients with a score >2 than in those with a score <2 at 12 months after RT (ICRURP, 71 Gy $\alpha/\beta = 3$ vs. 66 Gy ($p = 0.02$); $D_{0.1cc}$, 93 Gy, vs. 85 Gy ($p = 0.04$); D_{1cc}, 80 Gy vs. 73 Gy, $p = 0.02$; D_{2cc}, 75 Gy vs. 69 Gy ($p = 0.02$)). The probability of a score >2 showed a significant relationship with the DVH parameters and ICRURP (ICRURP, $p = 0.03$; $D_{0.1cc}$, $p = 0.05$; D_{1cc}, $p = 0.02$; D_{2cc}, $p = 0.02$).

A similar trend has been demonstrated by the Vienna group for 141 patients: the incidence of G1–G4 late toxicity for rectum was significantly higher when the D_{2cc} for the rectum was 75 Gy ($\alpha/\beta = 3$) (20% vs. 4%) as described above [46]. These findings were even more significant for the Vienna rectoscopy study in 35 patients [42]. In this study, rectosigmoidoscopy and rectal morbidity assessment were performed on 35 cervical cancer patients treated with EBRT and HDR-intracavitary brachytherapy. The total doses, normalized to 2-Gy fractions (EQD2, α/β = 3 Gy), in 0.1, 1.0, and 2.0 cm^3 ($D_{0.1cc}$, D_{1cc}, D_{2cc}) of rectum were determined by summing the EBRT and ICB plans. Correlation analysis between clinical symptoms (LENT/SOMA) and rectoscopic changes (Vienna Rectoscopy Score, VRS [41]) was performed. For dose–response analyses, the logit model was used. Mean follow-up was 18 months. LENT/SOMA score was 1 in 4 patients, 2 in 8 patients, 4 in 136 patients. Telangiectasia was found in 26 patients (74%); 5 had ulceration corresponding to the 0.1 -m^3 volume (anterior wall). Mean values $D_{0.1cc}$, D_{1cc}, and D_{2cc} were 81 ± 13 Gy, 70 ± 9 Gy, and 66 ± 8 Gy, respectively. The ED_{50} values for VRSP3 and for LENT/SOMAP2 significantly increased with decreasing volumes. D_{2cc} was higher in patients with VRSP3 compared to VRS < 3 (72 ± 6 Gy vs. 62 ± 7 Gy; $p < 0.001$) and in symptomatic versus asymptomatic patients (72 ± 6 Gy vs. 63 ± 8 Gy; $p < 0.001$). VRS correlated with the LENT/SOMA score. This study confirmed that rectosigmoidoscopy is sensitive in detecting mucosal changes, independent of clinical symptoms. The localization of these changes corresponds to the high dose volumes as defined by imaging. The development of mucosal and clinical changes in the rectum seems to follow a clear dose effect and volume effect. Based on these two studies we recommend a dose limit of 70–75 Gy EQD2 for the rectal dose constraint.

Sigmoid. For the sigmoid, dose–volume constraints applied to date have not been linked to clinical outcome. In the Vienna series with 141 patients with a threshold of 75 Gy, 9% (2/22) compared to 1% (1/119) had sigmoid toxicity ([46]). However, in the Vienna rectosigmoidoscopy study, the frequency of telangiectasia was 3 of 29 (10%) in the sigmoid (mean dose, 65.97 Gy) compared to 26 of 35 (74%) in the rectum (mean dose, 66.98 Gy) to the 2 cc volume [43]. In a recent small study by Sturdza et al. [44], 15 of 22 patients had major sigmoid interfraction variation. Therefore, due to underlying uncertainties for assessing the dose to the sigmoid colon (e.g., movement), the total calculated dose using the "worst case assumption" has to be handled with caution. Another interesting finding is that in different series published so far the dose to the sigmoid seems to be significantly different for a comparable dose to the HR CTV: for example, 63 Gy in Vienna [45] versus 69 Gy in Aarhus [5], both using the tandem-ring applicator and the same method for reporting. The reasons for these differences need to be elucidated.

Bladder. For the bladder, the overall situation for dose–volume assessment applying 3D-based parameter (2 cc, 0.1 cc) is still under investigation due to the insufficiency of clinical evidence. This is in line with the difficulty of showing dose effects for cervix cancer BT for the bladder in the past [38]. For centers changing from radiography to 3D-based dose–volume assessment it has been striking that in the past high doses have been applied in small volumes on a regular basis, often far beyond what has been shown by the ICRU bladder point. However, even in the Vienna series with 141 patients, no clear bladder dose effect could be shown for this large series applying different cut-off levels for small volumes. There is still controversy regarding the location of the high-dose area in the bladder. In a small retrospective study in Vienna of symptomatic and asymptomatic patients (n =34) receiving a dose of 90 Gy (EQD2, α/β of 3) the location of the high-dose volume was investigated as an additional parameter. The posterior bladder wall was divided into a low and a medium segment (including and excluding the bladder neck). In 18 patients with a high dose in the medium segment, only 3 experienced bladder side effects, whereas 16 patients with a high dose in the lower segment suffered from late adverse bladder side effects (Munandar A et al., unpublished material).

These findings indicate that an additional parameter may be useful in future clinical research to increase the value of "pure" DVH parameters for assessing bladder morbidity.

Vagina. For the vagina, no dose–volume parameters have been recommended by the Gyn GEC ESTRO group. High uncertainties in dose assessment exist [43, 47]. Furthermore, no clinical evidence had been reported. In a recent study of vaginal morbidity in Vienna, telangiectasia, bleeding, fibrosis, and shortening correlated to different dose levels in absolute D_{2cc} volume [47]. Innovative research approaches will be necessary to better understand the underlying mechanisms and to define parameters and a model which may be feasible for predicting outcome.

References

1. CTCAE, Common Terminology Criteria for Adverse Events. 2006.
2. Soma L. LENT SOMA tables. Radiother Oncol. 1995;35:17–60.
3. Portelance L. IMRT reduces small bowel, rectum, and bladder doses in patients with cervical cancer receiving pelvic and paraaortic irradiation. Int J Radiat Oncol Biol Phys. 2001; 51:261–6.
4. Vistad I et al. Postradiotherapy morbidity in long-term survivors after locally advanced cervical cancer: how well do physicians' assessments agree with those of their patients? Int J Radiat Oncol Biol Phys. 2008;71(5):1335–42.
5. Tait DM et al. Acute toxicity in pelvic radiotherapy; a randomised trial of conformal versus conventional treatment. Radiother Oncol. 1997;42(2):121–36.
6. Mutic S et al. PET-guided IMRT for cervical carcinoma with positive para-aortic lymph nodes-a dose-escalation treatment planning study. Int J Radiat Oncol Biol Phys. 2003;55(1):28–35.
7. Aoki T et al. Clinical evaluation of dynamic arc conformal radiotherapy for paraaortic lymph node metastasis. Radiother Oncol. 2003;67(1):113–8.
8. Mundt AJ et al. Initial clinical experience with intensity-modulated whole-pelvis radiation therapy in women with gynecologic malignancies. Gynecol Oncol. 2001;82(3):456–63.
9. Brixey CJ et al. Impact of IMRT on acute hematologic toxicity in women with gynecologic malignancies. Int J Radiat Oncol Biol Phys. 2002;54(5):1388–96.
10. Mell LK et al. Dosimetric comparison of bone marrow-sparing intensity-modulated radiotherapy versus conventional techniques for treatment of cervical cancer. Int J Radiat Oncol Biol Phys. 2008;71(5):1504–10.
11. Chen MF et al. Adjuvant concurrent chemoradiotherapy with intensity-modulated pelvic radiotherapy after surgery for high-risk, early stage cervical cancer patients. Cancer J. 2008;14(3):200–6.
12. Esthappan J et al. Treatment planning guidelines regarding the use of CT/PET-guided IMRT for cervical carcinoma with positive paraaortic lymph nodes. Int J Radiat Oncol Biol Phys. 2004;58(4):1289–97.
13. Mundt AJ, Roeske JC, Lujan AE. Intensity-modulated radiation therapy in gynecologic malignancies. Med Dosim. 2002;27(2):131–6.
14. Beriwal S et al. Early clinical outcome with concurrent chemotherapy and extended-field, intensity-modulated radiotherapy for cervical cancer. Int J Radiat Oncol Biol Phys. 2007; 68(1):166–71.
15. Salama JK et al. Preliminary outcome and toxicity report of extended-field, intensity-modulated radiation therapy for gynecologic malignancies. Int J Radiat Oncol Biol Phys. 2006;65(4):1170–6.

16. Barraclough LH et al. External beam boost for cancer of the cervix uteri when intracavitary therapy cannot be performed. Int J Radiat Oncol Biol Phys. 2008;71(3):772–8.
17. Potter R et al. Clinical impact of MRI assisted dose volume adaptation and dose escalation in brachytherapy of locally advanced cervix cancer. Radiother Oncol. 2007;83(2):148–55.
18. Chargari C et al. Physics contributions and clinical outcome with 3D-MRI-based pulsed-dose-rate intracavitary brachytherapy in cervical cancer patients. Int J Radiat Oncol Biol Phys. 2008;74:133–9.
19. Perez CA et al. Tumor size, irradiation dose, and long-term outcome of carcinoma of uterine cervix. Int J Radiat Oncol Biol Phys. 1998;41(2):307–17.
20. Eifel PJ et al. Time course and outcome of central recurrence after radiation therapy for carcinoma of the cervix. Int J Gynecol Cancer. 2006;16(3):1106–11.
21. Eifel PJ. Concurrent chemotherapy and radiation therapy as the standard of care for cervical cancer. Nat Clin Pract Oncol. 2006;3(5):248–55.
22. Chan P et al. Dosimetric comparison of intensity-modulated, conformal, and four-field pelvic radiotherapy boost plans for gynecologic cancer: a retrospective planning study. Radiat Oncol. 2006;1:13.
23. Georg D et al. Image-guided radiotherapy for cervix cancer: high-tech external beam therapy versus high-tech brachytherapy. Int J Radiat Oncol Biol Phys. 2008;71(4):1272–8.
24. Lim K et al. Cervical cancer regression measured using weekly magnetic resonance imaging during fractionated radiotherapy: radiobiologic modeling and correlation with tumor hypoxia. Int J Radiat Oncol Biol Phys. 2008;70(1):126–33.
25. Lee CM, Shrieve DC, Gaffney DK. Rapid involution and mobility of carcinoma of the cervix. Int J Radiat Oncol Biol Phys. 2004;58(2):625–30.
26. van de Bunt L et al. Motion and deformation of the target volumes during IMRT for cervical cancer: what margins do we need? Radiother Oncol. 2008;88(2):233–40.
27. Beadle BM et al. Cervix regression and motion during the course of external beam chemoradiation for cervical cancer. Int J Radiat Oncol Biol Phys. 2009;73(1):235–41.
28. Pötter R et al. Recommendations from gynaecological (GYN) GEC ESTRO working group (II): concepts and terms in 3D image-based treatment planning in cervix cancer brachytherapy-3D dose volume parameters and aspects of 3D image-based anatomy, radiation physics, radiobiology. Radiother Oncol. 2006;78(1):67–77.
29. Potter R et al. 3D conformal HDR-brachy- and external beam therapy plus simultaneous cisplatin for high-risk cervical cancer: clinical experience with 3 year follow-up. Radiother Oncol. 2006;79:80–6.
30. Viswanathan AN et al. Final results of a prospective study of MR-based interstitial gynecologic brachytherapy. Brachytherapy. 2008;7:148.
31. Mahantshetty U et al. MRI-guided high-dose-rate intracavitary brachytherapy in cervical cancers at Tata Memorial Hospital: the initial clinical outcome. Brachytherapy. 2009;8(2):112.
32. Narayan K et al. Comparative study of LDR (Manchester system) and HDR image-guided conformal brachytherapy of cervical cancer: patterns of failure, late complications and survival. Int J Radiat Oncol Biol Phys. 2009;74(5):1529–35.
33. Tan LT et al. Clinical impact of computed tomography-based image-guided brachytherapy for cervix cancer using the tandem-ring applicator – the Addenbrooke's experience. Clin Oncol R Coll Radiol. 2009;21(3):175–82.
34. Charra-Brunaud C, Peiffert D. Preliminary results of a French prospective multicentric study of 3D pulsed dose-rate brachytherapy for cervix carcinoma. Cancer Radiother. 2008;12(6–7):527–31.
35. Gerbaulet A et al. The GEC ESTRO handbook of brachytherapy. Brussels: ESTRO; 2002.
36. Koom WS et al. Computed tomography-based high-dose-rate intracavitary brachytherapy for uterine cervical cancer: preliminary demonstration of correlation between dose-volume parameters and rectal mucosal changes observed by flexible sigmoidoscopy. Int J Radiat Oncol Biol Phys. 2007;68(5):1446–54.

37. ICRU. Dose and volume specification for reporting intracavitary therapy in gynaecology. Bethesda: International Commission of Radiation Units and Measurements; 1985.
38. Potter R et al. Definitive radiotherapy based on HDR brachytherapy with iridium 192 in uterine cervix carcinoma: report on the Vienna University Hospital findings (1993–1997) compared to the preceding period in the context of ICRU 38 recommendations. Cancer Radiother. 2000;4(2):159–72.
39. Potter R et al. Survey of the use of the ICRU 38 in recording and reporting cervical cancer brachytherapy. Radiother Oncol. 2001;58(1):11–8.
40. Koom WS, Sohn DK, et al. Computed tomography-based high-dose-rate intracavitary brachytherapy for uterine cervical cancer: preliminary demonstration of correlation between dose-volume parameters and rectal mucosal changes observed by flexible sigmoidoscopy. Int J Radiat Oncol Biol Phys. 2007;68:1446–54.
41. Wachter S et al. Endoscopic scoring of late rectal mucosal damage after conformal radiotherapy for prostatic carcinoma. Radiother Oncol. 2000;54(1):11–9.
42. Georg P et al. Correlation of dose-volume parameters, endoscopic and clinical rectal side effects in cervix cancer patients treated with definitive radiotherapy including MRI-based brachytherapy. Radiother Oncol. 2009;91(2):173–80.
43. Berger D et al. Uncertainties in assessment of the vaginal dose for intracavitary brachytherapy of cervical cancer using a tandem-ring applicator. Int J Radiat Oncol Biol Phys. 2007; 67(5):1451–9.
44. Sturdza AE et al. Uncertainties in assessing sigmoid dose volume parameters in MRI-guided fractionated HDR brachytherapy. Brachytherapy. 2008;7(2):109.
45. Kirisits C et al. Dose and volume parameters for MRI-based treatment planning in intracavitary brachytherapy for cervical cancer. Int J Radiat Oncol Biol Phys. 2005;62(3):901–11.
46. Georg P et al. Dose-volume histogram parameters and late side effects in magnetic resonance image-guided adaptive cervical cancer brachytherapy. Int J Radiat Oncol Biol Phys. 2010 Apr 10 (epub).
47. Fidarova EF et al. Dose volume parameter D(2cc) does not correlate with vaginal side effects in individual patients with cervical cancer treated within a defined treatment protocol with very high brachytherapy doses. Radiother Oncol. 2010 Jun 17 (epub).

Index

L

MIX
Papier aus verantwortungsvollen Quellen
Paper from responsible sources
FSC® C105338

If you have any concerns about our products,
you can contact us on
ProductSafety@springernature.com

In case Publisher is established outside the EU,
the EU authorized representative is:
Springer Nature Customer Service Center GmbH
Europaplatz 3, 69115 Heidelberg, Germany

Printed by Libri Plureos GmbH
in Hamburg, Germany